SCHOOL HEALTH EDUCATION

HARPER'S SERIES IN SCHOOL AND PUBLIC HEALTH EDUCATION, PHYSICAL EDUCATION, AND RECREATION

DELBERT OBERTEUFFER
EDITOR

SCHOOL HEALTH EDUCATION

FIFTH EDITION

A TEXTBOOK FOR
TEACHERS, NURSES, AND OTHER PROFESSIONAL PERSONNEL

DELBERT OBERTEUFFER
Ohio State University

ORVIS A. HARRELSON
Tacoma Public Schools

MARION B. POLLOCK
California State College
at Long Beach

HARPER & ROW
PUBLISHERS NEW YORK EVANSTON SAN FRANCISCO LONDON

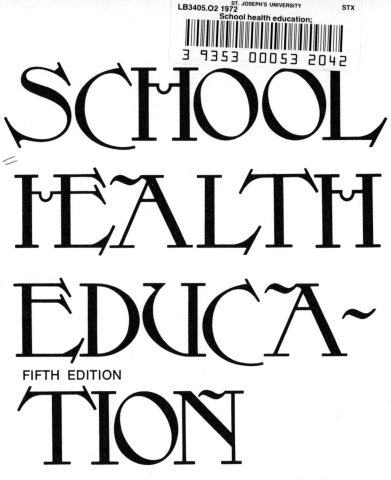

SCHOOL HEALTH EDUCATION, FIFTH EDITION

Standard Book Numbers: 06-044872-5 (Clothbound Edition)
06-044873-3 (Paperback Edition)

Library of Congress Catalog Card Number: 76-174523

TO
TED OBERTEUFFER
JULIE, DAVID, AND BOB HARRELSON
CHARLES DAVID FORREST

CONTENTS

INDEX

FOREWORD TO THE FIFTH EDITION

This fifth edition gives, as did its predecessors, extensive treatment to the new insights and concepts in curriculum development, teaching strategies, and professional services in school health education. Health education is conceived not only as a broad curriculum embracing all of the elements relating to the improvement of the quality of life, but as a series of health-related experiences under the direction of physicians, nurses, dentists, teachers, and other professional personnel.

The text has been completely rewritten. Marion B. Pollock has contributed most of the material in Part One and Orvis A. Harrelson, from his experience as medical director in a public school system, has developed Part Two. The book is intended for college and university students, including nurses, teachers, administrators, and others preparing in the health sciences, who will assume responsibility in educational programs. It will be useful to physicians who relate themselves to the school program and to public health personnel who cooperate in its development. The chapters are designed to range over the whole field of school practice involving instructional, administrative, environmental, and service aspects of a school health program and the program as seen in relation to the community forces from which it springs.

The book is divided into two parts. Part One, Foundations of Curriculum and Teaching, describes those problems or circumstances that make the study of health education an important part of a child's education. Special attention has been given to conceptual teaching and a description of the development and use of behavioral objectives. Part One describes the processes of curriculum and teaching common to any discipline with careful attention to applications particular to health education. There are chapters on planning and organizing for teaching, on teaching strategies stressing innovation and student involvement, on patterns of health instruction, and on methods and techniques of evaluation of instruction. Controversial and categorical issues in health education, especially education regarding drug abuse and sex, are the subject of the final chapter.

Part Two deals with foundations of administration and organization involving the promotion of health, disease controls, programs of appraisal, nutrition activities, specific problems of school-age development, and administration and community relationships.

New material has been added throughout. New illustrations of teaching units, integration plans, appraisal activities, and program evaluation are included.

The authors are indebted to many professional associates who taught them much about coordinated and cooperative programs, and to others who have given their consent to quote passages from their writings in support of material here. We are grateful to Dr. Elena M. Sliepcevich for the opportunities to explore conceptual teaching and to Mrs. Anne Fleming and Mrs. Roy Murphy for manuscript preparation.

Delbert Oberteuffer
Orvis A. Harrelson
Marion B. Pollock

PART ONE
FOUNDATIONS OF CURRICULUM AND TEACHING

CHAPTER 1
THE NEED

The existing atmosphere of change, challenge, and dissent is by no means a recent phenomenon. Every generation has been challenged by and yet has managed to absorb changes that evolved from earlier times, other struggles. What is different today is the rapid acceleration of change, pushed along not only by social forces, but also by an unprecedented increase in knowledge and technology. Established patterns of education are no longer serviceable as a means of transmitting what is known. Textbooks and other materials are out of date almost before they can be published. New educational systems are necessary today, for health education as well as every other discipline in the curriculum.

In an increasingly complex, urbanized society, perhaps the greatest educational imperatives for the next several decades will be man's need to learn who he is and to achieve some greater degree of self-actualization. We live in times disturbed by racial tension, alienation between young and old, and shifting perceptions of acceptable moral codes and value systems. At the same time that we are more and more clustering together in urban societies and enjoying marvels of speed in communication and transportation, each of us is more alone than ever before in history—not physically set apart from our neighbors, but emotionally isolated.

The task of the school, therefore, is to devise curricula that can help students discover their own humanness and how they may live effectively with their fellow human beings. In speaking of this crucial issue confronting schools for the 1970s and 1980s Boulding says:

"It must never be forgotten that what any society is producing is people . . . the educational system is producing men, not manpower; people, not biologically generated nonlinear computers." Educational systems, he continues, must be means, not ends, serving man rather than technology.[1]

Educators have not been deaf to this argument. Humanizing the school environment is the focus of the current publication program, "Schools For the 70's—And Beyond," of the National Education Association's Center for the Study of Instruction. Another approach is found in the Association for Supervision and Curriculum's 1970 Yearbook, *To Nurture Humaneness. Commitment for the '70s.*[2] Never before has health education had such powerful allies, and perhaps never has there been a greater need for a dynamic kindergarten through twelfth grade curriculum in school health education. A curriculum that encourages the student to develop skills of critical thinking and problem solving, rather than focusing on memorization of facts about anatomy and physiology or disease. A curriculum that views health as a continuum of well-being and recognizes the interrelationships among physical, social, and mental-emotional forces influencing an individual's position on that continuum at any one point in time. A curriculum that recognizes human health as a means enabling man to make the most of his potential, rather than as an end in itself. Most important, perhaps, a curriculum that motivates the individual to seek new information as a lifelong commitment.

What is known about health science and human behavior that tends to promote well-being is useless without the assistance of education as a means of communicating that information. Western civilization embraces a firm belief in the worth and dignity of the human being. Extensions of this belief have been the lifting of man from ignorance, the removal of many of the shackles of disease, the improvement of the conditions of his existence, and the extension of his expected lifetime. The result has been to improve the vitality of many people and to free them for the creative life. They have been liberated from the restraints of poverty and illness and have found new and hitherto unexpected worth in themselves.

This improvement is the product of the union of science and education. Wherever civilization is most advanced, wherever the quality of man's living is best, it is more than coincidental that programs of school and public health education have flourished. These programs have interpreted scientific knowledge and used scientific practice not only to conserve life but to give life a chance for fullest development.

THE DEVELOPMENT OF SCIENTIFIC KNOWLEDGE The volume of available information resulting from scientific research and development is growing at so rapid a pace as to test man's ability to store it, let alone absorb it. It is estimated that today the entire amount of nonredundant information stored in the world's libraries amounts to 1 quadrillion bits. By 1980, at present rates, this amount will be doubled. Man may not learn fast enough how to use so much new information to his advantage even for his preservation. There are those who fear that science may eventually destroy man as he too enthusiastically accepts and applies its discoveries with little thought or perhaps ignorance of possible ecological implications.

Ecology, the study of how living organisms and the nonliving environment function together as a whole, is rapidly becoming a science of survival. What most worries many ecologists is man's failure to recognize his own absolute dependence on all his ecosystems, such as the oceans, forests, and grasslands. Only as a balance is maintained among these ecosystems can man survive. A study of "human ecology" is emerging as perhaps more aptly descriptive of the issues to which the health educator must address himself today.

Pesticide residues in unborn babies and in mothers' milk are at danger levels. The amounts of DDT present in the soils of Sweden, for example, are greater than the total quantities ever used in that country. The constant threat of total atomic bomb destruction not only of mankind but of all life-supporting ecosystems is a modern nightmare. Biological warfare, nerve gas, the use of psychological techniques such as brainwashing, and indiscriminate use of herbicides and defoliants are other examples of possible irreversibly destructive applications.

Alas, the problem is not simply one of discovery of new technology. The problem is fundamentally one of developing a synthesis of *all* science so as to understand nature's processes in relation to man, and then to utilize what the synthesis discloses for man's *development* rather than his *destruction.* A synthesis of the sciences can not only reveal more of each science to the others, but can provide guidelines to the means whereby science can be applied to benefit mankind.

THE USE OF SCIENCE IN LIVING The more effectively man can learn to apply the knowledge science is steadily accumulating, the greater facility he will have in understanding and solving his problems. His world will become easier to control, his objectives easier to attain, and his life safer, if more complicated. From laboratories all over the world have come discoveries that have been useful to civilization—discoveries of new surgical techniques, such as the transplanting of human kidneys, corneas, and even hearts; mechanical devices to replace failing human organs; new immunizations and vaccines; ways to preserve food, heat houses, and purify water; and ways to correct hormonal imbalances and prevent human ovulation, as well as hundreds of other innovations.

Opportunity to use scientific knowledge is unending. If we used present knowledge about the detection, control, and treatment of cancer, more than 50,000 deaths could be prevented annually. Death from cervical cancer could be substantially reduced in incidence if a simple test were routinely sought by women on a periodic basis and treatment begun where indicated. The crippling effects of rheumatic fever could be reduced or prevented. The emotionally disturbed and the mentally ill could be helped to return to a useful life. With early detection, effects could be arrested and blindness from glaucoma prevented. Lung cancer could be virtually eliminated. Venereal disease could be controlled. A lifetime protection against tooth decay could be developed. Loss of sound teeth due to periodontal disease could be prevented. These are but a few of the benefits to the individual and the community that would result if the union between science and education were fully implemented.

But it is not sufficient that this knowledge be used merely for preventive purposes. To be free of the illnesses, disabilities, and discomforts imposed by new man-made environmental insults and adverse changes in American life styles is highly desirable, of course. But man can come into his own and reach his fullest potential only when he learns to live *creatively* and *constructively.* When science can be an instrument of change for the better, helping him to live beyond a level of ordinary effectiveness, beyond mediocrity, at a level where he functions at his best, then we will have made the most of life.

If man were to use what is known about ways to improve the functioning of the human body, he could learn to see better, to have greater strength, and to possess greater emotional and physical resilience with which to carry on the work of the world. He could expand his perspectives and make sounder judgments, and thus he could enhance his sense of well-being and satisfaction. He could get more work done during the day. He could, if he wished, be wiser in the selection of a mate, and produce better results in the rearing of his children. He could find stimulation and rewards in new intellectual and recreational pursuits. These are but a few of the things that man could enjoy if he would *use* what is known to science. Until that time comes, or until the individual uses science in that way, we live *in* an age of science but we are not *of* it.

THE ROLE OF SCHOOL HEALTH EDUCATION

It is at this point that school health education becomes of greatest service. In both its protective and developmental or creative aspects health education concerns itself with application of knowledge to the processes of life and living. It seeks to promote skills of problem solving and decision making based upon the rational rather than the irrational or emotional impulses.

In the broadest sense, much of man's scientific achievement affects his development and survival. Because the school is the principal medium for transmitting man's cultural heritage, all the school's efforts may be viewed as having a bearing on man's growth, development, and preservation. Hence, broadly speaking, education in the processes and purposes of living, in protection and promotion of health, and in the means of most effectively utilizing one's resources occupies much of the school's time. Health education so conceived becomes a major function of general education.

Health education for the seventies and beyond will need to clarify, sharpen, and develop curricula and organizational patterns that are acceptable not only to teachers but to learners. The subject matter and teaching strategies of the future must bear a higher degree of relevance to the tempo of the times and to the lives of students than has been the case in the past. And, as in every other area in the school's curriculum, a conceptual approach to the growing body of knowledge encompassed by health education is not just an innovation but a necessity. The ultimate goal in every discipline seems to be shifting from the means by which current information is transmitted to the *use* to which it is put in the organization of one's life. The lag between scientists' discoveries and public acceptance and usage of knowledge can no longer be dealt with solely during school years.

The goal of health education, therefore, whether it be in a school or community setting, is to give man the tools by which his potential strengths, energies, and social, physical, and mental-emotional effectiveness can be fully realized. Decisions and actions founded upon application of such tools become more deeply satisfying and constructive.

– the obligation of the school

The school, as a confining and structured institution receiving its pupils, by law, at the tender age of six (and even earlier in Headstart and nursery school programs), must continually look to the quality of that experience.

Children are required to attend school five or six hours a day, thirty weeks a year, for twelve years or more. No other social institution enjoys such certainty of patronage. Having received a healthy child, then, the school has the responsibility of contributing positively to his total growth and development during his school days and turning him out at the end not only undamaged, but improved mentally, physically, emotionally, socially, and spiritually. The young adult who has completed his education must have come through that experience with a strong feeling of self-respect as well as an ability to treat other people successfully and respectfully. There can be no defense for a school system which, having received a child wholesome and well-adjusted at six, sends him out twelve years later damaged and diminished in self-esteem and spirit because of his school experience. There can be no excuse for a school system that is inattentive to the disturbed psychological state of some of its employees who produce children in their image—nervous, insecure, maladjusted. Society has no right to compel attendance in firetraps, or to ask that twelve years of a child's life be spent in dirty, overcrowded, or antiquated buildings. The environment of the school must promote health and be good for life, not destructive of it.

– the readiness of the learner

But the obligation is even broader than that. The main business of the school is to teach, to facilitate learning. When one asks, "What conditions must prevail if learning is to take place?" he discovers that four interrelated conditions are necessary.

First, there must be good teaching. The teacher needs to be skilled. He must possess a basic understanding of generally accepted principles of learning, behavioral characteristics of learners, motivation, and teaching techniques. Equally important, he must be able to differentiate between teaching and imparting information, and he should be oriented to the first as his goal. He must know how to select content that is meaningful rather than trivial.

Second, the facilities, the materials for teaching must be good—good books, good laboratories, good equipment, good materials and audio-visual aids.

But it must be said, because it is inescapably true, that the best teachers in the world using the best equipment and materials available will fail unless the learner is ready to learn. *The quality of learning depends upon the quality of the organism doing the learning.*

Hence the third and fourth conditions—the genetic or hereditary potential of the student and the quality of the organism as it is at the time it arrives at the school. These are basic to all learning. Learning simply cannot go on acceptably unless the last two conditions are conducive to it. Teachers, administrators, parents, guidance counselors, personnel in testing offices, and particularly critics of education must understand this.

This is the basic thesis of the scientific vis-a-vis the "academic" point of view: there is a biological understructure for education. Man can learn only in proportion to the quality of his biological base, and whatever the demands of the future, education must be planned with the biological base in mind.

The evidence supporting acceptance of the biological base of intellectual potential is ample, even commonplace. For example, students suffering from some organic or functional disorder are handicapped not just physically but also socially and mentally. Emotional disturbances not only reduce mental and social effectiveness, but also inflict pain and physical damage upon the organism. Physicians estimate that as much as 70 percent of their medical practice is in treatment of malfunctioning and disease that is psychosomatic in origin.

An increasing number of modern educators are taking this holistic view of the individual. A child is a complex organism whose functions cannot be dealt with separately. He cannot be helped to grow and develop if he is thought of as a composite of discrete elements—the intellectual, physical, social, emotional, psychological, spiritual, or political self.

Man is *not* a composite of separate entities, such as body, mind, and spirit, arranged in some sort of hierarchy of importance. He is a multidimensional unity, with each component existing within a complex of interrelationships.

Irreversible impairment of intelligence can follow severe early malnutrition, especially protein deficiency. Borderline malnutrition in children retards scholastic progress. Who has not felt the mental slump that arrives midmorning following a skipped or skimpy breakfast or experienced the mood-altering satisfaction of a good dinner at the end of a hard day's work? Those who deprecate the poor in our society for lacking the ambition to accomplish as much as they might fail to remember that energy depends upon adequate food and that insufficient nourishment diminishes man's ability to function in all aspects of living. A combination of the debilitating effects of disease and malnutrition among adults as well as children is a world health problem of giant proportions. Until this problem is solved, educational progress, or progress of any kind whatever, will be difficult if not impossible in many developing countries.

Education is a function of the educatee. The educator can only provide him an array of opportunities to react to new experiences and grasp new ideas. If the learning child is handicapped in any way, even by lack of love, so is his potential for learning and change. Socrates said that "Even in the process of thinking, in which the use of the body seems to be reduced to a minimum, it is a matter of common knowledge that grave mistakes may often be traced to bad health."

WHAT IS HEALTH?

There are many definitions of health. One with widest official acceptance, perhaps, is that adopted by the member nations of the World Health Organization (WHO). Health has been described by WHO as "a state of complete, physical, mental, and social well being, and not merely the absence of disease and infirmity."[3] Certainly this was a step toward a holistic notion of man and an approach that begins to define health from a positive view rather than describing what it is not. Nevertheless, this definition prescribes a condition literally impossible to attain. No one is *completely* well in all three aspects, even assuming that there *are* only these three. In addition, the WHO statement suffers from a certain circularity in that it defines health as a state of well-being, which is to say that health is a state of health. Halbert L. Dunn speaks of health in terms of high-level wellness, which is defined as "an integrated method of functioning which is oriented toward maximizing the potential of which the individual is capable." He sees wellness as a "direction of progress" rather than as an optimum point of attainment.[4]

The School Health Education Study defines health as a comprehensive generalized concept—"a quality of life involving dynamic interaction and interdependence among the individual's physical well being, his mental and emotional reactions, and the social complex in which he exists."[5]

From these points of view, one can see health in terms relating neither to physical things alone nor to the status quo. Health can describe man only in function and in total. It can be thought of as the

> . . . optimum functioning of the human organism in all its complexity from the subtle processes of metabolism to the most sensitive perception of beauty or truth or love. When any significant aspect of this functioning goes awry then the quality of human life is threatened. The extent of the threat depends upon the nature and the degree of the malfunctioning. Advanced illness whether centered in body, mind, or soul rapidly destroys the effectiveness and meaning of all of life. These three aspects of man are so related and interdependent that serious malfunctioning in any one rapidly affects the others.[6]

Health as a state of being may, of course, be bad or inferior, or less than good. In that case, health can perhaps more accurately be understood as an index, a measurement, not of status but of function. Then health can be defined as the condition of the organism that measures the degree to which its aggregate powers are able to function.

To educate in health, therefore, is to equip the individual with the concepts and behaviors fundamental to sound and consistent decisions and choices that tend to promote his well-being and that of his family and neighbors. The goal of health education is to help each person seek that pattern of behavior which moves him toward an optimal level of health rather than the reverse and to give him the ability to avoid many of the imbalances, diseases, and accidents of life.

– the integrating experience

The purpose of going to school is to become educated, not, as it seems sometimes, to get through the prescribed course work. How much the business of going to school contributes to the toll of personality problems and general ill-health is difficult to assess. Children are sent off to school in varying stages of readiness, usually at a point in time mandated by a formula locked to date of birth. After that, for five or more hours a day, five days a week, thirty weeks a year, he will be exposed to the influence of teachers, classmates, and administration; to curriculum, method, and environment, whatever and however they may be. The experience is bound to leave its mark, and, in many ways, other than anticipated or intended. We are all the victims or the beneficiaries of our school life—probably both in most cases. Schooling can be helpful or harmful, promote child development or retard it, be a disintegrating or an integrating experience.

In the United States, the individual is traditionally the unit around which we build our social structures. Yet the schools and the educational establishment are under heavy fire these days from students who complain that they have been forgotten. They are not content to be passive recipients of what educators decide is essential for them, nor with evaluations based upon ability to give back what has been presented as "truth." These students demand that the schools be more directly concerned with the real world and with helping them discover satisfying answers to the question that nags us all, Who am I? An added problem facing school people is one of selecting from the rapidly increasing body of knowledge in every discipline the information and skills most relevant to student needs and demands.

The following statements, an outcome of a recent conference exploring educational trends, reflect the same concerns:

> To be part of today's world, the educational program and system—the institution—must prepare persons to solve problems on the level in which they are involved. . . . The demands for change now being made by the young people and underprivileged persons of this country are not new, but the qualitative dimension of the demands is real and is going to upset the life of every individual. The school must be prepared, therefore, to give this generation a

> chance to have its bout with thinking, accepting, respecting, and considering what has gone on in human life. If past and present older generations have been guided by a real set of values, today's youth and future generations will come to similar conclusions; but these conclusions will be their own, be accepted, and be relevant to their needs. If we can't accept this test, we really have very little to teach.[7]

However, nothing in education becomes particularly significant until the individual recipient sees the value in knowing it and wishes to involve himself in the learning experience. It is he who must do the integrating, and teaching must not only encourage him to do so but provide opportunities that allow him to learn and achieve purposes he sees as important. A curriculum designed to give children learning experiences commensurate with their developing abilities and interests is, next to the teacher, the most important influence upon their school experience. Learning how to learn, how to solve problems, think critically, what it is to be a human being, are integrating experiences when they are founded upon the child's needs and interests and when the welfare of the child comes first.

NEEDS AS A BASIS FOR INSTRUCTION

What does it take to achieve a creative and vital adaptation to one's world? What forces in the world support the effort to live well, and what forces deter it?

Today's school health education reflects the philosophy that curriculum must be based upon human needs. Not just needs that may be identified as gaps between present status and desirable norms, but also physical needs such as those for food, water, and warmth; social needs such as for self-respect and feelings of belonging; and integrative needs, such as for identifying a personal value system—in short, the total needs of man as a continually growing, developing, striving organism. School health education also considers interests in making curriculum decisions. No one would argue that interests alone should dictate curriculum decisions or emphasis. Still, interests are in many ways reflections of needs, as well as strong indicators of timeliness and relevance. Careful studies have identified the kinds of interests shared by students at any level of schooling. The prototype for such surveys was developed in the state of Ohio school system in 1930. A similar study was conducted in Denver, Colorado in 1947. Recent replication of those investigations found that only 25 percent of the compared items showed a marked shift in interest over a fifteen-year period. A host of clues to ways to teach health so as to help children develop and clarify their values for use in integrating the experiences they are having can be inferred from these kinds of data.

If we accept the thesis that man is constantly trying to satisfy his needs, then learning experiences which aid in that process are valuable materials for health education. As one of the subcommittees of the World Health Organization has put it:

> The urges to satisfy certain fundamental human needs, such as survival, food, love, and social approval, are the mainsprings of human behavior. But people strive for many other things which are no less important to them, though less vague. Their interests are seldom concerned with such abstractions as "life" and "health", but are usually more defined, e.g., striving to prevent sickness from certain diseases, or getting along with people, or overcoming some physical handicap. People are interested in doing those things which seem to help them to achieve something they want, or to cope with their own specific personal problems.[8]

There should be no confusion about the purposes of modern health education. It aims to improve the quality of living. It is not just classroom instruction in watered down anatomy or physiology. It does not depend upon fear as a motivating force influencing behavioral choices. It is not organized about a series of categorical health problems with little else than their life-shortening possibilities to tie them together. Rather it is based upon integrating relationships among the powerful concepts identified as representative of the body of knowledge encompassed by health education.

The focus of health education is not knowledge for the sake of knowledge alone, but the individual as he grows and develops throughout his school years with his special needs, his special goals. Today's health teaching actively involves the student in identifying the things he wants to know and the ways he goes about learning them. Teaching strategies are designed to give him practice in behaviors related to real-life concerns. Behaviors and skills internalized in this way cannot fail to influence the individual's choices among alternatives, not only in the classroom but outside—not just choices that improve health when this is necessary in the remedial sense, but day to day choices that contribute to well-being rather than the reverse.

It is not an easy task to plan and implement an educational program as dynamic and meaningful as that described here. The health teacher must be equipped with a sound background in a wide array of behavioral and physical sciences. *He must also have an accurate picture of the problems man must face today.*

– health status of the population

What is the status of the people in the United States and in the world? Ideally we would like to see all people living at a high level of wellness, creatively productive at the level of their full potential, and unhampered by adverse environmental or other conditions. It is difficult to determine the ratio between reality and that ideal, however. Statistics that show us how many people are living at peak performance do not exist. Data *do* exist from which some meaningful inferences can be made. We can determine problems. We can analyze man's needs and pinpoint those essential for effective living and survival. Fact finding is prerequisite to the development of a valid program of health instruction. Before any intelligent action can be taken to improve the quality of life, the present status must be established.

A study of the individual himself and in relation to his many communities (the many social groupings in which he works, enjoys recreational activities, and lives with others) will reveal personal and aggregate needs. Some can be met by individual action. Others require group effort expressed in public health measures and programs.

PROBLEMS AND SOURCES

Scientists around the world—in laboratory, hospital, medical practice, classroom, and in the field—are constantly investigating the problems and forces that threaten life or cause debility. The great killers of yesterday, such as malaria, yellow fever, cholera, and plague, have slowly been defeated wherever the results of that research are available and used. Yet, as each destructive force is countered, others emerge to demand attention. And so physicians, engineers, chemists, ecologists, educators, sociologists, and a host of other technologists continue to work to find better ways to solve old problems and to meet new problems sometimes resulting from solutions to old problems. Man must learn ways to improve his life and then put into practice what he discovers to be effective.

– our civilization not an unmixed blessing

People in the United States take pride in the industrial, social, scientific, and educational leadership that they have achieved. Never has the combination of American wealth and American know-how more dramatically impressed the world than in man's first landings on the moon. We enjoy the highest per capita income in the history of the world. The United States has the greatest Gross National Product of any country in the world. Yet in the midst of such affluence and power, millions of Americans live in poverty. The steady trend toward urbanization has produced delinquency, family disintegration, increased rates of mental illness, and inner-city degeneration. Our streets are choked with automobiles spewing noxious fumes and transporting people whose idea of a walk is from car to curb. Americans, not too long ago proud of being the most vigorous people in the Western world, typically today try to stay in shape by taking pills, or practicing controlled starvation, or paying to be pummeled or manipulated by machines that exercise their muscles for them! W. Raab, in an article in the *Journal of Sports Medicine,* paints this depressing picture:

> Physical mass degeneration is one of the ominous features of Western civilization. The detrimental effects of lack of exercise, combined with those caused by socio-economic emotional pressures and tensions, are widely recognized as contributing to neuroses, incapacitating conditions of the muscular and gastrointestinal systems, metabolic disturbances and insidiously developing functional and structural cardiovascular disorders.
>
> In this country, more than one-half of all deaths are caused by heart diseases, and the nation's economy is drained by sickness, early invalidism, and the cost of belated rehabilitation procedures.[9]

Many of the health problems of the affluent society have their origins in our too rich diet and too effortless life styles. Do you wish to get from the first floor in an office building to the second or third? Enter an elevator and push a button. It is not so much that we do not choose to walk rather than ride, it is that so few even think of walking as an alternative. Do you want the car window lowered or the radio aerial raised? Push a button. We can push a button to wash our clothes and dry them, to wash the dishes, to whisk away the garbage, and to open the garage door. Obesity is the disease of civilization. Fat-doctors, fat-farms, and reducing-aid manufacturers are amassing vast fortunes by serving those who wish to eat their cake and not have it, too.

In the relentless growth of the megalopolis, little or no attention has been devoted to the recreational needs of people. Houses, factories, apartment complexes, and stores have all been built in close proximity, and rarely has space been left for open air, parks, playgrounds, swimming pools, and woods. City dwellers sometimes have to go miles in search of recreational areas. Long lines of cars stream out of the cities at the beginning of a weekend and clog the highways into the cities at the end. For those unable to afford any escape, the city has been aptly termed an "asphalt jungle." An estimated 2 percent of the general population in the United States is afflicted with major mental illness. Estimates for the concentrated urban areas run as high as 10 percent.

The National Institute for Mental Health illustrates the kinds of mental health concerns common among American communities with the following statistics which can be expected in a hypothetical community of 500,000.

> Nearly 10,000 children—over 7 percent illegitimate—will be born into the community during the year. At least 2000 will require some form of mental health service during their lifetime, 40 percent in mental hospitals.
>
> More than 99,000 adolescents and adults in the community have no more than an eighth grade education; among the children in high school, 6 percent will drop out next year.

> Of the 4000 draftees screened last year for military duty, 1485—nearly 40 percent—were rejected; a third of these because they were mentally or emotionally unfit.
>
> Each year, within the community, over 6600 serious crimes—an average of 19 a day—are handled by the police. The crimes include 26 murders, 56 rapes, 528 assaults, 1240 auto thefts, and 2996 burglaries. Nearly 3300 youngsters 10–17 years of age are brought before the juvenile courts annually.
>
> Also during the last year, nearly 2700 persons were admitted to inpatient psychiatric facilities.
>
> Living in this "average community" are 1980 schizophrenics, thousands of people suffering from depression, nearly 13,000 alcoholics, 9900 homosexuals, 165 narcotic addicts, and 1300 mentally ill children.[10]

These figures, be it remembered, tend to understate the urban condition, since mental illness and social problems are greater than the national average in urban areas.

THE STRUGGLE FOR STABILITY

Problems of tension, frustration, boredom, and monotony resulting from sedentary and confined living conditions are universal. Emotional disorders such as chronic anxiety, depression, insecurity, and lack of self-esteem or confidence probably affect everyone at one time or another. Most of us manage to adjust to stress and maintain a reasonable balance. There are many mood ameliorating methods, but, increasingly, we are becoming a nation of drug abusers in our efforts to cope with these unpleasant feelings. However "uptight" you may be, there is a substance you can eat, drink, inject, or inhale that will help make life more bearable—not so much the illegal substances either, but those quite acceptably used socially and assiduously promoted by commercial enterprise.

Alcohol and tobacco are both drugs, although we sometimes seem to forget this fact. Alcohol, in a wide array of flavors and recipes, is used by the majority of the adult population, and two-thirds of them began drinking while in high school or earlier. There are at present somewhere between 6 and 8 million alcoholics in the country. According to a study made by the United States Department of Transportation, one of fifty drivers on the road is drunk. Not just comfortably relaxed as a result of a drink or two, but drunk! Cigarette smoking, for its stimulating or tranquillizing effects, is so widespread a practice as to make the smoker confident that his need to smoke supersedes the nonsmoker's right not to be forced to breathe second-hand fumes. At the same time, medical evidence convincingly links cigarette smoking with a wide range of conditions leading to premature death.

Coronary and other cardiovascular diseases are no longer the exclusive affliction of the aging but strike down 40- and even 30-year-old smokers these days. The number one cause of death from cancer for men is that of the lungs and bronchi; the incidence of this type of cancer increased from 18,313 in 1950 to 45,838 in 1964, and is rising rapidly. The mortality rate for smokers with chronic bronchitis and emphysema is doubling every five years. However, something seems to be happening that might halt this trend. The latest Public Health surveys show that among the 17 to 24 age group, only 37 percent are smokers compared to 48.5 percent for the 25 to 44 group. In population numbers this difference amounts to about 12 million fewer smokers among the younger group.

Appropriately labeled a medicated society, we place enormous confidence in pills and contentedly consume billions of them annually in an effort to cure or alleviate ills that are real or to palliate our stress-associated pains and tensions. In 1966 a reported 18 billion aspirin tablets were manufactured, plus billions of buffered and other forms of salicylates. About 8 billion amphetamines are produced in a year, enough to provide every man, woman, and child with thirty-five 5 mg doses. The House of Representatives Crime Committee estimates that 8 percent of all doctors' prescriptions last year were for these stimulants. Yet amphetamines, according to informed sources, are the drug of choice for only two rare diseases—so rare that about 1 percent of our annual production would take care of all real needs. The rest is sold illegally or misused in some way. About 3½ billion barbiturate capsules or tablets are turned out by American pharmaceutical manufacturers, and this amount is augmented by more imported from European manufacturers. It is believed that fully half of these dangerous drugs, too, go into illicit channels of sale and that those obtained legally are often abused. At last reports 1,400,000 pounds of tranquillizers were being dispensed yearly. Nonprescription sleep inducers and antihistamine cold tablets are made of virtually the same chemicals. Yet millions of Americans regularly dose themselves with cold tablets in ignorance of their sleep-inducing potential. The significance of this for an automobile-dependent society is frightening.

No one seems to grow into adulthood without some degree of emotional stress. Adolescents, whose earlier dependence on parental authority is more and more reduced, are at the same time beset with anxiety, frustration, and fear of failures. Young people are experiencing new freedom, strong sexual urges, but increased responsibility. Many are not easily able to handle these opposing pressures and find drugs a means to ease their problems and at the same time provide a feeling of belonging to a group. Many hard-core addicts began to use dangerous drugs as a means of defying authority or modifying an unpleasant feeling when they were teenagers.

Statistics on the use of hard-core narcotics—heroin, codeine, morphine—are difficult to ascertain accurately. However, the Bureau of Narcotics and Dangerous Drugs in 1969 estimated that there were about 64,000 addicts in this country, 52.2 percent of whom were in New York. The next worst problem areas were California, Illinois, and New Jersey. These people are able to adjust to life only by escaping via the depressant effects of the drug upon which they are totally dependent.

It is nearly as difficult to say how many people are marijuana smokers, although those who smoke it seem to talk about it more freely these days. Most statistics are based on estimates: for example "it is estimated that nationwide 35–50 percent of high school and college students may have tried marijuana." Of course we could as safely say that 100 percent *may* have, because this is a most ambiguous claim. The casual reader does not interpret it that way though and sees it as 50 percent *have* tried marijuana. A 1970 survey in Maryland, described as "the most comprehensive ever conducted in the United States," found that use of marijuana was less prevalent than had been estimated by "one recognized expert, less than most students themselves expected, and less than the public apparently believed." Less than 7 percent of the 56,000 students surveyed admitted its use, and just 5 percent more said they had tried it only once.[11] Nevertheless, it can probably be said that next to alcohol and tobacco it is the most widely abused drug and certainly generates the most concern of the three. Stanley Yolles, National Institute of Mental Health Director, estimated in 1970 that 12 to 20 million Americans were using marijuana. An 8 million plus or minus factor notwithstanding, that is still a lot of drug consumption.

Maintaining a balance among the individual's needs and the demands of his world is not always a problem simple enough to be solved by using some kind of drug or other coping behavior. When these fail, or when dependence on them makes the user unable to function acceptably in society, outside help is needed. About 1.2 percent of the total population, or 2,392,761 separate individuals, needed this kind of help in 1966 and were treated in psychiatric hospitals or clinics. Many of these patients were narcotic or alcohol dependent, but the basic problem was mental or emotional. Although there is a definite continuing downward trend in mental hospital resident populations over the age of 24, patients in the age group under 15 and 15 to 24 have been increasing at annual rates of 9.5 percent and 5.3 percent, respectively. This fact has special significance for school health education.

Juvenile delinquency as a manifestation of instability in many cases has been steadily increasing. In large part this increase is attributable to the social changes reflected in urbanization and inner city blight. Although admittedly the largest subgroup among delinquents are those occasional normal youngsters who have participated in an act of vandalism, usually as part of a group, the others are genuinely maladjusted, recidivistic, and in need of rehabilitation that recognizes the emotional problems involved. "Young people between the ages of 16 and 23 in 1964 represented 12.9 percent of the population but accounted for 27 percent of the arrests made that year. They were responsible for 26 percent of all murder and nonnegligent manslaughter; 34 percent of all manslaughter by negligence; 50 percent of all forcible rape; 49 percent of all robbery and breaking and entering; 36 percent of all larceny; 53 percent of all auto thefts; and 36 percent of the prostitution."[12] The years of adolescence are critical to these young people who must learn to function effectively in this changing world, and critical also to those who could help them.

What about college men and women? Emotional problems are cited most often by students as their number-one concern, especially in relation to the struggle to find out who they are. The third ranking cause of death among college students is suicide, the rate being about ten times that of the same age group not in college. Surprisingly, the major factor in student suicides is not pressure to obtain grades and succeed but, as in all age groups, the loss of or separation from a loved one.[13] About half of college dropouts are attributable to emotional problems of one kind or another.

An effective index of the health status of young men is an outcome of the Selective Service Act.[14] Every year over a million draftees are given preliminary physical and psychological examinations, testing their qualification to serve in the armed forces. In 1968 a total of 1,164,912 registrants were examined. The percentage disqualified increased for the second year in a row to 42.1 percent. More than 93,000, or 8 percent, failed the mental test, and almost 350,000, 29.9 per cent, were medically disqualified.

These are but some of the problem behaviors reflecting the inability of the individual to function effectively in the world in which he lives. Health education in the schools is designed to help him find ways that are constructive, both for himself and for those around him. The challenging problem is: How can we begin to restructure a society so that intolerable pressures are removed and yet order and reason prevail?

Everyone must learn to gear his own needs, desires, ambition, likes, and feelings to the real world. Socialization is the child's primary learning task. No one is born with these psychological or social adjustments built in. We *learn* all of our attitudes and behaviors. The fact that so many fail to make effective adjustments is evidence that some have not been taught how to achieve and maintain stability, or that appropriate learning has been made virtually impossible due to adverse environmental circumstances.

PEOPLE, POLLUTION, AND ECOLOGY

It took millions of years for the world population to reach its 1930 figure of 2 billion. By the year 2000, only 70 years later, this figure is expected to reach a staggering total of 7 billion! In the United States, for the first time, overpopulation is becoming a matter of concern. Currently we are growing at the rate of 3 million a year—a quarter of a million people every month—the equivalent of a city the size of Dayton, Ohio! There are some who regard this rapid increase of people as a sort of environmental pollution, "popullution."

Paul Ehrlich, Stanford University ecologist, says the problem is not so much where to put all the people, but how we are going to feed them and where we are going to put their junk. And how we are going to find water, power, and air for them.

> It is already too late to avoid famines that will kill millions, possibly by 1975. We are playing environmental roulette, overbreeding, putting crud in the environment, poisoning our water, killing our fish, sloshing pesticides which kill the insects that kill the pests, heading straight into the worst crisis mankind has ever seen."[15]

It is predicted by some British scientists that this overpopulation and the spread of technology will cause a true increase in both anxiety states and neurotic depressive states. Soon, they say, nearly everybody will be taking psychotropic medicines either continuously or at intervals. Many predict that either a successful program of population control will be developed, or death by stress will control and balance population growth. Maybe so, but nobody has yet come up with any real solution to the other kinds of pollution.

What has been called the affluent society might as aptly also be called the effluent society. Our cities are drowning in oceans of trash and garbage! Current estimates are that the average city dweller discards five pounds of trash a day, and the rate is increasing. Add to that the junked automobiles and household appliances, cast-off plastic containers, aerosol cans, the virtually indestructible "disposable" bottles, aluminum beverage cans whose discarded pulltags glitter underfoot everywhere, and a thousand other marvels of our technological advances. It amounts presently to a colossal 350 million tons costing about $4.5 billion a year to hide. We are already running out of ways and places to do so, and the annual amount of refuse is expected to double at least within the next twenty years.

The nation's rivers for generations have been burdened with the task of absorbing the cities' accumulation of raw sewage and industrial wastes. Rivers are no longer figuratively, but literally, cesspools in many cases. Even large bodies of water such as Puget Sound, Lake Tahoe, and Galveston Bay are threatened by pollution that may completely destroy the food and biological chains necessary to support marine life. Lake Erie already is nearly dead, because the oxygen demand of pollutants has reduced the oxygen level to zero, breaking the cycle of natural events that maintains the self-purifying ability of the surface waters. Indeed, it has been predicted that within the next decade, owing to pollution, the oceans themselves will no longer be capable of supporting marine life.

These problems are not ours alone, but world-wide.

Joseph Wood Krutch has said, "What it comes down to is this: Science and technology are creating more problems than they're solving—and yet we go right on with it."[16] Pollution, of Earth's skies, waters, and soil with poisons, man-made radioactivity, photochemical smog, asbestos, detergents, defoliants, and a host of other organic compounds threatens man's ability to survive on this planet. Man himself will have to take the steps essential to reverse this situation before it is too late. To do so he must not only be awakened to the problem, but informed enough to participate constructively in solving it.

ATOMIC PROBLEMS Radiation from nuclear reactors and other sources of atomic energy is a fearful byproduct of scientific advances. The horror of Hiroshima not forgotten, we still have stockpiled around the world enough atomic bombs to destroy civilization. Atomic bomb testing continues to rock Earth's mantle and pollute Earth's atmosphere. It has even been suggested that we test an atomic bomb on the surface of the moon! The constant threat of the potential outcome of such testing, to say nothing of total nuclear war, is a mental health problem almost immeasurable in its impact.

The use of radioactive isotopes in treatment of cancer, in preserving food and medical research; the use of nuclear reactors as a source of power, and a host of other valuable applications are tremendous plus factors favoring continued development of nuclear science. However, the price may eventually be greater than we would like to pay, unless preventive action is taken.

Radioactive fallout and safe disposal of atomic waste materials have been serious problems from the first. Early predictions that man's need for power sources would be forever filled by the construction of atomic ships, vehicles, and power plants have been tempered by some problems not at first apparent. United States nuclear submarines provoke storms of protest from the people who live in the countries they visit and who fear possible contamination of their harbors. Nuclear plants suck in millions of gallons of cooling water every minute, adding 10 to 20 degrees to the sea water temperature before pouring it back into the sea. The resulting overheated coastal water destroys marine life and becomes a form of effluent in itself. In a suit against the Florida Power and Light Company for thermal pollution of the waters of Biscayne Bay, the United States government also hopes to prevent the completion of two new nuclear plants under construction. Science will have to tell us how to control radiation so that it is not destructive of health while it is being used to promote technology and industry.

SUPERSTITIONS AND MISCONCEPTIONS

There is nothing new about man's attempts to avoid disease and death, nor in his having on hand a store of beliefs about their cause and treatment. There have always been, even before recorded history, some more skilled than others in aiding the sick and injured, and these people have used a wide range of sometimes effective and sometimes useless and even loathesome substances in doing so. Thus from the sorcerers of ancient civilizations with their potions and incantations, through the Greeks and Romans with their many gods of healing, Hippocrates and the four humours theory of disease, Galen, Paracelsus, and on to such milestone figures as Pasteur, Jenner, Koch, and Ehrlich, medical knowledge and practice has changed and progressed at an ever more rapid pace. Accompanying the knowledge and practice of the experts in any one period there have always been the folk practices and the conventional wisdom about the thing to do for illness.

Many of these folk practices and beliefs persist over a long period of time even when they are dangerous or potentially injurious when applied. Hundreds of such beliefs have been identified and probably direct some of the health behavior of even highly educated people. These are the kinds of things that "everybody knows" are true and that are learned almost without design. "Feed a cold and starve a fever." Why? "Brown eggs are more nutritious than white eggs." "Plenty of hot, strong, black coffee will sober a drunk." "One beer is not as intoxicating as one standard highball." "Aches and pains in children and adolescents are only normal growing pains." "Venereal disease is inherited." The list is endless.

The danger in basing decisions about health problems on superstitions or misinformation is not so much that the treatment may be harmful as that valuable time may be lost. Harmful or fatal neglect of self or family may result from the misconception that health is the absence of physical disease or infirmity. To believe that physical health is unrelated to what goes on in the mind or in society is to deny oneself the advantages of what has been learned that might prevent or ameliorate health-destroying conditions. At the same time, to believe as firmly in either of the other two aspects of health as being the only source of ill health is equally dangerous.

THE WAR WITH DISEASE Western civilization has been characterized by an unremitting fight against disease and other forces threatening life. Medical and scientific achievement and progress are unquestionable, but much yet remains to be done. As yet little is known about the control and treatment of the hundreds of disease-causing viruses that scientists have identified. Even what is known about disease is not as helpful as it could be because too great a lag exists between what is discovered and its general acceptance or application. Education is the only real means of bridging this gap.

In 1900 the three leading causes of death in this country were communicable diseases: the influenzas and pneumonias, tuberculosis, and gastroenteritis. Together they accounted for about one-third of all deaths that year. By 1960 the combined death rate for these same three categories was less than 5 percent. New drugs—the antibiotics, steroids, psychotropics, and others developed through research—have given physicians strong weapons against infection, arthritis, heart disease, high blood pressure, emotional disorders, hormone imbalance, and many other crippling or fatal conditions. New vaccines such as those responsible for the virtual elimination of polio, measles, and soon mumps, and improvement in established immunizations and procedures add to the armamentarium of preventive medicine. Modern techniques of water purification, sanitation, and vector control have diminished the reservoir of disease-causing organisms.

The results have been spectacular. In the past few years some diseases such as polio, smallpox, meningitis, diphtheria, and scarlet fever have been virtually wiped out, whereas others such as measles, undulant fever, tuberculosis, tetanus, tularemia, typhoid fever, and whooping cough have been greatly reduced in incidence in this country. Despite this impressive record, communicable diseases are still a public health concern. In 1968, tuberculosis killed 3300 persons; influenza and pneumonia, still the sixth leading cause of death, took the lives of 34,000 Americans, and about as many died from arteriosclerosis. Some diseases such as syphilis and gonorrhea, which could be eliminated if what is known about their control and treatment were fully applied, are actually increasing in incidence. Infectious hepatitis is another communicable disease on the increase. The common cold implacably takes its annual toll of human health and production despite an army of researchers' efforts and the application of hundreds of so-called cold remedies and treatments. A related problem has been the appearance of drug-resistant bacteria contributed to in part by years of low-level routine dosing with antibiotics in a shotgun therapy approach to conditions not serious enough or appropriate for their use. The effectiveness of penicillin in the treatment of syphilis and gonorrhea is diminishing for this reason. The bacillus of tuberculosis is becoming resistant to the drugs that have been so successful against it in recent years.

The triumphs that modern medicine has won over communicable disease and organic dysfunction through chemotherapy and surgical advances has led to an increase in chronic disease figures. A larger proportion of the population survives to the older ages, for one thing, when the likelihood of chronic disease is greatest. The accompanying table lists the top twenty-five chronic conditions in the United States.

Selected Chronic Conditions Causing Limitation of Activities, July 1963–June 1965

Condition Causing Limitation of Activities	*Estimated number of cases*
Tuberculosis, all forms	148,000
Malignant neoplasms	260,000
Benign and unspecified neoplasms	227,000
Asthma, hay fever	1,152,000
Diabetes	571,000
Mental and nervous conditions	1,767,000
Heart conditions	3,619,000
Hypertension without heart involvement	1,369,000
Varicose veins	535,000
Hemorrhoids	243,000
Other conditions of circulatory system	758,000
Chronic sinusitis and bronchitis	621,000
Other conditions of respiratory system	461,000
Peptic ulcer	550,000
Hernia	556,000
Other conditions of digestive system	958,000
Conditions of genito urinary system	1,071,000
Arthritis and rheumatism	3,481,000
Other diseases of muscles, bones, and joints	785,000
Visual impairments	1,285,000
Hearing impairments	461,000
Paralysis, complete or partial	923,000
Impairments (except paralysis) of back or spine	1,769,000
Impairments (except paralysis and absence) of upper extremities and shoulders	401,000
Impairments (except paralysis and absence) of lower extremities and hips	1,325,000

Note: The National Health Survey Division obtains data on chronic conditions reported to have caused or contributed to limitation of activities. The estimates shown above include conditions limiting major activities such as working, keeping house, going to school, as well as those causing lesser limitation not related to major activity. Statistics for the prevalence of chronic conditions in institutional populations are not included, and therefore the survey may considerably underestimate rates for the total population.

Source: U. S. Department of Health, Education and Welfare, Public Health Service, *Vital and Health Statistics,* "Chronic Conditions and Activity Limitations, United States, July 1963–June 1965," Series 10, no. 51 (February 1969), p. 20.

Notice that only one is directly attributable to a bacterium, a reflection of man's victories over these organisms, but also of the fact that communicable diseases are seldom chronic in nature. The latest figures available, reporting the period of July 1965 to June 1966 estimate that 93.7 million persons, or almost half of us, had one or more chronic conditions in that year. Among these persons, about 21.4 million had some degree of activity limitation. About 4 million were unable to carry on the major activity of their age-sex group, and 17.4 percent were seriously limited in work or play activities.[17]

Much of the chronic disease that middle-aged and older people must counter is not necessarily degenerative in origin. The term "*degenerative*" is not often accurately applied. It connotes a change for the worse, lessened efficiency, an alteration in function that almost always has serious consequences. Medical or surgical intervention is often necessary in order to correct or compensate for the change. Among those reporting chronic activity-limiting conditions, many are victims of one or more such diseases that might have been avoided or postponed had the individual based his health-care decisions upon sound health information.

If the leading causes of death in our populations in 1968 are examined, striking opportunities for improvement and prolongation of healthful life are apparent if the potential outcomes of health education are realized.

Deaths and Death Rates for the Ten Leading Causes of Death in 1968, and Death Rates for Similar Causes in 1900

Rank	*Cause of Death and Category Numbers of the Eighth Revision of the International Lists (1968)*	*Number of Deaths in 1968*	*Rates per 100,000 Population*	
			1968	*1900*
1	Diseases of heart	745,350	372.9	137.4
2	Malignant neoplasms	318,910	159.6	64.0
3	Cerebrovascular disease	209,420	104.8	106.9
4	Accidents	111,460	55.8	72.3
5	Influenza and pneumonia	69,750	34.9	202.2
6	Certain causes of mortality in early infancy	42,460	21.2	62.6
7	Diabetes mellitus	38,470	19.2	—[a]
8	Arteriosclerosis	33,350	16.7	—
9	Bronchitis, emphysema, and asthma	33,130	16.6	—
10	Cirrhosis of liver	28,910	14.5	12.5
	All causes	1,923,000	962.2	1,719.1

[a]Not obtainable because of change in classification.

Source of 1968 data: U. S. Department of Health, Education and Welfare, Public Health Service, *Vital Statistics Report,* Annual Summary for the United States, 1968, p. 3.

Source of 1900 data: U. S. Department of Health, Education and Welfare, Public Health Service, *The Facts of Life and Death,* Washington, D.C., U. S. Government Printing Office, 1968.

Cardiovascular disease has been termed the greatest epidemic of all time. However, heart disease is clearly susceptible to prevention through weight control, diet choices eliminating foods rich in cholesterols and saturated fats, and elimination of cigarette smoking. Coronary heart disease, the most common form of heart dysfunction, causes more than half the number of related deaths. There are more than 14 million people living who still suffer disability due to one or more forms of heart and blood vessel disorder.

People must be educated to avoid infections that might lead to heart damage; to seek qualified medical care on a routine, preventive basis, and to adopt a life style that avoids harmful excesses of any kind. This will not guarantee freedom from heart disease but will go far toward increasing both the length and the quality of one's life.

In 1900 cancer was eighth among the leading causes of death, killing 64,000 of the population. In 1968 it ranked second, and took the lives of 318,910 people. Except for accidents, cancer is the leading cause of death among schoolchildren. However, even though cancer mortality is rising, hope for patients is better than ever before. If treatment is begun early enough, two out of six patients will survive, one in six will die who *could* have been saved, and three will die of cancers that cannot yet be controlled. Certainly the incidence of incurable cancer would be reduced if people were to take early action when certain symptoms appeared, or if preventive tests were sought on a routine basis. The curriculum that does not provide students with information about cancer and its control is not concerned with present-day reality and needs.

THE TOLL OF ACCIDENTS

Accidents could be dramatically reduced if each of us were committed to the concept of safety as a means to increased enjoyment of activity rather than as a curb to pleasure. The National Safety Council reports that there were 56,400 deaths and 2 million disabling injuries in 1969 from highway accidents alone. An estimated 51.8 million persons in the civilian population were injured during the year July 1966–June 1967. By far the greatest proportion of these—22.6 million—occurred in the home, although of course those occurring in moving vehicles resulted in much more serious injury. Accidents are the fourth leading cause of death at all ages, and first among the 1 to 36 age group.

Death as a result of automobile collision could be diminished by at least 5000 a year were driver and passengers to *use* the seat belts that manufacturers are compelled to install for their protection. Most people let their belts lie in a useless jumble behind the seats. Many rear seat belts have never been unwrapped from their factory packaging. Some use seat belts only when on long drives, or on the highways, or when visibility is poor or roads slippery. Yet most accidents occur during daylight hours, when the roads are dry and the car is traveling in residential areas. The fact that those in the age group 17 to 24 have by far the highest injury rate in auto accidents, three times that of other age groups, indicates how much might be done to lower this rate were enough attention given to automobile safety in the curriculum.

Substantial reductions have been effected in industry, in recreational areas, and in public transportation as a result of intensive safety campaigns (education) and imposition of carefully planned safety measures. Much remains to be done in home safety and automobile safety. The economic waste resulting from accidents of all kinds is estimated to be more than $15 billion annually. The heartbreaking loss of human life and human talent is beyond estimation.

Accidents do not need to happen. Somebody or something causes them. School health education approaches this problem, as all others, by giving the student an opportunity to formulate a plan of future action that will tend to avoid accidents and promote the safety of all.

MATERNITY, INFANCY, AND THE BIRTH RATE There were 3,470,000 live births registered in the United States in 1968, the smallest number since 1946 and the lowest rate ever observed when underreporting of earlier years is considered. There were 75,300 deaths of infants under 1 year of age, resulting in a mortality rate of 21.7 per 1000 births. This is the seventh successive year in which the infant mortality rate in this country has reached a record low. Nevertheless, this rate still is one of the highest among the nations of the Western world. The maternal death rate in the same year was 27.4 per 100,000 live births, decreased from 1967's rate of 28.9. These downward trends are encouraging, but both figures could be dramatically lowered. Many of these deaths are from causes we know how to prevent or treat. If pregnant women knew more, were better prepared for motherhood in their school years, they would seek better care during pregnancy, avoid use of substances dangerous to the developing fetus, and know better how to care for their babies after birth. Infection, maternal diets, secondary complications like heart or kidney disease, and fears or tensions are the principal causes of disaster involved in pregnancy and maternity. Adequate education could do much to lower the unnecessarily high infant and maternal death rates.

Much attention is being given to the birth rate not only in the United States but all over the world. Overpopulation is perceived as a serious threat to the ecology. Use of contraceptive devices and preventive hormones is being promoted, studied, and ceaselessly debated by church, physicians, politicians, and laymen. It has been proposed that the United States Congress prepare legislation empowering the government to regulate family size, or that income tax deductions for dependent children be limited to no more than two or three. For the first time, the notion that any woman has the right to decide whether or not she wishes to allow a fetus to develop to term is being given serious consideration. Abortion laws are being rewritten in more and more states to permit doctors more freedom to perform abortions as women request them.

Thoughtful young people are seeking genetic counseling before planning marriage in situations where there is risk of transmitting hereditary defects. Students want to know about the Rh factor and its role in child development, and they are interested in the function of DNA in cell growth and reproduction.

Adolescents turn more often to their peers for information than to their parents. In doing so, they more often learn half-truths and misconceptions than sound information, and almost nothing about the social and emotional aspects of family or its many responsibilities and how to meet them. Often peer-educated themselves, many parents admit that they feel inadequate to the task of teaching their children what they need to learn about the nature of the sexual drive, its control, and its relationship to the structure of the family as the social unit that serves to fulfill these needs. A well thought out health education program can offer great opportunities for young people to obtain the information they need and plan for a reasoned, in part at least, rather than an emotion-based selection of a marriage partner. The problems associated with the rising birth rate are a real-life concern of young people in secondary schools today.

FOOD AND DIET

American boys and girls today tend to be taller and heavier than were their parents and grandparents, and are becoming physically and sexually mature six months to two years earlier than earlier generations. This trend is no longer a phenomenon unique to the United States but is beginning to be seen world wide. For example, Japanese children born since World War II show a dramatic increase over height and weight averages typical of Japanese people for centuries. Many factors have contributed to such changes; control of many diseases, more interbreeding due to increased population mobility, and better health care. Most important, however, is the improvement in nutrition. Modern food preservation techniques have eliminated seasonal nutritional deficiencies that once had to be endured. More is known about the function of nutrients in supporting essential body needs. In the richer countries, particularly, meat is easily obtained, and other good sources of protein are abundant. A wide variety of vitamin-rich foods and plenty of milk and other dairy products are prepared and marketed under controlled standards of quality.

And yet in the midst of this fortunate situation, the nutritional problem in this country is considerable. For one thing, people just do not choose the foods they need for optimum growth and repair. Low income makes it difficult for at least one-fifth of our population to obtain proper balance among nutrients.

Some of us overeat because of patterns of consumption learned during childhood years when activity and growth requirements necessitated a higher calorie diet. Some of us are "foodaholics," who eat to satisfy needs based on emotional tension. Diet-food production is big business. Harvard researchers in nutrition Jean Mayer and Johanna Dwyer demonstrated that in attempting to cut down on food consumption, too often people rely on folk beliefs about food values that are inaccurate. Need for improved education in nutrition was demonstrated by the School Health Education Study, whose 1964 survey reported that, on the average, less than half of the questions asked about nutrition were answered correctly at the twelfth-grade level.[18]

A panel recommendation of President Nixon's White House Conference on Food, Nutrition, and Health includes the following statement:

> The buying habits of the food purchaser, whether rich or poor, are not always based on adequate knowledge of the nutritional value of specific food products. Nutrition education programs, therefore, are essential ways to improve the nutrition of all Americans, but education by itself provides no substitute for insufficient food.[19]

Dietary practices of young people, especially girls, become increasingly worse throughout teen years. Typically they are deficient in Vitamins C and A and lack needed calcium and iron. There is a pattern of inadequate breakfasting and overdependence on carbohydrates in the form of sweet foods, french fries, and cola drinks.

Other forces shape nutritional practices. Advertising and food packaging play major roles in directing food selection habits. In advertising campaigns food processors and distributors have seized upon the health-promoting qualities of food more effectively than has education in most cases. Cultural patterns of eating and food selection influence some people to choose diets that may not be best for their particular needs. Perceptions of figure ideals, problems with teen-age acne, or a desire to conform to current peer-group behaviors motivate adolescents to choose or reject certain foods more powerfully than do any requirements for sound nutrition. Education needs to recognize these forces and turn them to good use. A teen-ager is far more interested in learning what foods will help him become what he wants to be than in memorizing the four food groups or in hearing that certain foods are "good for you."

Although dental health is stressed in all grades from kindergarten through the twelfth grade, tooth decay is one of our most prevalent diseases. It is estimated that there are over 1 billion unfilled cavities in the teeth of American men, women, and children, and one out of five Americans has lost all of his teeth by the time he is 50 years of age. The impact of dietary deficiencies on the incidence of dental disease is inescapable. In order to build strong tooth enamel the body must have calcium, protein, and Vitamin D, plus trace elements of other minerals such as fluoride. If any one is missing, tooth development is hindered. Vitamin C is absolutely essential for strong gums, and more teeth are lost because of periodontal disease than from caries. A large proportion of the population get inadequate amounts of this important vitamin.

Food is available to most people in the United States. The problem of improving health through improved nutrition involves education virtually as much if not more than it does capacity to buy. Students need to learn how to analyze their needs and how to apply scientific facts about nutrition in satisfying those needs.

CONSUMERS AND HEALTH CARE

In a society characterized by a burgeoning economy supported by easy credit, installment buying, and planned obsolescence, consumers face critical problems. Consumer crusader Ralph Nader has waged almost a one-man fight to prod reluctant giant corporations into reforms on pollution, auto safety, and product warranties. In doing so, he has given a great deal of visibility to the problem. Both state and federal offices of Consumer Education and Protection are working toward the same goals. In the final analysis, however, it is the consumer himself who is most powerful as he decides to buy or not to buy, chooses one service over another, or accepts or rejects information offered him.

A daily exercise in judgment is required even of a child, coin clutched in grubby little fist. Few of these judgments involve a product, service, or information that does not bear directly or indirectly on health. The responsibility of education then is to help students develop and use sound criteria for making such judgments. Whether one is choosing a breakfast cereal, an automobile tire, a toothpaste, or a physician, certain questions need to be asked. Decisions about the choice of one or another product need to be based on facts rather than on hearsay and motivated by reason rather than emotion. Choices should be consciously rational rather than manipulated by advertising. A concurrent responsibility is to educate people to differentiate between the kinds of decisions that they are competent to make and those that they are not.

Over-the-counter drug sales amount to more than $1 billion every year. Almost all of these purchases were self-prescribed and taken without any kind of medical supervision. Vitamin sales have been so effectively promoted that many mothers have been brainwashed into believing that child neglect is synonymous with failure to provide a daily vitamin pill. Actually, vitamins for normal diet needs are best obtained through a balanced diet. Painkillers, plain and fancy; laxatives, quick or gentle; sleep inducers; tonics whose regular use, it is inferred, make the user feel younger and more energetic and virile; hair dyes that promise similar benefits; skin creams that will "banish" wrinkles or ugly blemishes; in short, if there's something you'd like changed for the better there's a product guaranteed to help you!

The enormous amount of money wasted in buying these products aside, the greater danger is that in self-dosing, significant symptoms may be masked and qualified medical advice delayed until too late.

Americans have the right to choose their own physicians. We are free to go anywhere to seek care, whether it be to a faith healer, a chiropractor, a witch doctor, a quack, or a medical doctor. A goal of health education is to see that students know the kinds of training and competencies expected of a given practitioner, as well as how to determine the educational preparation of anyone who calls himself "Doctor."

As a concern of health education, the selection and use of professional health services has three aspects: the education of people to seek such help, the education and distribution of sufficient health personnel throughout the population, and education empowering people to discriminate between qualified health personnel and quacks. Quackery should be defined not only in terms of substandard training but also of substandard ethics or practices.

Health information is also an area of analysis and judgment. The alert consumer is one who is sensitive to what is happening in the world that affects his own health and that of his family. Considerable study has been directed not only to the safety but also the efficacy of drugs developed for human consumption. A host of over-the-counter drugs have been barred from sale as a result. Government agencies have also been fighting for some time to prohibit the sale of many prescription drugs. For example, some ninety combinations of antibiotics or antibiotics with sulfa, it is claimed by the Food and Drug Administration, endanger not only patients who receive them, but entire populations. It is found that excessive use of these germ-killing agents allows resistant strains of bacteria to multiply. This situation in turn creates the possibility of epidemics of infections that resist treatment.

The thalidomide babies, whose pathetic, limbless bodies resulted from use of a new sleeping pill compound during the first trimester of pregnancy, offer terrible proof that drugs may injure as well as cure or control. Other negative effects include lowering of normal body defense mechanisms, injuries to cells, imbalance among essential body materials, genetic changes, chemical carcinogenesis, and, as mentioned before, changes in microbial ecology. The mixed antibiotics have been ruled hazardous as well as ineffective for the purposes claimed and are thought to double the risk of adverse reactions in the patient.

Another drug, chloramphenicol, produces an irreversible and fatal suppression of bone marrow, resulting in aplastic anemia. The risk of contracting this disease within a year of taking this drug is thirteen times that for persons not so exposed. Yet chloramphenicol continues to be widely prescribed for both sound and trivial reasons.

Why would a qualified physician prescribe dangerous drugs for his patients or prescribe a brand-name drug no more effective than one available under its generic name but costing several times as much money? It could be that possible benefits far outweigh the risk of any adverse effects. It may be that it just is not possible for a busy physician to keep up with all the drugs turned out every year. Between 1940 and 1969, there were 858 basic new drugs developed! Dr. Edward R. Pinckney, former editor of the *Journal of the American Medical Association,* is quoted thus:

> The references cited in ads which were intended to indicate general clinical testing, acceptance and success of a drug—in order to influence the potential prescription for that drug—were not at all what they implied. And unless the doctor-user of the drug traced down the multitude of references, he naturally assumed widespread support for the advertised product.
>
> Thanks to the restrictive educational policies of the profession, there aren't enough doctors. The ones we have must work fifty and sixty hours a week and have no time to go to medical libraries and authenticate the claims made for the medicine they prescribe.[20]

Another physician, Richard Burack, in his useful little book that details generic names and comparative prices for most drugs in common use, says that "Most doctors' efforts to keep up to date have been expended in listening to detail men representing pharmaceutical manufacturers. Or in reading glowing advertisements in medical journals in which the claims are stated in large print and the much greater amount of copy listing contraindications (as required by law) is in very small hard to read print."[21]

The consumer himself should accept some part of this responsibility by asking questions about the drugs prescribed for him so that he knows what they are and why they are prescribed in his case. He should also be careful to take them *only* as directed, as *long* as directed, and no longer. And he should continue to be sensitive to health-related information available to him in reports announced by authoritative individuals and agencies. In order to do this, he also needs to learn what constitutes an authoritative source.

Figures on health care costs show that between 1950 and 1966, total national expenditures for health services and supplies (hospital costs, physicians' fees, and drug costs) increased from $11.9 billion to $41.8 billion. In the same period of time, expenditures for out-of-hospital drugs rose from $1 billion to $3.2 billion. In fact, the Social Security Administration reports that health care expenditures are growing faster than any other element in the nation's economy. In the fiscal year 1969, the figure was reportedly a record $60.3 billion. Health insurance is virtually a necessity, as health-care costs sky-rocket beyond the ability of any but the wealthiest to afford major ill-ness expenses. The cost of a hospital stay in even a four-bed room is about $60 a day, with minimum nursing care and treatment, and an average of $100 a day is predicted in a year or two.

It generally is acknowledged that at least some kind of health protection is currently owned by 70 percent of the population. In addition, two types of Medicare insurance plans administered by the Social Security Administration are available to persons over 65.

Public Health surveys have shown that individuals and families owning health insurance are far more apt to seek medical care for health problems than those who lack this protection. The ideal of preventive medical care may become more nearly a reality when everyone is protected by some kind of health insurance plan. Health education can provide meaningful opportunities for students to examine the comparative costs and benefits of health insurance so that value judgments can be based upon thoughtful analysis of facts.

HEALTH EDUCATION FOR TODAY'S WORLD

The needs for health education are clearcut and compelling. They are the needs of people as they seek to learn who they are, to find some degree of self-fulfillment in the world in which they live, and to develop their unique capabilities among others not always agreeable to their aims. They are the needs of man to know how to live, how to protect and rear his family, and how to use his growing fund of knowledge to his own and others' best interests.

– health education as part of general education

Does organized education in the United States have a commitment to curricula meeting these needs? Only partially, and only in some places. There are well established curriculum entities such as biology, life science, social studies, and others that touch on some of these problems, but it is necessary to come to grips with them in a direct fashion rather than peripherally or indirectly. Students today are demanding that their studies be relevant. This is what good programs of health education have been doing for years. Health education, human ecology if you like, considers not just the academic *things* of man's existence, but man himself.

John Gardner says of general education:

> All education worthy of the name enhances the individual. It heightens awareness, or deepens understanding, or enlarges one's powers, or introduces one to new modes of appreciation or enjoyment. It promotes individual fulfillment. It is a means of self-discovery. . . . In the deepest sense it enables one to live more fully in the dimensions that are distinctively human.[22]

Arno Bellack strikes a similar note when he says:

> The goal of general education is not to train students as specialists in mathematics, geography, biology, or whatever other subjects they might study. Rather, the goal is to make available to students the intellectual and aesthetic resources of their culture in such a way that they become guides for intelligent action and help students create meaning and order out of the complex world in which they find themselves.[23]

These statements express the goals of health education as well: to educate for self-fulfillment and to help students create guides for intelligent action and develop a framework of values to provide meaning and order to their world.

– is it a discipline? Whether or not health education is a discipline depends upon the way we perceive the meaning of the term "health education." It certainly is not a pure science in the sense of chemistry or physics. It is an applied science that draws upon the physical, biological, medical, and behavioral sciences for its body of knowledge. It is a discipline that synthesizes concepts and theories of these several areas and interprets them in the context of human needs, human values, and human potential. It is deeply concerned with the promotion of personal effectiveness and the quality of life.

What are the concepts basic to health education? The School Health Education Study identified three key concepts that express the most powerful ideas relative to health, serve as unifying threads of the curriculum, and characterize the processes underlying health:

1 Growing and Developing
A dynamic life process by which the individual is in some ways like all other individuals, in some ways like some other individuals, and in some ways like no other individuals.

2 Interacting
An ongoing process in which the individual is affected by and in turn affects certain biological, social, psychological, economic, cultural, and physical forces in the environment.

3 Decision Making
A process unique to man of consciously deciding to take or not

take an action, or of choosing one alternative rather than another.[24]

What is the mode of inquiry that is most representative of this discipline? Problem solving—the lifelong process that each of us needs to master in order to function effectively as a person and as a member of society. Health education stimulates the learner to examine, analyze, question, compare, and search out significant data. Important outcomes of these activities are internalization of concepts, which serve as powerful organizers of data as the individual continues to accumulate information, and formulation of a system of values by which he can live most effectively and contribute positively to his own life and that of those around him. Health education helps man to find out who he is by studying man himself.

– preventive or developmental?

Perhaps the popular view of health education is that it seeks to prevent disease. The traditional, outmoded hygiene and fact-centered approach of the past has been to teach about health by teaching about disease. In some areas this has not changed much. The National Institutes of Health, for instance, are really National Institutes of Disease. Mental health clinics are really concerned with mental illness of one degree or other. A truly preventive view, however, is not just a finger-wagging warning that disease or injury may be the outcome if certain procedures are not followed. A preventive view should be one that anticipates and removes possible conditions that might result in injury or disease; that applies measures to counter sources of potential illnesses; and that compensates for present handicaps to the end that the school may be a place where progress is possible for every child to the limit of his potential.

But the goal of health education is not limited by the notion of prevention. To improve the human condition, a developmental view is also necessary. Not the protection and promotion of the physical health of the individual alone, but the social, emotional, and spiritual aspects, as well, need to be allowed to grow and prosper. This holistic view of man recognizes and builds upon the innate need for self-fulfillment and self-actualization which lives within every person, can we but reach it.

SUMMARY

The point of view of this chapter has been that health cannot be viewed as a one-dimensional nor a static quality. Physical and mental health are inseparable and cannot be talked about as separate with any more logic than they can be ministered to as discrete entities. Things happen to or are done for the whole person, not just for his body or for his mind. A man is not a collection of organs held together by a suit of skin and directed in his movements by a ghost who lives in his skull. He is a complex being of intricately interrelated and interdependent parts and functions. Health has physical, social, mental, spiritual, and emotional components, and what affects one affects them all in some way. Health is a functional state of capability, a dynamic rather than a static quality. It is not mass, but function. It is not an end to be achieved, but a means to achievement of meaningful goals.

Health education for the seventies and beyond will need to define and sharpen its basic concepts. Subject matter and teaching methodology will need to be geared to the needs and capabilities of the new generation with their special demands for relevance as they perceive the world.

The philosophy of today's health education is that human beings are feeling, thinking, behaving organisms who are required to function effectively in a society ever more perplexing in its changes and complexity. In a technological world in which knowledge increases with such bewildering speed, not content but process—ways of dealing with knowledge—is the essential skill. But perhaps the imperative outcome of health education must be a student who knows who he is, who has been helped to discover his own humanness, and who has built a meaningful system of values by which he can order his life.

To help the student acquire a meaningful health education, the school must join with the family and the community, with health agencies, and with medical programs in both their preventive and constructive

The Health Needs of the School and Community Population May Be Met by:

A Program of Instruction and Environmental Control	and	A Program of Service and Environmental Control
which is founded upon		which is founded upon
An Appraisal of Individual and Social Needs		An Appraisal of Community Needs
and from which is derived a		and from which is derived a
Curriculum		Medical, Dental, Psychiatric, Educational, and Sanitation Program
requiring		requiring
Skilled Health Educators		Skilled Health Personnel
who constantly seek an		who constantly seek an
Evaluation of Outcomes to determine whether		Evaluation of Outcomes to determine whether
The Needs Were Met and, where necessary, Replan		The Needs Were Met and, where necessary, Replan

aspects. The total program of health education thus evolved becomes the responsibility of everyone, and perhaps most significantly of the student himself.

The essence of a modern health education program is described in the chart on the facing page.

The chapters that follow will discuss the problems fundamental to such a program and the principles and processes that seem indicated in the solution of those problems. The program seeks to (1) help students learn how to discover the information they need to make decisions about their behavior; (2) help develop children who are fit to learn; (3) give them an opportunity to develop skills of problem solving and critical thinking; and (4) secure for them a school environment that favors and promotes their growth and development. If these purposes can be achieved, the school will have made a powerful and lasting contribution to the health of the nation.

NOTES AND REFERENCES

1 Kenneth Boulding, "Expecting the Unexpected: The Uncertain Future of Knowledge and Technology," *Prospective Changes in Society by 1980,* Denver, Designing Education for the Future, Citation Press, 1967, p. 213.

2 Association for Supervision and Curriculum Development, *To Nurture Humaneness. Commitment for the 70's.* Washington, D.C., NEA.

3 Constitution of the World Health Organization, *Chronicle of the World Health Organization,* 1 (1947), 29–43.

4 Halbert L. Dunn, *High Level Wellness,* Arlington, Va., B.W. Beatty, 1961, p. 4.

5 School Health Education Study, *Health Education: A Conceptual Approach To Health Education,* St. Paul, 3M Education Press, p. 10.

6 Earl V. Pullias, "The Education of the Whole Man," *Quest,* Monograph I, December 1963, p. 41.

7 Joe Bales Graber, "A Melding of Minds," *Human Potential in a Dynamic Environment,* School Health Education Study, Airlie House Conference, Washington, D.C. 1968.

8 Expert Committee on Health Education of the Public, First Report, World Health Organization Technical Report Series, no. 89, Geneva: World Health Organization, October 1954, p. 9.

9 W. Raab, "U.S.A. Needs Mass-Conditioning Against Diseases of Civilization," *Journal of Sports Medicine,* 1 (June 1962), 117.

10 U. S. Department of Health, Education and Welfare, National Institute of Mental Health, *The Mental Health of Urban America,* April 1969, p. 4.

11 Richard M. Cohen, "Social Survey Reveals 12 Percent Used Marijuana, Few on Heroin," *Washington Post,* March 11, 1970, p. A1.

12 President's Commission on Law Enforcement and Administration of Justice, *Task Force on Juvenile Delinquency and Youth Crime,* 1967, p. 120.

13 Michael L. Peck, "Suicide Motivation in Adolescents," *Adolescence,* 3, 9, (Spring 1968).

14 Medical Statistics Agency, Office of the Surgeon General, Department of the Army, Washington, D.C., June 1969, p. 3. *Health of the Army, Results of the Examination of Youths for Military Service,* 1968.

15 M. Savoy, "Too Late Now To Avoid Famines, Expert Claims," *Los Angeles Times,* Feb. 13, 1970, part 4, p. 1.

16 Haynes Johnson, "Poison Ravages Desert's Life Cycle," *Washington Post,* February 13, 1970, p. A8.

17 U. S. Department of Health, Education and Welfare, Vital Health Statistics, *Limitation of Activity and Mobility Due to Chronic Conditions,* July 1965–June 1966, series 10, 45, May 1968.

18 Elena Sliepcevich, *A Summary Report,* Washington, D.C., School Health Education Study, 1964.

19 Jean Mayer, "Chairborn Obesity a 'Disease of Civilization,'" *Washington Post,* November 30, 1969, p. B4.

20 Nicholas von Hoffman, "Drug Ads," *Washington Post,* November 26, 1969, p. B7.

21 Richard Burack, *The Handbook for Prescription Drugs,* New York, Pantheon Books, 1967.

22 John Gardner, *No Easy Victories,* New York, Harper & Row, 1968, p. 73.

23 Arno Bellack, "The Structure of Knowledge and the Structure of the Curriculum," New York, Teachers College Press, 1964, p. 29.

24 School Health Education Study, *Health Education: A Conceptual Approach to Curriculum Design,* St. Paul, 3M Education Press, 1967, pp. 16–17.

SELECTED READINGS

Association for Supervision and Curriculum Development, *To Nurture Humaneness. Commitment for the 70's,* Scobey Mary-Margaret, and Graham Grace (eds.), Washington, D.C., NEA, 1970.

Breslow, Lester, "The Urgency of Social Action for Health," *American Journal of Public Health,* 60, 1 (January 1970), 1–16.

The Brookings Institution, *Agenda for the Nation,* Garden City, N.Y., Doubleday, 1969.

Byler, Ruth, Gertrude Lewis, and Ruth Totman, *Teach Us What We Want To Know,* Connecticut State Board of Education, 1969.

"Curriculum Change in Health Education," Bulletin of the National Association of Secondary School Principals, 326, Washington, D.C. (March 1968).

Daedalus, "Toward the Year 2000: Work in Progress," *Journal of the American Academy of Arts and Sciences,* 96, 3 (Summer 1967).

Dubos, Rene. *Man Adapting,* New Haven, Conn., Yale University Press, 1965.

———, *Man, Medicine, and Environment,* New York, Praeger, 1968.

———, *The Torch of Life: Continuity in Living Experience,* New York, Simon & Schuster, 1962.

Dunn, Halbert L., *High Level Wellness,* Washington, D. C., R. W. Beatty, 1961.

Designing Education for the Future, An Eight State Project, "Implications for Education of Prospective Changes in Society," Edgar L. Morphet and Charles O. Ryan (eds.), January 1967.

Ewald, William R., Jr. (ed.), *Environment for Man.* Bloomington, Indiana University Press, 1967.

Foreign Policy Association (eds.), *Toward the Year 2018,* New York, Cowles, 1968.

Fortune, "The Environment: A National Mission for the Seventies," February 1970.

Fraser, Dorothy McClure, "The Changing Scene in Social Studies," *Social Studies Curriculum Development: Projects and Problems,* Washington, D. C., National Council for the Social Studies, 1969, pp. 1–32.

Gardner, John W., *Self Renewal: The Individual and the Innovative Society,* New York, Harper & Row, 1964.

Ginzburg, El (ed.), *Values and Ideals of American Youth,* New York, Columbia University Press, 1961.

Heilbroner, Robert L., "Priorities for the Seventies," *Saturday Review,* January 3, 1970, pp. 17–19, 84.

Hilleboe, Herman E., "Public Health in the United States in the 1970's," *American Journal of Public Health,* 58, 9 (September 1968), pp. 1588–1619.

Holt, John, "Why We Need New Schooling," *Look,* January 13, 1970, pp. 52.

Joint Committee on Health Problems in Education of the NEA and the AMA, *Health Education,* 5th ed., Washington, D. C., NEA, 1961.

———, *Why Health Education?* Washington, D. C., NEA, 1965.

Kahn, Herman, and Wiener, Anthony J., *The Year 2000,* New York, Macmillan, 1967.

Kime, Robert E., *Health: A Consumer's Dilemma,* Belmont, Calif., Wadsworth, 1970.

Lerner, Monroe, and Odin U. Anderson, *Health Progress in the United States: 1900–1960,* Chicago, University of Chicago Press, 1964.

Long, Barbara Ellis, "Where Do You Learn To Be People Now?—In School?" *American Journal of Orthopsychiatry,* March 1969, pp. 291–93.

Means, Richard K., *A History of Health Education,* Philadelphia: Lea & Febiger, 1962.

Remsberg, Charles, and Bonnie Remsberg, "Why You Really Can't Get Good Medical Care," *Good Housekeeping,* February 1970, pp. 68–71, 140–142.

Smithsonian Annual II. The Fitness of Man's Environment. Washington, D.C., Smithsonian Institution Press, 1968.

Szasz, Thomas S., *The Myth of Mental Illness,* New York, Dell, 1961.

U. S. Department of Health, Education and Welfare, *Toward A Social Report,* Washington, D. C., Government Printing Office, 1969.

CHAPTER 2 PLANNING FOR LEARNING

Effective planning for teaching or learning depends in the final analysis upon the validity of the stated goals. Valid goals cannot be based upon an instructor's personal preferences, nor prescribed by conventional wisdom at any level of jurisdictional remoteness from the learner. If they are, they will be merely word exercises, for such goals are not likely to be known to, much less motivate, those whose future behavior they are supposed to reflect.

Goals should be derived from a synthesis of data gathered through careful analysis of three principal sources. These are (1) the needs, interests, and concerns of the learner himself; (2) the body of knowledge and logic of inquiry through which new knowledge is generated in a field; and (3) the society and the world in which the learner must live and function as a citizen. These are the sources fundamental to curriculum decisions in any field. Nowhere are these sources more crucial than in health education. Valid goals of health teaching cannot be determined except from an analysis of the learner's needs. One more procedure is appropriate, however, to make certain that the results will be acceptable to the learner. If he is himself involved in setting the goals, his commitment to them is more likely. His own value system and his own need perceptions have functioned in the process of selection.

By definition, goals are long-range plans. No one lesson or single course can assure their attainment. Nevertheless, they do provide stability to an educational program, permitting objectives expressed at course- or lesson-planning levels to be responsive to what is now, and what is relevant to a particular group, while at the same time contributing to achievement of the broader aims. Yet, whatever the learning activities selected, however unique they appear to be in a given teaching situation, certain similarities among goals are inescapable. Whether all or only some of them are evidenced by an individual's behavior at any given time, the following description of a health-educated person illustrates achievement of goals that can logically be inferred from analysis of data presently available in connection with these sources.

THE GOALS OF AN EDUCATED PERSON

An educated person tries to live his life and make health-related decisions in terms of what he has learned to be dependable information. He not only knows but values the basic facts about health and disease, and promotes his personal effectiveness through their application. He can evaluate claims and products advertised or offered to him and distinguish between those that are serviceable and those that are either harmful or useless. He can apply valid criteria to the selection of a qualified health advisor. He prefers a life of abundant, vital, creative energy, which can lift him above the commonplace and which offers the greatest potential for high-level being and achievement.

Such a person is not content with merely the absence of disease as his criterion of personal health, but actively seeks superior health, superior performance. He is not content with mediocrity, but practices a superior pattern of daily living that finds its reward in energy allowing him to live most with what he has to live with.

The educated person knows who he is and accepts his inadequacies along with his capabilities. The degree to which he is self-reliant, responsible for his own safety and dignity as well as that of his fellows, or conversely deprecates himself and relies upon his family or friends to make his decisions for him, will determine his growth as an effective citizen. If the educated person may be described as one who assumes some responsibility for local and community affairs, then a health-educated person would feel personal responsibility for measures established for the betterment of the health of all people.

He is capable of change and of thinking critically about health matters. He can distinguish scientific fact from political issues as for example in decisions about fluoridation of public water supplies. If new knowledge about nutrition, the influence of heredity, or immunization, or heart disease becomes available, he no longer holds unthinkingly to earlier teaching, but is flexibly receptive to change. Flexibility is particularly important to acceptance of health information because health education is so dynamic a field, bringing to the learner so much rapidly advancing research from the life sciences. Those who cannot bring themselves to accept change as a continuing, lifelong process quickly lose touch with what is current and therefore risk bigotry.

The health-educated person does not fear but feels secure in the face of change. He can react reasonably and effectively in new and disturbing situations, whether they be new threats of war, discovery of more powerful and terrifying weapons, new social problems and changes, or new disease threats. He has won the sort of self-confidence and stability that enables him to adjust to and derive enjoyment from living in the midst of our ever changing and often frightening world.

To help individuals work out their goals, conceptualize them, and then work toward them, and to help students become educated in the terms we have just described is not a simple task. As a matter of fact, it becomes extremely difficult for some people because to be successful at it may require an adoption of quite a different attitude toward education. The essence of the matter is in humanizing the curriculum. The curriculum presented in health education from the early grades through college should not be something foreign to students, the substance of which is chosen merely because it is there and may have some bearing upon life. On the contrary, the curriculum in health education *is* life—it is continuous with experience and has no values and seeks no ends other than those which are inherent in the process of living. This is what we mean by humanizing the curriculum—making it relevant to life. Material chosen to be taught lies along the path of needs, is related to needs in a very intimate way, has no values other than those inherent in the revealed need, or, better yet, is *demanded* by the student in order to satisfy a revealed and felt need. He *wants* to know because *knowing* is important to him, so the teacher helps him find the answers. Teaching in health education is essentially a *human* experience, not a textbook one nor an experience in "learning for learning's sake." The teacher must never forget this human aspect or health education will lose all its meaning and become just another subject to be studied.

When we speak of personal *goals* or *desires* or *needs,* we are speaking of things which are fundamental to all living beings. We are not referring to whims or passing fancies. We are suggesting that for the teacher or any other "outsider" to *guess* what is going on in a child's mind (rather than to attempt to find out), and proceed to base the curriculum upon such guesses is to risk error and waste energy. If he realizes that goal seeking and directiveness in organisms are a basic fact and life's most characteristic quality, the teacher will seek out these personal goals and purposes and select the instructional material in relation to them. If this is done successfully, the impetus to learn need not and will not come entirely from the teacher. The learner will be *drawn* to the lesson rather than *driven* to it.

But why is anybody drawn to anything? And how much effort will a person expend to arrive at his goal? These are questions important to the teacher. They involve motive, reason, purpose, ambition. A Freudian might say we are drawn to something, want it, and want to learn about it because it *gives pleasure.* Adlerian psychology would stress the *will to power;* people learn because they want the power that comes with learning. Viktor Frankl describes what he calls the *will to meaning* as being of equal, if not more, importance than power or pleasure:

> In my opinion man is dominated neither by the will-to-pleasure nor by the will-to-power, but what I call man's will-to-meaning, that is to say, his deep-seated striving and struggle for a higher and ultimate meaning to his existence. This is his mission in life—his unique task—for there is a personal task waiting for each personality to be realized exclusively by him and by him alone.[1]

Others have described these drives, inner compulsions, and goals as *ego motives,* or the desire to maintain and bolster self-esteem and prestige among others. There is agreement among psychologists that a dominant force in learning is our need for security and for success, and surely much of what is taught in school is accepted or rejected in terms of its relation to our own "security operations." If learning about heart disease bolsters our esteem, or gives us a feeling of knowing something important, then we are much more likely to learn it than if it bores us or has no meaning or if no one else cares about it.

There is pride in learning. Our society respects the learned person. Teachers can, with frequent success, relate health material to the student's personal desire to know a little more than the next fellow. Or, in terms of the desire for security, the teacher or physician will have taught well whenever he has assisted the learner to fulfill that desire. We feel secure in knowledge, especially knowledge that leads us to effective action.

THE SOURCES OF THE HEALTH CURRICULUM

To plan a curriculum likely to help individuals become educated in this way and achieve personally meaningful goals is difficult, and so is devising teaching-learning situations relevant to present issues. Added to this difficulty is the curriculum makers' perennial dilemma—how to create an educational system that is relevant for *all* students and that can prepare them to make a place for themselves in a society whose requirements are many and diverse, and, perhaps, some of them still unknown.

The sort of education that can facilitate development of human capabilities must be directly concerned with the real world. Curriculum decision-making, to be relevant, must be based upon relevant data. The questions to be asked are: Who is the person to be educated? What does he need to know? What does he *want* to know? What are the most powerful ideas or concepts believed by the specialists in a field to be representative of its body of knowledge? How can these concepts be communicated to serve as means of ordering new information as it is accumulated? What skills are needed and what behaviors are expected by the society in which the learner will live and function as a citizen?

THE LEARNER AND HIS NEEDS

A primary source of data from which educational goals may be inferred is the learner himself—his needs, interests, concerns, stage of maturity, and present abilities or lack of them.

Needs may be looked at in several ways. One point of view is the degree to which the present condition of the individual differs from some acceptable standard. An educational objective derived from this notion of need would be focused on a plan to provide learning opportunities designed to bridge such a gap. Another kind of need is reflected in the organism's innate urge to maintain a balance or equilibrium between internal drives and external conditions. Such needs, or disequilibria, may be physiological, emotional, or integrative in origin. The external conditions are those in the world around the individual that provide or limit the means available to satisfy his needs and restore balance. Physiological needs such as food, water, warmth; psychological or emotional needs such as those for affection, status, belongingness; and integrative needs such as the need for a feeling of identity, self-fulfillment, and self-respect are representative of this second kind of need.

The learner's interests and concerns might as logically be termed needs. If he is interested in something it is because the topic represents information or behaviors he wants to acquire. As such, it is a felt or expressed need. If he is concerned about a problem, then he seeks to learn about it as a means of coping with or solving it. Needs may be felt or not felt by the learner. The felt needs, interests, and concerns may be more easily quantified by the investigator because they are more readily apparent or perceived by the learner. The challenge to health education is to motivate the learner to become interested in needs that may be unfelt but no less imperative.

Considerable research already exists to tell us what needs are likely to be shared by children in our society, depending on their age, sex, and developmental level. Data relative to needs may be gathered in a number of ways: from medical and dental records; morbidity and mortality tables; observation of actual behavior such as personal health practices, food choices, use of tobacco and other drugs; records of critical incidents; and interviews with parents, teachers, or other significant adults. The best way to gather information is to ask the learner himself. Who knows better what his interests and concerns may be?

A number of standardized health-knowledge and health-behavior inventories are available and can be used to obtain additional useful information about the learner. Application of valid paper and pencil tests can yield data useful for planning and replanning instruction. Not only what the learner does *not* know, *but also what he erroneously believes to be true,* can be ascertained to the extent of what is sampled in the test. What is found to be already known provides a baseline for further sequential development of the concepts and inquiry processes selected as essential to his education.

The most extensive application of standardized tests in recent years was that carried out by the School Health Education Study in 1962.[2] A random sampling of students enrolled in large, medium, and small school districts across the country was conducted to investigate health knowledge and behaviors of those sampled in grades four through twelve. The resulting answer sheets were analyzed in terms of differences between sexes; differences among groups of school districts by size; strengths and weaknesses in knowledge about specific content areas; and misconceptions held by twelfth-grade students. Findings were tabulated and served as one basis for subsequent curriculum decisions basic to the Study's *Conceptual Approach to Health Education.* Some of the misconceptions typical of those revealed are the following:

Legislation guarantees the reliability of any advertised medicine.

Chronic diseases can be transmitted from person to person.

The purpose of fluoridating water is to purify it and make it safe to drink.

Venereal disease can be inherited.

Voluntary health agencies are supported by public funds.

A full time public health department provides complete medical diagnosis and treatment for any citizen.[3]

It was found that the average sixth-grade student could answer just over half of the questions he was asked! Dental health, mental health, and safety education were the weakest content areas. Ninth-grade students demonstrated least competence in the area of consumer health, followed by habit-forming substances, fatigue, sleep and rest, defense against disease, mental health, dental health, and safety and first aid, in that order. Ninth-grade scores on knowledge items were far better than those reflecting their practices.

Extensive needs and interests studies have been completed by many investigators, both in the United States and around the world. Most of these studies have been essentially adaptations or replications of the design developed to investigate the needs and interests of Ohio schoolchildren in 1932.

More recently a survey of the health interests, concerns, and problems of 5000 students in selected schools, from kindergarten through the twelfth grade, reported results categorized by topics in relation to age groups. It was discovered that the major topic, or basic health interest areas, were common to all students whether they lived in the inner city, rural, suburban, or high socioeconomic areas studied. Nevertheless, the researchers for this project warn that their findings should not be regarded as universals:

> Teachers or curriculum workers will still need to answer questions such as, what are the priorities in *my* class? And if, for example, three seventh graders out of twenty-five indicate they don't think drug education is at all necessary at this time, what are the implications of this for lesson planning?[4]

Finally, the curriculum worker must bring to his analysis of the needs of the learner what has been learned about the growth and development characteristics of children and youth in general, as well as what are believed to be acceptable theories of learning.

To base a curriculum in health education upon the needs, interests, and problems of students means that the teacher (or those who are developing teaching materials) must *discover,* not assume or estimate, the health problems of students; the felt and unfelt needs, the hazards that life holds (and of which the student may be unaware); the responsibilities and privileges of life; and the problems of the family and the many communities of people among whom they will live and work and about which they need to be informed. All of these can be material for teaching and learning. The important thing is to choose material to teach in health education that can be drawn from real life and that meets needs that exist whether the student recognizes them or not.

THE BODY OF KNOWLEDGE

Nearly every statement of the goals of education proposed since the 1917 *Cardinal Principles of Education* has placed health high on its list of priorities. The NEA Project on Instruction reiterated this commitment to the value of health education:

> The school, as the only social institution that reaches all children and youth, has responsibility for teaching the basic information and for helping young people develop the habits and attitudes essential for healthful living. Effective health education begins in early childhood and continues as a cumulative program through

> the elementary and secondary school years. It stresses the application of rational thought processes to health problems as well as the teaching of essential knowledge.[5]

The potential contribution of health instruction to the general education of all children is recognized by every key educational and medical association as well as by school administration and parent groups. But what is the essential knowledge fundamental to the application of rational thought processes to health problems?

Every discipline lays claim to some broad, but defined, range of principles, concepts, and generalizations that by agreement of its scholars is representative of its body of knowledge. Content identification processes and value systems are therefore inextricably tied one to the other. The question must continually be asked of the scholars, What knowledge is of most worth today? What knowledge does an educated man need to enable him to function effectively as a human being and as a member of his many communities?

There are two ways of looking at this question of identifying essential knowledge: first as the goal of general education and second as the goal of a specialist in the field. The difference between the kinds of knowledge is rather like the difference between the knowledge one needs to observe a football game, with sufficient awareness of the tactics being employed on the field as to follow them with appreciation and understanding, and the very special kind of knowledge one needs to be a skilled participant in a professional game. It is as a goal of general education that discussion of the body of knowledge unique to health education will be presented.

THE TRADITIONAL APPROACH

Health education has traditionally concerned itself with a series of content areas, each related to some aspect of health, usually a problem. The resulting list has, in effect, constituted an outline of what was viewed as the body of knowledge, or *scope,* of health education. Such a list of recommended areas of studies was proposed in the latest edition of *Health Education* (1961), prepared by the Joint Committee on Health Problems in Education of the NEA and the AMA. The recommendations of its authors, all recognized authorities, include the following:

> The content of health education might well include learning experiences selected from the following areas of study.
>
> 1 The human body—Its origins, structure, function, and control . . .
>
> 2 Biological needs of the human organism—Food, air, water, activity, rest, sleep . . .
>
> 3 Psychosocial needs of the individual—acceptance, security, recognition, achievement, affection, self-respect, adaptability . . .

4 Hazards to life and health—Hereditary and congenital anomalies, developmental disorders, disease-producing organisms, violence and injury, poisons, certain drugs, alcohol, chemicals, radiation, and other actual or potential causes of disability . . .

5 Progress in human health and the scientific bases for health care—Understanding and appreciation of the scientific advances that have been made in the achievement of a greater measure of health and longevity . . .

6 Health in the home and family—Meeting the biological and psychosocial needs of family members through understanding the nature and variations in health needs of husband, wife, infants, children, adolescents, and elderly people.

7 Health protection and promotion provided through community services—Pure water, safe food, clean air, sewage disposal, control of communicable diseases, healthful housing, fire prevention, accident prevention activities, health and hospital facilities, utilization of health and medical care . . .

8 State, national, and international needs, problems, and programs in health.[6]

The 1961–1962 School Health Education Study survey of the content of health education taught in institutions selected in a random sample of public school systems in the United States showed that the health topics that were emphasized by 50 percent or more of the respondent schools were as shown on the facing page.

Examination of most of the health textbooks and curriculum guides anywhere in the country reveals a total of forty or more separate subject areas that can be legitimately claimed as a part of this body of knowledge. All of these topics are drawn from the physical, biological, medical, and behavioral sciences (sociology, psychology, and anthropology) but are synthesized into a new science of healthful living. Which of these topics are included and emphasized in any one textbook or curriculum depends both upon tradition and the value systems of its authors, which lead them to perceive certain problems as of most social concern. In general, most of the topics already cited are considered representative of the body of knowledge and, hence, will be talked about in any book that purports to be "about" health.

CONCEPTS AS ORGANIZERS

Recently, however, some health educators have begun to realize that this fragmented approach to health teaching is not as effective as they would wish. Sparked by the pioneer efforts of two national study groups, most curriculum work today is focusing on the identification of concepts rather than upon factual information categorized by health topics.

Kindergarten Through Sixth Grade

Accident Prevention
Cleanliness and Grooming
Communicable Disease
Community Helpers
Dental Health
Exercise and Relaxation
Family Life
First Aid
Food Nutrition
Health Examinations and Appraisals
Personality Development
Posture and Body Mechanics
Rest and Sleep
Vision and Hearing

Seventh Through the Twelfth Grade

Accident Prevention; First Aid
Alcohol, Drugs and Narcotics
Boy-Girl Relationships
Cleanliness and Grooming
Communicable Diseases
Community Health Programs
Consumer Education
Dental Health
Environmental Hazards
Exercise, Rest, and Sleep
Mental Health and Personal Adjustment
Non-communicable Diseases
Nutrition
Parenthood (Tenth to Twelfth Grade Only)
Physical Changes During Adolescence
Posture and Body Mechanics
Preparation for Marriage (Eleventh and Twelfth Grades)
Smoking
Structure and Function of the Human Body
Venereal Disease (Tenth to Twelfth Grades)
Vision and Hearing
Weight Control[7]

Jerome S. Bruner speaks about the rationale underlying this movement in his book *On Knowing:*

> The history of culture is the history of the development of great organizing ideas, ideas that inevitably stem from deeper values and points of view about man and nature. The power of great organizing concepts is in large part that they permit us to understand and sometimes to predict or change the world in which we live. But their power lies also in the fact that ideas provide instruments for experience . . . . The structure of knowledge—its connectedness and the derivations that make one idea follow from another—is the proper emphasis in education.[8]

The identification of powerful concepts (words or ideas or generalizations that serve as organizers of related bits of information as they are received) to be used as a curriculum framework today offers the most logical and economical way to structure the study of any discipline. Similarly, then, the body of knowledge representing health education can be defined by identifying its most powerful concepts.

CONCEPTS AS CONTENT One approach to the problem of deciding what these most powerful concepts might be was that of the Curriculum Commission of the Health Education Division, American Association for Health, Physical Education, and Recreation.[9] This group first agreed upon certain health problems as those most crucial for the 1960s and 1970s. These were accidents; hazardous environmental conditions such as polluted water, air, chemicals, and radiation; inadequate teen-age diets; obesity; mental and emotional problems; sexual experimentation; early marriages; early parenthood; illegitimacy; abortions; changing roles of men and women; smoking; quackery; need for comprehensive health care; lack of fluoridation; periodontal diseases; venereal diseases; chronic and degenerative diseases and disorders; aging; exploding population problems; the need for disaster preparedness; and better understanding of international health problems.

Prominent scholars in fields concerned with these problem areas were asked to specify which were the most powerful concepts in their field of specialization. The resulting statements were refined and restated and supporting data developed for each. For example, the following concepts are those relevant to the problem of air pollution:

> Air may become polluted by certain materials and gases such as dusts, smoke and vapors. Most air pollutants are a nuisance problem and cause property damage, but some may affect health.
>
> The effects of air pollution on health are both direct and indirect. Much yet must be learned about the relationship between air pollution and health.
>
> With man's present knowledge, greater control of air pollution could be exercised in homes, in industry, and in the community at large.
>
> Air pollution control programs require community cooperation based on public understanding and support.[10]

For each of the concepts, in each of the problem areas, an outline of content was also provided. For example, relative to the last concept quoted above, the following content is supplied:

> Citizen groups can promote and support community efforts to find solutions for local problems.
>
> New laws may be needed to regulate human activity in home, industry, and community at large so as to prevent or minimize pollution problems.
>
> Individuals and groups need to be correctly informed of factors causing air pollutant problems and encouraged to take the necessary steps to control conditions affecting pollution. Community-wide programs of education and control contribute to this end.

Not concepts, however, but health *topics* or *problems* structure the information that represents the outcome of the commission's efforts.

The concepts were classified as generalizations of a lower order but supportive to the topics. As such, the result represents a sort of bridge between the traditional health content area and a conceptual approach to the structure of health knowledge. The authors do not claim that the problems or their concepts represent the total scope of health education.

The notion of using concepts as a means of defining content has been seized upon with growing enthusiasm by many health textbook authors and by curriculum developers at school, district, and state levels as well as some nonschool groups. Following a similar pattern, concepts have been used to describe *content* but always as supportive to or as an expansion of a topic or area of health instruction. The topics are generally indistinguishable from those representative of a traditional approach to the structure of the body of knowledge. Concepts are thus employed as means to the end of presenting factual information relevant to the topics to be studied.

– a conceptual framework The only curriculum development that has employed concepts as organizing elements with which to define the body of knowledge particular to health education is that of the School Health Education Study (SHES).[11] This innovative curriculum is structured upon a hierarchy of concepts with the most powerful concept, health itself, at the apex. Next in descending order of importance are three key concepts; *growing and developing, interacting,* and *decision making,* which exemplify the processes implicit in health behavior. At the third level of abstraction, ten concepts are identified as representative of the total curriculum in health education, kindergarten through the twelfth grade. Expansion of these powerful organizing elements of the curriculum results in a broader definition of the subconcepts and the supporting facts, principles, generalizations, and values comprising the body of knowledge encompassed by the discipline. In effect, the concepts are the ends rather than the means. They represent desired generalizations that depend upon the individual's personal organization of the perceptions afforded him by related learning opportunities. *In this context, then, concepts are not taught as such but taught toward instead.*

The ten concepts identified by the writers of the SHES conceptual approach as representative of the body of knowledge are these:

Growth and development influences and is influenced by the structure and functioning of the individual.

Growing and developing follows a predictable sequence, yet is unique for each individual.

Protection and promotion of health is an individual, community, and international responsibility.

The potential for hazards and accidents exists, whatever the environment.

There are reciprocal relationships involving man, disease, and the environment.

The family serves to perpetuate man and to fulfill certain health needs.

Personal health practices are affected by a complexity of forces, often conflicting.

Utilization of health information, products, and services is guided by values and perceptions.

Use of substances that modify mood and behavior arises from a variety of motivations.

Food selection and eating patterns are determined by physical, social, mental, economic, and cultural patterns.

It will readily be apparent that the ten concepts of the SHES conceptual approach do not represent any *new* areas of health knowledge, nor could they possibly, for they can only reflect the body of knowledge that exists. At first glance, it might even appear that they do not cover the total scope. Where is the concept for mental health? has been a·question often asked. The answer lies in looking further at the structure of this fresh look at curriculum design. Each of the concepts has been described, then broadenend through identification of several supporting subconcepts. Each of the subconcepts is further expanded to include an analysis of the physical, mental-emotional, and social implications of the statement as it relates to the health of the individual. For example, the first concept, "Growth and development influences and is influenced by the structure and functioning of the individual," is described further as follows:

Growth and development is a stage in the process of growing and developing. In this concept the individual is viewed as a complex interacting and decision making organism with certain hereditary potentials. Body functions, environmental conditions, the use of certain substances, and other factors may promote or hinder growth and development at any given point on the continuum of growing and developing.[12]

The first of the three subconcepts identified as supportive to this concept is "Heredity prescribes the potential for growth and development." The physical aspects of this statement are:

Each individual a unique biological pattern from the moment of conception (e.g., individuality resulting from the genes; physical features, size, and shape inherited; a biological basis for music, artistic, and mechanical abilities.)

The mental-emotional aspects are:

Heredity important in intellectual and emotional development (e.g., mental potential or native intelligence hereditarily determined;

superior mental traits found in persons with superior hereditary endowment.)

And the social aspects:

> Attainment of inherited potential environmentally or socially determined (e.g. strength, good looks, and robust health are socially advantageous).[13]

All three aspects are given equal emphasis in the development of every concept. None is taken by itself as being separately relevant, but each is viewed in dynamic interaction with the others. The holistic view of man and his health is thus explicitly delineated and built into the body of knowledge rather than left to chance interpretation. Mental health is not treated as an area of concern set apart from the others as a discrete topic, but is given major consideration in *every* concept. In the same way interrelationships among the concepts is planned and inescapable as they constantly interact with the processes of health behavior as symbolized by the three key concepts.

We have looked at the body of knowledge, then, as expressed by means of a list of topics or content areas—the traditional approach—by a list of problem areas expanded with a series of supporting concepts, and by a framework of concepts. Each approach is currently in use, and each has its disciples. However the body of knowledge is structured, it is an essential element for the making of curriculum decisions. The subject matter that is selected from this reservoir of information must be continually examined with the same rigor as is the learner and the society.

KNOWLEDGE AS PROCESS

But what about the logic of inquiry through which knowledge is generated in health education? As Bruner points out, process and the goal of education are really the same thing. If disciplined understanding is the goal, then that is the process as well. All disciplines consist not only of a fund of accumulated information but also of the processes used to acquire and apply that information. An important ingredient of this body of knowledge is specification of the processes implicit in health behavior.

Problem-solving skills, fundamental to decision making, are those by which the information has been accumulated and is most efficiently grasped and employed by the learner. He must know how to search out significant data, he must question, analyze, examine, compare, and consciously choose one alternative over another, based on what he discovers.

Learning lies in exploration, inquiry, and experimentation. A problem is realized, solutions are perceived, one or more of them is tried, and most of the time the solution is found. How much more effectively and economically problems can be solved when the learner can apply intellectual skills in connection with knowledge. Not knowledge accumulated through rote memorization but developed through discovery of material relevant to a problem.

Health problems are so many and so pervasive that to solve them requires learning in many areas of life. One learns about marriage, for example, not by studying some of the rudimentary phenomena of sexual behavior, but by examining factors that make for successful marriage. Economic, psychological, social, and spiritual forces are all significant. They are understood better when their relationship to the personal problems of marriage is apparent. Information needs to be intrinsic. *Material is intrinsic when it is relevant to a problem.* The processes employed in health teaching should be looked at with the same rigor as is the body of knowledge. Significant information can be rendered insignificant when the processes involved in its communication are trivial.

THE SOCIETY

We have said that health teaching, to be meaningful, must be based upon the needs and interests of the learner. The learner does not live in a vacuum but in the world. His needs and interests must be fulfilled in the world and are often reflections of the conditions of his world. In a democracy, the individual is called upon to make decisions as a voter on issues that are becoming increasingly complex. Therefore, the third major source of data influencing curriculum decision-making is the society. What does the individual need to know in order to achieve a rich, productive, satisfying life, both as a human being and as a worthwhile member of his communities? What are the skills and abilities he needs in order to make the kinds or judgments demanded of a participating member of society? The answers to these questions lie in an examination of social trends, issues, and problems.

Data abound. We need only look at the front page of any newspaper to find a wealth of information with implications for health education. Recently, an analysis of the quality of American life in terms of such aspects as health and illness; social mobility; the physical environment; income and poverty; public order and safety; learning, science, and art; and participation and alienation was prepared for the President by the Department of Health, Education and Welfare. A vast amount of data contained in this report has significance for curriculum making. Other current reports are the Panel Recommendations of the White House Conference on Food, Nutrition, and Health, and publications issued from the Office of Consumer Education and the National Vital Statistics System.

The American Association of School Administrators views the learner and society as two dimensions of the same purpose inasmuch as society is but the totality of individual lives, purposes, and actions. Analysis of the circumstances in which the youth of this generation must mature, become educated, and make a place for themselves in the world culminated in a statement of nine imperatives in education. Although they are not proposed as educational goals in themselves, all of them have significance in establishing the goals of health education. These carefully identified imperatives are: to make urban life rewarding and satisfying; to prepare people for the world of work; to discover and nurture creative talent; to strengthen the moral fabric of society; to deal constructively with psychological tensions; to keep democracy working; to make intelligent use of natural resources; to make the best use of leisure time; and to work with other people of the world for human betterment.[14]

Most of the specifics discussed so far that are relative to the need are also relevant to the study of society as a broad area of concern and will not be repeated here. However, there may be data of more immediate importance to a given school, neighborhood, or community that need to be looked at by a teacher or curriculum maker. Various ethnic or socioeconomic factors may be unique as data sources influencing curriculum decisions not so critical in other communities. For example, drug abuse may be a problem in an upper-class area, but for different reasons and of a different nature than the same problem in a ghetto. Nutrition may be less good among some groups of youngsters than among others, but for different reasons. Nutrition choices are often dictated by necessity or by cultural forces rather than by wilful neglect or ignorance of what is believed to provide balance in nutrients. The kinds of teaching strategies that can succeed with one group may be totally irrelevant to another.

POLITICS AND VALUES Obviously, the learner, the body of knowledge, and society are not mutually exclusive. Nor are these the only influences on curriculum making. Legislative and political factors have a powerful impact on curriculum. Crisis-oriented decisions are probably more often a source of curriculum emphasis for health education than in most disciplines. Health education for the 1970s will probably reflect the current national concern with teen-age drug abuse and also the crucial problems of environmental pollution and overpopulation. Unfortunately, the bandwagon approach is categorical and remedial, whereas a comprehensive kindergarten through twelfth grade curriculum looks at the total individual and the totality of social problems and is preventive in nature and intent.

Another source of influence is the values or philosophy of the teacher or other decision makers. It has been suggested that when educational objectives have been inferred from the data gathered from the learner, the scholars, and the society, the next step is to look at the objectives to see if they are in agreement with the philosophy to which the school is committed. This step is very nearly implicit in the act of identifying objectives, however. It would be difficult, if not impossible, for most educators to perceive objectives based upon such studies that were inconsistent with their value systems. It is possible, of course, that the value systems of those identifying objectives might conflict with those in some areas of the community. This kind of conflict is exemplified by controversial topics such as sex education and drug abuse. The crucial point to be emphasized here is that the curriculum must represent the values and valued content of *all* involved social groups, especially the students themselves as one of these groups.

FEASIBILITY OF OBJECTIVES

An equally critical issue is the question of feasibility. Can the objective be achieved in the allotted time and with the age groups for which it is intended? A fundamental consideration in planning for learning is the readiness of the student to receive what is taught.

Bruner's comment on readiness proposes that any subject can be taught effectively and honestly to any child at any stage of development. Given that this is true, what needs to be considered also is the point in time when such teaching will be most efficient. At the University Elementary School associated with the School of Education of the University of California, Los Angeles, some very interesting work is being carried out relative to this problem which indicates that the child's developmental stage is vital to the effectiveness and economy of learning.

Readiness is a function of maturation in association with experience and can also be an outcome of a need or interest to learn about something. In the first case, readiness relates to a child's present learning abilities—whether he can only work at a very concrete level of perception or whether he has the ability to grasp abstractions, to formulate and test hypotheses, and to conceptualize.

Readiness is also a matter of timing. For example, "Teach Us What We Want To Know" shows that interest in sex is acute by the seventh grade and even earlier.[14] Children at this age are asking to learn more about birth, birth control, and even abortion. The SHES survey revealed that some, but not all, of these topics are offered in many schools but not until the eleventh or twelfth grades.[15] The fact that twelfth-graders and many adults have accumulated so many misconceptions about sex and childbirth attests to their efforts to learn and the inadequacy of their "teachers," who are most likely to be their peers.

Readiness to learn *about* a health concern is not necessarily the same thing as readiness to *act* in accord with the information obtained. Facts alone will not be decisive in motivating desirable health behavior.

Godfrey M. Hochbaum's model of health behavior considers readiness in connection with an individual's motivation to take action.[16] The primary factors involved are that the individual must perceive himself susceptible to a health problem, he must believe that the health problem would have serious consequences for him if it should occur, and he must be aware that an alternative acceptable to him exists that will avoid the problem. The man who has suffered a painful coronary heart attack is far more apt to be receptive to education about the harmful effects of cigarette smoking than a vigorous young man who entertains no fears about the possibility of a heart attack.

Other factors influence readiness. Such factors as one's sex, nutritional status, energy level, visual acuity, strength, family relationships, attitudes, and beliefs—all these and more influence readiness to learn.

Readiness, the receptivity of the learner, varies not only among but within individuals in terms of timing, intensity, flexibility, and motivation. But it is basic to learning and requires of the health teacher an ability to determine his students' levels of development, experience, and value systems. He must try to arrange teaching strategies to suit the needs and readiness of each particular individual and group.

If teaching can be defined as the process by which changes in behavior are effected in an individual, it is helpful to know in advance what behavior is desired. A great deal of emphasis is being given therefore to the definition of "behavioral" objectives. It is usual for curriculum developers to formulate a set of objectives. What is not so usual is to find that the listed statements are properly stated or operational in design. How should a behavioral objective be stated, and what makes such a statement qualify as operational?

The importance of defining instructional objectives in terms of observable student behaviors was stressed at least as long ago as 1930 by Ralph Tyler. Tyler was involved in the development of achievement tests and argued then that plans for instruction should be based on statements which clearly stated what behavior would be expected from a student who had achieved an objective. These were the two-dimensional statements (a behavior and the content that the student is to deal with in practicing the behavior) whose value is increasingly accepted by educationists.

Much of the current rapid momentum in the use of behavioral objectives can be attributed to the advent of programmed instruction. Those developing such materials saw at once that in order to structure materials so that a specific answer opened the door to the next bit of learning, precision was essential in the selected objectives. If only one answer can be accepted, which is usual in programmed instruction, then the objective and its matching instruction must pinpoint that behavior and that content. This need for precision is similarly essential in the work of systems analysts, particularly those engaged in military training programs, and for those concerned with the development of educational technology. For the health educator, behavioral objectives derive their greatest potential from the stress placed upon behavior rather than information. Health education is in essence a behavioral science. It is not so much what the student *knows* about health as how he *behaves* that interests us. Behavior in this context refers to the kinds of actions he takes with reference to the protection and promotion of his own health as well as that of his family and fellows. If we are truly interested in changing health behavior, why not take the time to determine in advance of instruction what immediate behavioral changes can contribute positively to our goals?

HOW SHOULD EDUCATIONAL OBJECTIVES BE STATED?

Curriculum makers differ in their beliefs about how educational objectives should be stated. However, when the vast majority of educators agree on some practice, one can be fairly sure it is out of date, so that lack of accord is not altogether a misfortune. Whereas there is some agreement that an operational objective must describe a behavior that can be demonstrated in a classroom situation, there is less agreement about the exact level of specificity at which that behavior should be defined. Those who are oriented toward the programmed instruction model insist that the statement must include the exact criterion of its achievement. Those who model educational objectives on those suggested in the taxonomy developed by Benjamin Bloom and others are inclined more to classification of the content dimension with sometimes less precision in the behavior.[17]

A more flexible point of view is held by those who believe that the criterion or test of an objective's achievement can be inferred from the behavior called for and that objectives can be stated with more or less precision and still be properly termed "behavioral." For example, those who believe in the rigorously defined programmed instruction model might say: "Given a list of ten common foodstuffs, the student will be able to classify each according to its food group with 80 percent accuracy." The taxonomy model might be "Know that a food which is made of animal flesh belongs to the meat group." The moderates might state the objective like this, "Classify foods in relation to the four food groups." Those who prefer the last form argue that evaluation based upon the behavior called for (in this case, classifying) allows the teacher greater latitude. Also, when objectives are defined this broadly, individual instructors can use them as guides but choose their own way of accomplishing them since they are not so rigidly prescriptive as the programmed version.

Because there is much controversy relative to the form of a properly stated behavioral objective, let us look more closely at these three different points of view.

The cult of the so-called purist behavioral objectives writers has its origins in Robert F. Mager's book, which programs instruction in developing his brand of statement. The principal difference between Mager's objectives and other specific operational objectives is that Mager's carefully describe the conditions under which the learner will show mastery of the objective. In addition, some stage-setting "givens" are usually provided. For example:

> Given a human skeleton, the student must be able to correctly identify by labelling at least 40 of the following bones; there will be no penalty for guessing.[18]

It is claimed that by specifying only the lower limit of acceptable performance (that is, forty bones) each learner is free to surpass the others by naming more or all of them. The obvious conclusion is that we need not be concerned in the least *which* bones the student names as long as he can rattle off forty of them. Nor do we care if he really identifies specific bones or just makes lucky guesses. A problem implicit in any criterion specified objective (labeling at least forty bones) is that it must perforce be limited to teaching him to label bones, which is a dubious skill at best. When all objectives are developed in this way, there is no attention given to the affective domain, those objectives focused on changing attitudes and beliefs; and there is no notice of the fact that objectives can have more than one function in curriculum decision-making. They can and need to be developed as a means of structuring curriculum plans at the level of an institution, course, unit, single lesson, or even part of a lesson. Those objectives defined at the institutional or even course and unit level neither need nor should have the criterion included in the statement. Nevertheless, those who embrace the programmer's model sternly reject any other kind of statement as "lacking acceptable rigor" in form and therefore useless.

The other extreme of specificity perhaps is that proposed by Bloom and others. Considerable effort has been given to elaboration of instructional objectives to comply with the Bloom taxonomy or hierarchy of six categories or cognitive processes. One difficulty with this model is the ambiguity of the behaviors specified at the lowest, or *knowledge,* level of the hierarchy. This level also offers the most detailed analysis of the kinds of knowing there are. However, many of these classifications differ from one another only in terms of their content dimensions.

Two studies in health education illustrate what can happen when "kinds of things" to be known are classified as a means of identifying educational objectives. The first study applied the Bloom taxonomy to a selected area of health education. The result was a list of over 500 objectives concerned with nutrition alone. Of these, 448 were given the same student behavior, "to know." The rest of the objective consisted of a fact that was consistent with a taxonomy classification such as "terminology, classifications, specific facts, etc." The second study was closely patterned after that on nutrition and defined over 350 objectives related to alcohol use and abuse. Of these, 224 again called for only one student behavior, "to know." The student was required only to be "aware" of 53 more objectives, and the real classification always depended upon the accompanying *fact* and its place in the taxonomy. For example, one objective classified under the Bloom Hierarchy of Educational Objectives as "1.11 Knowledge of Terminology" might be "*Knows* that marijuana is usually the dried flowers and leaves of the female hemp plant" or "*Knows* that alcohol usually refers to a specific chemical compound, ethyl alcohol, which is a colorless, thin liquid with a mild, pleasant odor." We know exactly *what* the student is supposed to learn; the only problem is to decide what behavior we should accept as evidence that he "knows."

Two studies in health education give over 80 percent of their emphasis to the lowest level of the hierarchy, which is largely simple factual recall. Only the small remaining proportion was focused upon objectives concerned with processes or cognitive skills. Such an overemphasis upon factual recall is inconsistent with the goals of an educated person, which have been described as rational behaviors, not an accumulation of hundreds of facts. Still, if care were taken to give equal emphasis to the other more complex behaviors of the hierarchy, comprehension, application, analysis, synthesis, and evaluation, application of the taxonomy might be a useful tool for the development of instructional objectives in health education.

The third method of defining behavioral objectives lies somewhere between these two schools of thought, accepting any objective stated in operational terms (clearly describing something the student is to be able to do as a result of instruction) as a behavioral objective. The level of specificity of the behavioral term is neither so general as to be impossible to interpret nor so specific as to provide the teacher no alternatives.

No matter whose definition is accepted, however, a properly stated behavioral objective, most authorities agree, satisfies these criteria: (1) It is stated in terms of the learner, not in terms of the teacher's intentions; (2) it is operational, in that the learner can practice the behavior and measurably demonstrate his new ability or change in belief in the classroom; (3) it specifies a single behavior and a single content area. Whether it is broadly stated or narrowly defined depends upon its function in the curriculum plan.

– must all educational objectives be stated at the classroom level?

It is also agreed that objectives can and should be stated at varying levels of precision, depending on their distance from the learner himself. Clarity in expressing a target behavioral change is not the only function of specificity in stating educational aims, nor are the two terms necessarily synonymous. An attempt to define what is meant by a too general, albeit clearly stated objective, may result in hundreds of objectives for one unit of study. Too specific objectives can be as confusing as ones that are too general. An objective should be stated at the level of generality that describes the behavior the student is to master in connection with a given area of content. The content, too, may vary in specificity from concrete to abstract, depending on its distance from the learner.

David R. Krathwohl suggests that there are three levels at which objectives can be meaningfully defined.[19] At the most remote level are the broad, abstract, most general statements expressing educational goals for several years or a given total program. For example, "Knows that body parts, systems, and functions grow and develop at varying rates both among and within individuals." At the next level are the objectives defining the instruction for a single course. For example, "Analyzes the varied influences which initiate or modify individual patterns of growing and developing." Third, and closest to the learner himself, are the most specific, those upon which lessons or parts of lessons can be focused. For example, "Describes genetic determinants of given physiological traits." The abstract nature of the first two levels of objectives provides a relatively stable referent for choosing specific classroom objectives among possible alternatives. For example, although not everyone might wish or need to approach the subject of nutrition in exactly the same way, few would disagree that a student should know how to select foods for a meal that is nutritional and balanced. The broader statements, or goals, serve as guidelines, whereas operational objectives insure flexibility.

It is perhaps at the level of the long-range goal that statements concerning attitudinal change are most realistically developed. Like it or not, changing an attitude is a long-term project, and the effect of instruction may be delayed for many years. Attitudes are "caught" too early, and too many forces are in operation to make attitude modification the objective of a single lesson or even a series of lessons. And, as Krathwohl points out, many of the objectives in the affective domain, especially at the lowest, or "receiving" order, are indistinguished from those in the cognitive domain in any case.

John I. Goodlad urges that the term "objectives" be used to refer only to purposes stated in terms of the learner. When purposes for schools or teachers are discussed, only the terms "aims" or "goals" should be used, he says. He too defines three decision-making levels of remoteness from the learner, but somewhat differently than Krathwohl. Most remote is the *societal* level, which would include those goals determined by schoolboards, legislators, or federal authorities. Closer are the *institutional* goals, those set by teachers and school administrators for a school or for a school system. Closest to the learner is the *instructional* level, and only the statements written at this level should be termed behavioral or educational objectives.

Perhaps a fourth criterion needs to be added to those cited earlier to describe a properly stated objective. A behavioral objective should be stated at the classroom level. Whether it is broadly stated or narrowly defined depends upon its function at that level.

BEHAVIORAL TERMS

What kinds of terms may acceptably be used in stating behavioral objectives? A current science curriculum developed in 1969 by the American Association for the Advancement of Science states that there are basically only nine verbs that should be applied to behavioral objectives. These are *name, identify, order, describe, construct, distinguish, state a rule, apply a rule,* and *demonstrate.* Not so prescriptive, Mager considers that the verb used need only be clearly descriptive enough to communicate its meaning in like manner to the person who wishes to implement the objective. Most agree that this condition is fulfilled when the term is as unambiguous as possible.

– ambiguous terms

Ambiguous statements of objectives typical of many curriculum guides, lesson plans, and textbooks require that the students "know," "understand," "appreciate," "*really* appreciate" and so on. For example, we often see statements of this nature:

To understand the nature of alcohol and narcotics
To know how reproduction occurs and life begins
To appreciate the importance of good posture

But what will the learner be doing when he shows that he "knows" or "understands" or "appreciates"? For example, "understand" can be interpreted in many ways: (1) to learn indirectly as by hearsay (I *understand* that she is not well); (2) to be tolerant of the needs or problems or views of another person (There, there, don't cry, I *understand*); (3) to comprehend the meaning of symbols, sounds, forms, or language (I *understand* Latin); (4) to conclude, infer (Do I *understand* that you want me to read this chapter?); (5) to be able to follow directions (I *understand* this recipe for lemon cake). Which one is meant? Which one do we expect the student to learn and exhibit to tell us that we have helped him achieve the objective? What happens if *he* perceives the objective to be one thing and the teacher another?

– what's so good about behavioral objectives? Even the ambiguous "understands" kind of objective is at least a *kind* of behavioral objective, however, at a very general level of definition, and can be properly labeled so under the taxonomy. What is totally unusable is the kind of statement that may be a topic, a teacher intention, or a generalization, but not an instructional objective. Some examples of this kind of statement are:

Example 1

General Objective	Presentation of scientific information concerning alcohol.
Specific Objectives	The use of alcohol is a habit shared by many.
	In making your decision on whether or not to drink you might consider the latest scientific facts available.

The general objective is simply a vaguely stated teacher intention. The first of the so-called specific objectives is a generalization, and the second might more appropriately be termed advice to a would-be drinker. A teacher could simply read these statements to the class and instruct them to copy them in their notebooks for later contemplation. No activity is called for or any direction given for an implementing activity. It would be better to state objectives such as:

Explains reasons why many people drink alcoholic beverages.

Interprets scientific data relative to the effects of alcohol use

Example 2

To teach the students accepted techniques of how to solve their health problems

This is such a comprehensive goal that it would challenge the skills of a series of teachers. And it is not a behavioral objective. No student involvement is called upon here and very likely none will result. Evaluation based upon this objective should measure the teacher's success rather than the students'. Yet, as we have said, the purpose of teaching is to change the learner's behavior. This kind of statement tells the teacher what *he* is to do, but it does not give any idea of *how* he is to do it or what the student will be doing when he exhibits satisfactory achievement of whatever the teacher decides to do. A better statement would be:

> Applies accepted techniques in solving personal health problems.

Example 3

General Objective: To develop in the learner a sense of responsibility to himself and others in regard to the use of narcotics

Specific Objective: To help the student understand how narcotics affect the body

Although these objectives are decorative, they would not be much help in planning meaningful teaching activities or evaluation. Not only are the behaviors unclear, but they are teacher rather than student oriented. It is no wonder that teachers who look at such objectives end up telling students facts rather than helping them to learn. A better general objective would be:

> To conclude that decisions about the use of narcotics depend upon an individual's perceptions of his responsibility to himself and his community

And a more meaningful specific objective would be:

> Describes the effects of narcotics upon an individual.

Example 4

Develop an understanding and appreciation of the family in present-day America

Should understand that the roles of the family members change as society changes

Accept the fact that they have a responsibility to contribute continuously to a happy and effective family life

This is the mixed-bag sort of list of objectives often seen in curriculum guides. The first appears to be stated in terms of the student's behaviors, albeit ambiguously (notice that he will not only *understand* but also *appreciate* the family. A large order!) The next statement is a prescription, and the last is an assertion with prescriptive overtones. It would be better to say:

Illustrates family relationships that maintain and promote the health of its members

Relates changes in family roles to changes in a society

Concludes that the continuing efforts of every member are essential to a successful family relationship

Example 5

General Objectives: Reinforcing our personal health habits
Introduce new body parts with an appreciation of the relationship of the coordinated parts
Knowledge of facts basic to good hygiene
Evaluation of knowledge for use at specific times

This conglomeration of topics stated in various forms, and a teacher direction confounded with a student behavior (we must assume that it is the student who is supposed to appreciate the relationship of the coordinated parts, not the teacher who is introducing them) has been taken, as have all of these examples, from curriculum guides or textbooks currently in use. Given the last one, what would you do? What kind of a lesson could you devise based upon such a statement? Perhaps it would be better to list the following as objectives:

Discusses personal practices essential to good living
Demonstrates desirable habits of personal cleanliness

TERMINOLOGY, A PROBLEM

One of the problems involved in talking about an "objective" is that as a term, it has no universally accepted definition. An objective can mean whatever its formulator wants it to mean. Communication is less than perfect in such a situation, since, as we have said, subsequent discussion or uses may be taking place at different or even several levels of generality. Another problem results from the multiplicity of terms employed in speaking about instructional objectives. Depending on the source and often within the same source, an objective may be termed "behavioral," "performance," "student performance," "educational," "terminal," "enabling," "precise," "specific," "operational," "outcome," "behavioral outcome," "information," "planning," "expressive," or just plain "objective"! It has so long been the custom to decorate lesson plans and curriculum guides with some kind of suitably laudable purpose that no one really pays much attention to them, once they are proposed.

While it cannot be argued that good teaching is impossible in the absence of properly stated objectives, neither can it be denied that a behavioral objective vastly facilitates the teaching task. Ralph Tyler believes that decisions about objectives are the most important of all because objectives serve as the criteria for all the other decisions in curriculum making. If this is true, then it follows that carefully formulated objectives can provide direction and coherence to any educational program.

Robert M. Morgan states the following concerning the behavioral or performance objectives in a systems approach to education currently being carried out under the aegis of the United States Office of Education:

> Without performance objectives, there is no basis for deciding which learning intervention or teaching strategy would be most effective. When decisions on teaching strategies have been made without performance objectives, there is no empirical means for determining the degree of effectiveness of the strategy employed. Too often decisions about changes in instructional practices are made in terms of what someone *thinks* is the effect of the practice on what is *hoped* to be the result, without verification.[21]

The kinds of test items by which student achievement is measured reveal what a teacher's real intent has been. And it happens often that teachers do not themselves decide what their intentions (objectives) have been until after the hapless students have experienced the instruction. Analysis of typical teacher-made tests reveals that eight out of ten measure knowledge of specifics only. Yet in a world of rapid growth in the amount of factual knowledge known to man, it is conceded that knowledge of specifics is least important among educational goals. There is no rule that a teacher cannot decide what he is going to require his students to do in order to test their achievement *before* he does his teaching. For some people it is easier to think of the evaluation first and infer the objectives from that. Once they have been stated, they should be looked at carefully to see whether they in fact only seek the most simple cognitive skills such as recall, define, and describe isolated facts or structures.

There is, of course, no one set of objectives whose mastery is essential to achievement of a school's goals. If these were, it would be necessary that the objectives be continually evaluated and revised to meet new conditions, new needs. However, there are some very concrete advantages to use of such statements of objectives as a means of planning and implementing health teaching.

First of all, specifying educational objectives in terms of behaviors is the most meaningful and powerful way to analyze the instructional process, whatever the discipline. In doing so, the teacher is forced to examine his own intentions in advance of his lesson planning. Specifying objectives makes teaching a professional, decision-making function, rather than a potpourri of "discuss the book," "give a lecture, show a film." With specific objectives teaching becomes a rational procedure rather than an intuitive behavior. A teacher who knows exactly what he wants the student to be able to do (and why) when the instruction is completed can not only plan the most appropriate learning opportunities but also devise the most valid means of appraising student achievement. It is not surprising that a teacher guided by an objective such as "to help the student understand and appreciate the role of the family" tends to confuse teaching with telling.

Second, use of behavioral objectives precludes irrelevance and waste of time and materials and thus greatly facilitates many aspects of teaching. Selection of learning opportunities or teaching strategies appropriate to a particular group of learners is facilitated when both behavior and content are stated in advance. It is much easier to prepare a ticket for a traveler who knows exactly where he wishes to go and by what means than for one who does not. Evaluation is not only facilitated but is inherently valid if based upon a behavioral objective, because the student is asked to exhibit a behavior he has been practicing in connection with the subject matter stipulated in the objective. We would never ask a student to demonstrate ability to solve an algebraic equation as a result of having given him an opportunity to practice addition and multiplication. Yet some tests are just that irrelevant to what has actually been taught. When the expressed intent is that the student will "really appreciate the potential dangers of drugs" it is little wonder that the teacher is at a loss to devise means of measuring achievement of such an objective. The result is that the ability to recall factual information ends up as the criterion, the obvious assumption being that the higher the score, the greater the "appreciation." Fuzzily stated objectives can result in trivia more readily than precisely stated objectives.

Not evaluation of the learner alone but also evaluation of the teacher and the objective itself are facilitated when a behavioral objective is employed. When students cannot demonstrate satisfactory achievement of the target behavior and content, the teacher can devise new or different enabling activities to provide wider experience or increased practice. He may also discover that a given objective is not feasible for his group and therefore discard or restate it.

Supervision and inservice education are facilitated when what the teacher is attempting to accomplish is clearly specified in advance. The degree of success or failure is measurable, and strengths and weaknesses can be diagnosed when the criterion is established through operational definition of teaching intent.

Communication is facilitated, especially between teacher and student, but also between teacher and supervisor and one teacher and another. Carefully designed objectives, developed at increasing levels of complexity and abstraction from kindergarten through the twelfth grade, allow successive teachers to reinforce and build upon expected competencies. Each teacher can see the significance of the objectives for his class to those that will follow. When behaviors are stated clearly and unambiguously enough to provide like meanings to any teacher, then whatever means are chosen, the same ultimate behavioral changes should result. Students who are actively involved in the learning process (and behavioral objectives are far more facilitative of this kind of teaching strategy than the "knows" and "appreciates" kinds of statements) are more apt to internalize the behaviors basic to positive health attitudes than students who are passive recipients of information.

Current research seems to support the potential contribution of behavioral objectives to the effectiveness of health education. Dalis found that it was possible to enhance achievement in health education among high school students by providing them with objectives prior to instruction planned to implement the behaviors.[22] Eiseman found that instruction based upon a learning opportunity and a related behavioral objective resulted in greater student involvement in the teacher-learning.[23] Walbesser found that knowledge of a behavorial objective not only increased the learner's rate of achievement but differentially affected the rate of forgetting. Students in the experimental group on retest made better scores than they had immediately following instruction, whereas the control group did not score as well as before.

OBJECTIVES IN THE AFFECTIVE DOMAIN

Whereas the discussion of instructional objectives so far has largely dealt with those in the cognitive domain, this does not mean that no consideration should be given to those in the affective domain. These are the objectives concerned with changes in attitudes, values, and interests. Those who have developed the taxonomy of the affective domain believe that the term "internalization" is best defined by the description of its categories. In general it refers to the inner growth that occurs as the individual becomes aware of and then adopts the attitudes, personal codes, and values that become a part of his system of beliefs and shape his behavior. The categories range from the nearly cognitive level "awareness," "responding," "valuing," "organization," to the level "characterization by a value or value concept." Achievement of an affective objective is as difficult to measure as it is to plan. For this reason, some behavioral objective writers do not attempt either to formulate this kind of statement or to consider an attitudinal objective necessary or feasible. Yet the goals of health education are strongly committed to changes in attitudes. To assume that these changes will occur in connection with cognitive behaviors without any more direct attention to them is both illogical and slipshod teaching. Learning activities *can* be devised to help students identify their beliefs and make a reasoned analysis of alternatives as a basis for eventual commitment to a value system that can promote personal and community well-being in a host of ways. Objectives to this end can be stated in the same way as cognitive behaviors. An example of such an objective might be: "Volunteers to work for improvement of health facilities" or "Formulates a statement of responsibilities appropriate for his age group."

EXPRESSIVE OBJECTIVES

Generally speaking, certain curriculum areas, by their nature, are more difficult to break down into specific quantifiable outcomes. Like art and music, health education is such a subject. Its goals are behaviors that may be varied yet still acceptable as a solution to an individual problem. Many of these behaviors will require lifelong modification. Eisner suggests that objectives which are not so prescriptive as evocative, and which simply identify an educational encounter or task to be completed, should be added to any set of educational objectives as a separate category. He terms these "expressive" as opposed to the instructional or behavioral objectives.[25] Planning for learning should not focus on cognitive objectives alone, but should include affective and expressive objectives as well.

SELECTION OF CONTENT

To decide what knowledge is of most value to any generation of students has perhaps never been quite the mind-boggling task it is today. It is no longer possible even to guess what kind of world today's children will inhabit as adults or what their problems will be. Many students in schools today will take up careers, the tools, skills, and needs for which do not now exist. Change is a phenomenon more accepted in technology than in social institutions, however. And therein lies the educator's dilemma: How are we to provide young people with the knowledge and skills they will need tomorrow, within the framework of a social institution as resistant to change as the public schools traditionally have been?

A new and growing humility among educationists forces acknowledgment that there are no absolutes, and what has been called "truth" is only a word that describes something a society perceives as desirable because it seems to work. Specific content can no longer be the desired end in education. Goodlad, in his brilliant little essay "Some Propositions in Search of Schools", relates the following:

> In curriculum planning, disciplined choice must replace the leisurely, often whimsical, cumulative processes of the past. The selection of most significant bits of content no longer is difficult: it is impossible. Consequently, teachers and pupils must seek out those fundamental concepts, principles, and methods that appear to be most useful for ordering and interpreting man's inquiries.[26]

During the past several years much emphasis has been given to curriculum reform. In nearly every discipline, an attempt has been made to identify the powerful ideas and principles that describe the *structure* of its body of knowledge. To learn structure, says Bruner, is to learn how things are related.[27] Once a student grasps the fundamentals of a discipline, he is able to broaden and deepen his knowledge about it because the meaning of each new idea has relevance for him. Learning how to learn, then, becomes the imperative in education, not simply for use in the schoolroom but as a lifelong activity. Mastery of isolated bits of information about selected diseases or the physiology of man has been the traditional emphasis in health education. Facts in isolation from their reference to the self and to man's health are quickly forgotten, for they are meaningless even though they may be based upon careful studies of the learner's needs and interests. The new school of health education does not view students as a group of captives sentenced to receive passively what the experts decide it is desirable for them to know. Nor does health education confine itself to physical aspects of health, but considers them only as in dynamic interaction with social and mental-emotional aspects of human behavior. Health-related facts in such a context are not the imperatives in education, but only data useful in decision making and problem solving.

The key concepts and principles of health education are abstractions representative of the fundamental, hence relatively stable, components of its subject matter. They are not written out and taught as statements to be learned in and of themselves. Instead, they are used as organizing elements toward which the learning opportunities are oriented. Conceptualization is the result of the individual's personal interpretation of these experiences and is an internalizing process. With the internalization of concepts, the individual can handle new data and apply them in new situations as a rational process without having to sort back through all the facts and perceptions that contributed to his grasp of the fundamental involved.

Perhaps the greatest priority in health education today is process. Human beings are feeling, thinking, acting organisms functioning in a society that is becoming increasingly complex. It is not so important that specific facts be learned as that *ways* of discovering them be mastered. Knowledge is the vehicle rather than the destination in a process approach to learning. The teacher becomes a facilitator of learning rather than communicator of facts. Teaching can go on in a classroom without any learning happening at all. In a process-centered classroom, learning can be an absorbing, even exciting, experience. To focus upon mastery of processes rather than upon information is to equip the learner with cognitive skills useful in other situations throughout his lifetime. Standard information can be dealt with more intelligently in the present, and new information can be discovered and applied when necessary in the future.

Concepts are useful as a framework for ordering facts and generalizations. Generalizations help the student construct some kind of consecutive whole out of his world. It is not enough to consider the effect of calorie control in weight reduction, but the whole problem of metabolism should be explored to make sure that the principles involved in energy interchange are understood. Bruner explains the importance of a conceptual framework very well:

> Teaching specific topics or skills without making clear their context in the broader fundamental structure of a field of knowledge is uneconomical in several deep senses. In the first place, such teaching makes it exceedingly difficult for the student to generalize from what he has learned to what he will encounter later. In the second place, learning that has fallen short of a grasp of general principles has little reward in terms of intellectual excitement. The best way to create interest in a subject is to render it worth knowing, which means to make the knowledge gained usable in one's thinking beyond the situation in which the learning has occurred. Third, knowledge one has acquired without sufficient structure to tie it together is knowledge that is likely to be forgotten.[28]

THE AIMS OF HEALTH INSTRUCTION

In planning for effective teaching and learning, a clear definition of the teacher's aims is essential. The principal aim of school health instruction is to promote favorable behavior in situations involving the individual's health as well as that of his fellows. Broadly put, the aim of health instruction is to help people to learn to live well—to live scientifically, efficiently, economically, and with satisfaction. Behavior is what counts. It is what we do that counts. As Durant says, "We become what we do."

At the same time, the acquisition of knowledge and the development of attitudes about health behavior are also of great importance. To impart knowledge is the simplest thing to be done in the classroom. Students can be given information, tested for retention, and given more information. Whether the results are influential in a pattern of living depends in part on the way the knowledge was acquired and also upon a variety of other intervening variables over which the teacher has little or no control. The teacher knows that it is not enough to learn about immunization. To be immunized against those diseases for which such controls exist is the essential outcome. All the knowledge in the world will not protect against smallpox, diphtheria, measles, or tetanus. But knowledge, meaningfully gained, is the first step in motivating a person to seek immunization.

Attitudes about health and health behavior help to determine what an individual does in a given situation. It has been said that attitudes are self-reports. They can usually be discovered only by asking a person how he feels about something or some action. The response is often mediated, sometimes unconsciously, by what the person questioned perceives as the way he *ought* to feel. The way he ought to feel in turn is an outcome of a wide variety of variables as well, such as the individual's sex, age, socioeconomic status, ethnic or cultural background, education, group pressures, and influences of communications transmitted via the mass media.

That attitudes are learned there is no doubt, and they can be modified by later learnings. Knowledge that seems vital to the learner as something that has potential impact on his desired life style or his personal goals is far more apt to develop positive attitudes toward health behavior than knowledge that seems unrelated to real-life concerns.

The goals of school health instruction might be outlined as follows:

1 To promote health behavior (action, conduct, habits) favorable to high-level wellness and the quality of life

2 To promote development of a well integrated personality, allowing enjoyment of life based upon a realistic acceptance of one's limitations as well as capacities

3 To clarify misconceptions and superstitions, and provide accurate information about personal and public health matters

4 To facilitate the development of a feeling of security based upon acquisition of sound information, positive attitudes, and scientifically wise behavior

5 To contribute to the life of the community through the development of health educated citizens who know the advantages and necessity of supporting health measures designed for the common good

6 To develop ability in students to see cause and effect, to take preventive or remedial steps, and thus to lengthen life and improve the quality of living

SUMMARY

The principal sources of the goals and instructional objectives of health education are (1) the learner, his needs, interests, concerns, and present knowledge and abilities; (2) the body of knowledge and the methods used by the scholars in the field to generate new knowledge; and (3) the issues and requirements of the society and world in which the learner lives and must satisfy his needs. Careful investigation and analysis of a wide array of data derived from these sources are essential to the formulation of valid goals.

The emphasis in planning teaching should be on process, or ways of discovering and using health information, rather than on transmission of facts. The concepts, powerful ideas, or generalizations that appear to structure the body of knowledge can be used as a framework for instruction. They thus serve as organizing centers for a series of learning opportunities planned to help the learner in his progress toward their realization. The teaching strategy is to focus upon specific problems or interests of the student, all of which build toward a selected generalization. Then the generalization will become the learner's personal organization of the data and perceptions he has experienced rather than merely passive memorization of a meaningless statement. As he begins to classify the specifics, his notion of the overarching generalization begins to shape itself in his mind. The learner formulates his own concepts, whether as a result of school activities or real-life interactions. The schools have the opportunity and the obligation to see that his concepts are based upon scientifically sound information rather than hearsay, misinformation, or advertising claims.

Concepts, then, represent goals rather than a point of departure in teaching. Goals describe the broad purposes of health education. Statements inferred from the goals to structure short-term enabling activities are most useful when they are stated in terms of the learner, stipulate what the learner is to be able to do, and with what area of the subject matter he is to be able to deal.

If students are to be helped to discover their own humanness, and participate meaningfully in real-life situations to that end, relevant educational goals need to be developed and their achievement carefully planned. Upon the care with which these two tasks are carried out depends the success or failure of the schools in fulfilling their responsibility both to the learner and to society.

NOTES AND REFERENCES

1 Viktor E. Frankl, "The Search for Meaning," *Saturday Review,* XLI, 37 (September 13, 1958), 20.

2 Elena Sliepcevich, *School Health Education Study—A Summary Report,* Washington, D.C., 2, 1964.

3 Sliepcevich, *School Health Education Study,* p. 6.

4 Ruth Byler, Gertrude Lewis, and Ruth Totman, *Teach Us What We Want To Know,* Connecticut State Board of Education, 1969, p. ix.

5 Dorothy Fraser, NEA Project on Instruction, "Deciding What To Teach," Washington, D.C., NEA, 1963, p. 114.

6 The Joint Committee, *Health Education,* Washington, D.C., NEA, 1961, pp. 76–78.

7 *Ibid.*

8 Jerome S. Bruner, *On Knowing.* Cambridge, Mass., The Belknap Press of Harvard University, 1963, p. 120.

9 AAHPER, *Health Concepts,* Washington, D.C., AAHPER, 1967, p. 4.

10 *Ibid.,* pp. 31–32.

11 *Ibid.*

12 SHES, *Health Education A Conceptual Approach,* St. Paul, 3 M Education Press, 1967, p. 21.

13 *Ibid.,* p. 36.

14 American Association of School Administrators, *Imperatives in Education,* Washington, D.C., American Association of School Administrators, 1966, p. i.

15 Sliepcevich, *op. cit.,* pp. 34–36.

16 Godfrey M. Hochbaum, "The Professional and the Lay Side of the Coin," *International Journal of Health Education,* X, 4 (1967), 4 (reprint).

17 Benjamin Bloom *et al., Taxonomy of Educational Objectives, Handbook No. I: Cognitive Domain,* New York, McKay, 1956.

18 Robert F. Mager, *Preparing Objectives for Programmed Instruction,* San Francisco: Fearon, *1962.*

19 David R. Krathwohl, "Stating Objectives Appropriately for Program, for Curriculum, and for Instructional Materials Development," *The Journal of Teacher Education,* 16 (March 1965), 83–92.

20 American Association for the Advancement of Science, *Science, A Process Approach,* Washington, D.C., American Association for the Advancement of Science, 1967, p. 41.

21 Robert M. Morgan, "Es-70—A Systematic Approach to Educational Change," *Educational Technology,* 9, 9 (September 1969), 50.

22 Gus Dalis, "The Effect of Precise Objectives Upon Student Achievement in Health Education," unpublished doctoral dissertation, Los Angeles, University of California, 1969.

23 Seymour Eiseman, "An Approach for Student Involvement in Health Education Classes," *Journal of School Health,* 39, 6 (June 1969), 408–411.

24 Henry Walbesser, "Behavioral Objectives and Learning Hierarchies," Symposium, American Education Research Association, 1970 Annual Meeting, Minneapolis, Minn.

25 Elliott Eisner, "Instructional and Expressive Educational Objectives: Their formulation and Use in Curriculum," *AERA Monograph Series on Curriculum Evaluation,* Chicago: Rand McNally, 1969, pp. 1–31.

26 John I. Goodlad, "Some Propositions in Search of Schools," Washington, D.C., NEA, 1962, p. 29.

27 Bruner, *op. cit.,* p. 7.

28 Jerome Bruner, *The Process of Education,* Cambridge: Harvard University Press, 1960, p. 31.

SELECTED READINGS

American Association of School Administrators, "Health Education," *Curriculum Handbook for School Administrators,* Washington, D.C., 1967.

AERA, "Instructional Objectives," American Association of School Administrators, *Monograph Series on Curriculum Evaluation,* Chicago, Rand McNally, 1969.

"America the Inefficient," *Time,* March 23, 1970, pp. 72–80.

Association of Supervision and Curriculum Development, *What Are the Sources of the Curriculum?* Washington, D.C., Association of Supervision and Curriculum Development, 1962.

Berman, Louise, *From Thinking to Behaving,* New York: Teachers College Press, 1967.

Bloom, Benjamin, *Stability and Change in Human Characteristics,* New York, John Wiley, 1964.

Bruner, Jerome S., *On Knowing,* Cambridge, Mass., Belknap Press of Harvard University, 1963.

Eisner, Elliott W., "Educational Objectives: Help or Hindrance?" *The School Review,* Chicago, University of Chicago Press, 1967, pp. 250–282.

Eiss, Albert F., and Mary B. Harbeck, *Behavioral Objectives in the Affective Domain,* Washington, D.C., National Science Supervisors Association, 1969.

Erikson, Erik H., *Childhood and Society,* 2nd ed., New York, Norton, 1963.

Fabun, Don, *The Dynamics of Change,* Englewood Cliffs, N.J., Prentice-Hall, 1967.

Fraser, Dorothy McClure, "The Changing Scene in Social Studies," *Social Studies Curriculum Development: Prospects and Problems,* Washington, D.C., National Council for Social Studies, 1969, pp. 1–32.

Gagné, Robert M., "The Analysis of Instructional Objectives for the Design of Instruction," in Robert Glaser (ed.), *Teaching Machines and Programmed Instruction, II, Data and Directions,* Washington, D.C., NEA, 1967, pp. 21–65.

———, *The Conditions of Learning,* New York, Holt, Rinehart & Winston, 1965.

Goodlad, John I., *Planning and Organizing for Teaching,* Washington, D.C., NEA, 1963.

Lindvall, C. M. (ed.), *Defining Educational Objectives,* Pittsburgh, University of Pittsburgh Press, 1964.

Macmillan, C. J. B., and Thomas W. Nelson, (eds.), *Concepts of Teaching: Philosophical Essays,* Chicago, Rand McNally, 1968.

Melching, Wm. H., Harry L. Ammerman, Paul G. Whitmore, and John A. Cox, *Deriving, Specifying, and Using Instructional Objectives,* Professional Paper 10–66, Alexandria, Va., George Washington University, The Human Resources Research Office, 1966.

Morphet, Edgar L., and Charles O. Ryan, (eds.), "Implications for Education of Prospective Changes in Society," *Designing Education for the Future: No. 2,* New York, Citation Press, 1967.

Solleder, Marian K., *Evaluation Instruments in Health Education,* Washington, D.C., American Association for Health, Physical Education, and Recreation, 1969.

Tyler, Ralph, *Basic Principles of Curriculum and Instruction,* Chicago, University of Chicago Press, 1969.

U.S. Department of Health, Education and Welfare, *Toward a Social Report,* Washington, D.C., Government Printing Office, 1969.

CHAPTER 3 ORGANIZING THE HEALTH CURRICULUM

To organize is to plan the coordinated functioning of related activities in such a manner as to achieve an ordered total program. Organizing the health curriculum entails a number of problems, roughly divided into two sets: first, those problems about which decisions are usually made at the school administration level and, second, those problems that are the responsibility of the teacher at the classroom level. Both sets of problems require decisions centered about the questions What? When? For whom? and How? but at different levels of generality or distance from the learner himself.

Change in curriculum is not new to our schools but is often more noticeable in method than in organization or substance. Content continues to be central. Only the basis for its selection has changed from time to time. Old content has sometimes been replaced as new knowledge has emerged; new courses have appeared that tend to have more practical application, such as typing and driver education, and some old courses, such as Greek and Latin, have been dropped in some places. Related courses have been combined, such as English and literature into language arts, but in general, patterns of school organization have remained traditional in terms of specific content.

Classrooms have been customarily occupied by thirty or so students and a teacher for fixed periods of time. The school year continues to be based upon the needs of an agrarian society no longer typical of our communities. Completion of secondary school requirements is still based upon the Carnegie unit in most school systems. All of these factors impose a certain degree of uniformity and rigidity in curriculum decision-making.

Education has been equated with "covering" fixed amounts of information, generally as contained in a textbook and supplemented by the teacher's accumulated fund of knowledge. Competition and grading have been assumed to be the significant motivational devices for learning. Evaluation and subsequent progression through the graded school have depended upon the student's ability to take in the information he is provided and to give it back on examinations whether digested or not.

In the subject-centered, content-specific, graded curriculum, there are traditionally three organizational alternatives for health education at the institutional or school administration level of decision making. These are integration, the specific course, and correlation. The problem at this level may involve the total curriculum for all students at any one grade; or it may be in connection with a given subject area as it will be organized vertically from kindergarten through the twelfth grade. We will look first at organizing for teaching health education in terms of these three traditional approaches. Later we will look at some changes in organization that are emerging in answer to the dynamics of our rapidly changing social and technological environment.

CURRICULUM PATTERNS IN HEALTH INSTRUCTION

A curriculum is usually described as all of the organized learning experiences that take place under the direction or responsibility of the school. The curriculum supposedly reflects the values of a society—and an answer to the question, What knowledge is of most worth? If those responsible for the administration of a school or school system believe that a comprehensive health education program should be provided, or if local or state boards of education require health instruction, then it will be a part of *what* is taught—a part of the school's curriculum. *When* it is taught depends again upon decisions at the administrative level. Some school administrators believe strongly that it is essential that health instruction be provided every year, from kindergarten through the twelfth grade. Some schools organize the teaching of health education in courses planned for all students in one or more specified grades. Still other administrators limit health instruction to those areas of information mandated by law or demanded by crisis-oriented pressure groups. The many crash drug-abuse education programs begun in 1970 are of the latter nature, although curiously enough drug-abuse education has been required in nearly every state since the Temperance Movement days.

Whatever the range of health issues and problems selected for school health education, decisions regarding *how* it is to be organized as part of the overall curriculum result traditionally in one or more of the three patterns. Some schools use one, some use two, and in some places all three are in operation since the three are not mutually exclusive but interrelated. Ideally, every teacher should know enough about the science of health to be a reasonably competent health teacher. In the elementary schools each teacher *is* usually responsible for all of the health teaching that goes on in his class.

The pattern of organization most often used at the elementary level is termed the "integration" or "core" curriculum. In the secondary schools, health may be taught as a separate course, "direct teaching" and by a health teaching specialist. Health may also be taught as part of a broad field of instruction such as biology or social science, or taught along with a series of related subjects. This pattern is called correlation.

For example, health education is sometimes taught along with physical education under the assumption that inasmuch as physical educators and health educators have similar goals, their preparation and interests must be the same. Thus a good physical education teacher might, during the physical education periods, teach a great deal about the significance of exercise, diet and training, isometrics, and the relation of exercise to resistance to disease. In such instances health information is correlated with physical education. Whatever the host area, however, health instruction is the responsibility of a teacher whose prime interest and preparation is not health but his own specialty.

What are the special characteristics of these three patterns of organization? How is each organized at administrative and classroom levels? What are the strengths or weaknesses of each pattern?

INTEGRATION AS A PATTERN OF CURRICULUM

To integrate is to relate the parts of something to the whole. To employ integration in planning for teaching and learning is to seek relationships, generalizations, or concepts that tie experiences or facts together to make a meaningful whole. As a process, integrating functions as a part of *any* effective teaching-learning program, however it may be organized. As a curriculum plan integration refers to the means by which a subject area is introduced and treated in a given educational situation. Generally typical of the elementary school, integration may also be effectively employed as planned reinforcement of other patterns of health teaching in the secondary schools.

> The word *integration* is used to refer to both a *state* and a *process*. As a *state* it implies the attainment of perfection, completion, or wholeness. Integration in this sense is a goal toward which every individual and social group presumably should strive. As a *process*, however, integration refers to the means used to achieve this state of perfection. Integration can also refer to the manner in which the interdependent parts of a larger whole relate or are brought into harmonious relation with each other.[1]

Or integration may mean an inner harmony among the individual's beliefs, attitudes, and character; it may mean simply the discovering of relationships between specialties, such as accounting and physics, for example; it may mean the adjustment of the individual to his culture; it may mean the adjustment of the various cultures of the world to one another; or it may mean a set of assumptions about nature, humanity, and the universe that transcend cultural differences and therefore could presumably be accepted by all men the world over.[2]

Integration involves the adjustment of parts to a whole; all the parts work smoothly together with no friction and nothing out of step; thus they function with maximum efficiency. To integrate is to relate parts to the whole—it makes no difference what the "whole" or purpose is. A well-integrated automobile is one in which all parts—carburetor, spark plugs, tires, chassis, driver, battery, and all the other thousands of parts—work smoothly together to provide safe, economical, and pleasurable transportation. If the battery goes dead, the spark plugs become fouled, or the driver becomes intoxicated, disintegration sets in. The "wholeness" of safe transportation is not achieved.

A well-integrated battle requires complete and efficient interrelationship among all branches of the service involved and a complete meshing of individuals within those branches. The price of disintegration in battle is lives. A well-integrated gang of thieves functions smoothly in their antisocial activities by having each member coordinate his activities with the others to the end that the big bank robbery is accomplished without a hitch. Integrating is a process or a state of affairs, but neither demands that its "wholeness" or its purpose be bad or good.

To seek integration in learning is to seek relationships, concepts, the "big ideas," the putting of things together. In traditional educational patterns from elementary school through college, learning is diversified and specialized. A student in college may not see any relationship between a course in the philosophy of education and one in general methods, and yet the two courses may be related in their fundamental viewpoints. Physics and chemistry courses may be so taught as to represent completely separate areas of knowledge; thus the student may miss the "big idea" of the physical basis for human life.

Integration, as a curriculum design, came into being in the 1920s. There was a great deal of resistance to it at the time on the grounds that it smacked of the much maligned progressive education in its view of student needs as basic to planning, and involvement of the students in the planning procedures. Some of the problems that occurred were an outcome of the very novelty of this sort of curriculum. Knowledge, until then entirely subject centered and categorical, had never been organized in such a way as to make it an easy task for youngsters to find the information they needed in order to solve the problems that interested them. Teachers had not been taught those skills themselves and, therefore, were not equipped to help students learn them. Ability to generalize and to synthesize information gathered from a wide range of disciplines was required. It was difficult and threatening for teachers, trained in a subject-centered curriculum, to accept or attempt teaching that was not textbook oriented. This problem still exists, to some degree. There is a homely saying, "We tend to be down on what we're not up on"; unwillingness to work with new ideas was a powerful hindrance to the acceptance of integration as the vital curriculum plan it can be.

Today, however, the swing to identification of key concepts that appear to give structure to a discipline promises to make integration newly appealing and useful. As Phenix has said, the process of concept formulation appears to offer the one way in which man's intellect can help him order the confusing multiplicity of experiences that continue to bombard the senses.[3] Organization of learning experiences in an integrated curriculum can help students to order relationships among facts gathered from as many subject areas as are relevant to a problem. Today's emphasis on process, rather than content, is an additional integrating force since learning skills, or cognitive processes, are universal tools, timeless in their usefulness and limitless in their application. Problem-solving skills, once mastered, can be applied as long as the intellect can function and there are resources upon which to draw.

The term most often associated with integration is the "core curriculum," in which content and learning experiences are focused upon a central theme without reference to the conventional subjects or disciplines. Such a central theme in the elementary school core curriculum might be *transportation.* In learning about the problems and issues associated with transportation, the students begin to examine the implications for health that are inescapably involved. Questions may arise concerning how transportation is related to availability of foods, preservation of perishable food products, safety of passengers, transmission of disease agents, accessibility of health care, air and noise pollution, housing problems, and so forth. While students are learning about transportation, they are also studying and learning about history, mathematics, reading, composition, art, music, and other subjects—not as discrete, unconnected topics nor as ends in themselves, *but as contributions to the study of transportation.*

A concept is an even more effective means of organizing and integrating health instruction. Cushman concludes that "the greatest contribution of the conceptual approach to health education will be that it better identifies our discipline, and gives us the needed framework for knowledge and ordering our learning experiences".[4] Concepts serve not only to structure a body of knowledge, but also as organizing centers for the activities that are planned to build competences in language and problem-solving skills as well as broadening comprehension of other areas of general education.

For example, teaching toward the concept, "There are reciprocal relationships involving man, disease, and environment,"[5] or any other similarly broad generalization used as an organizing center, engages the student in activities requiring the whole array of cognitive skills and affective behaviors as he progresses from kindergarten through the twelfth grade. As the student works with the learning opportunities he is also learning related history, vocabulary, spelling, art, literature, audio-visual techniques, drama, legislation, and ecology to mention a few subjects. Most important, he participates actively in meaningful activities related to his own needs and those of the communities in which he lives. He learns about living and ways of choosing relevant information from the ever-increasing stream of information that pours in on us from the world and even the universe today. These are the kinds of learning he must have if he is to live in the world and find meaning in his existence.

Gardner points out that the pressing need today is to educate for an accelerating rate of change.

> Education, at its best will develop the individual's inner resources to the point where he can learn (and will *want* to learn) on his own. It will equip him to cope with unforeseen challenges and to survive as a versatile individual in an unpredictable world. Individuals so educated will keep the society itself flexible, adaptive, and innovative.[6]

An integrated curriculum is designed to develop the versatile man.

The strength of the integration model of curriculum is its potential for this kind of education. Integration is implicit in Goodlad's proposal for a fresh emphasis on general education in the elementary school.[7] Integration is also compatible with the emerging, sought for, humanistic curriculum. The planned use of data and techniques of other disciplines as they are discovered in relation to the health issues being investigated reinforces learnings already gained and growing in the subject areas considered part of the general education program. Development of knowledge of self, knowledge of others, how to acquire knowledge, and other aspects of the humanistic curriculum are outcomes particular to the skillfully developed integrated curriculum in health education.

To develop a core curriculum requires some variations and talent not always found in traditional subject-centered plans. In the first place time must be provided. Core curriculum is frequently scheduled two or three consecutive hours a day for at least four days a week. Core teachers need to be versatile, skilled in handling discussion, helpful in finding resources, and patient. The school library needs to be fairly well developed to supply the needs of students seeking out the answers to problems developed within the unit. The faculty must be committed to the idea of allowing students to plan with them for the work to be covered. Individual and group guidance is an important aspect of core, and teachers should be ready to spend time helping individuals and small groups with their quests. Evaluation is a constant process; the class will want to know about their progress from time to time, and individual effort will need constant appraisal.

But above all the learning must be solid, substantial, and to the point. Much of the criticism of this kind of curriculum arrangement has come from those who want only those components of a traditional discipline taught without any particular effort made to seek relatedness or meaning. Geometry, they say, is good for geometry's sake and never mind how it fits into man's relation to his world. In his discussion of the selection of subject matter, Bruner makes the following statement:

> What then of subject matter in the conventional sense? The answer to the question, "What shall be taught?" turns out to be the answer to the question, "What is nontrivial?" If one can first answer the question, "What is worth knowing about?" then it is not difficult to distinguish between the aspects of it that are worth teaching and learning and those that are not. Surely, knowledge of the natural world, knowledge of the human condition, knowledge of the nature and dynamics of society, knowledge of the past so that it may be used in experiencing the present and aspiring to the future—all of these, it would seem reasonable to suppose, are essential to an educated man. To these must be added another: knowledge of the products of our artistic heritage that mark the history of our aesthetic wonder and delight.[8]

THE USE OF RESOURCE PEOPLE, INCLUDING THE HEALTH EDUCATOR

Another of the major requirements of successful core development is the availability and use of people other than the core teacher. He should not be expected to "go it alone."

The health educator in all probability will not be the core teacher but will be a resource specialist. As Stratemeyer and others point out:

> A flexible but well planned pattern of experiences at the elementary school level allows for using specialists when needed. The entire class might seek help on an area of common concern, or a group might ask for special assistance during a laboratory period, or an individual might schedule time for rather extensive exploration. The proposed curriculum design makes many special demands on the time schedules of specialists, on systems of grouping learners, on the availability of materials. The entire school must be responsive to . . . the demands placed on personnel and resources.[9]

This is particularly important to personnel from the health sciences. Local physicians, dentists, public health workers, sanitarians, hospital administrators, people from voluntary health agencies, and many others are useful in supplying ideas, experiences, and information to core teachers either in building the resource unit or in conducting the study unit itself.

Naturally, the school health educator is interested in the amount of understanding about health that can be developed from such integrating studies. As indicated earlier, the amount of material from health education and its related fields varies with the unit and with the core teacher's skill and imagination. Teachers unprepared in health education will be less likely to give a full treatment to the possibilities for learning about health inherent in the unit.

Where such integrated plans exist, the health educator should:

1 Make available suggestions for problems rich in health material
2 Assist with the discovery of resources for data on the problems
3 Suggest a wide variety of student activities of pertinence to the solution of the problems
4 Arrange, if invited to do so, to bring resource people or teaching aids to the school
5 Be available himself for group leadership in the exploration of phases of the problems
6 Assist when needed with the development of the unit

A weakness of integration is that it depends so heavily upon the interest, motivation, and skill of the individual teacher. Elementary teachers are prepared to be generalists, and they do a remarkable job of teaching all of the subjects for which they are responsible. Few, however, are given much or any preparation for the health instruction for which they are the primary source during the vital first years of school. If the teacher feels insecure in his grasp of health information or uncomfortable about teaching youngsters about matters that may be very personal or controversial, he will not be eager to find time for very much health teaching. If the teacher perceives "health" as human anatomy or physiology, what will be taught will not be health but the structure and functions of the human body. Further, in the absence of a qualified and interested health coordinator, there is seldom a supervised plan to ensure a comprehensive health curriculum. Without such coordination, even effective health teaching can be fragmented and repetitive. So many youngsters have been instructed year after year in the proper method of brushing the teeth that some leave the public schools unable to recall that health instruction included anything else. To understand one's body becomes too frequently the object of the health course rather than to understand *oneself.* Physical education personnel, especially in dance, are forever talking about body control, body movement, my body, and your body, without, seemingly, the slightest concern for the dichotomy such usage fosters. The body is perceived as a machine apart from the mind or the soul. Digestion deals with food and peristalsis, not with behavior and the interrelationships among social, emotional, and bodily functions; thus digestive upsets are only related to "something I ate."

In health education we are trying to help people understand themselves as total personalities within the totality of their environment.

It is easy to teach health piecemeal—dental health today, family and marriage tomorrow. We forget that neat, but unrelated, capsules of information are seldom of more use than to pass the next test (if it is not too far removed in time). But facts that fit into a whole or that can be ordered according to a class of ideas which have significance for an individual in his own life are absorbing and are not only retained but serve to increase the student's power to generalize and discriminate among new facts as they are encountered.

Present evidence indicates that (1) students who have had experience in core programs do as well on standardized tests that measure knowledge of subject matter and vocabulary as students in traditional programs; (2) teachers and administrators who organize teaching in core curricula find that students show greater evidence of growth in ability to think critically than those taught by traditional methods; (3) the interrelatedness of the physical, social, and emotional aspects of health behavior is more readily grasped by students in core programs than those taught by the conventional approach; and (4) development of positive health behaviors is more apt to be an outcome since the objectives of the integrated curriculum focus not upon facts but upon process and vital concepts of healthful living.

THE SPECIFIC COURSE Perhaps the most familiar of the three patterns of curriculum organization is direct teaching in a regular class period devoted entirely to health instruction. This is the usual format for a "course" in health. Research indicates that this may also be the most effective of the three as a means of positively affecting health behavior. In a growing number of schools health is a required course. In some it is elective. Either way, the effective teacher makes it a dynamic experience, in which health content is the vehicle for learning rather than the goal. The skills and abilities developed through such a course should enable students to discover new knowledge as it is needed throughout life and to apply that knowledge as it is relevant to immediate problems. A health teacher needs to select the knowledge that can contribute to the student's need for self-acceptance and to his understanding of other persons and their needs, and most especially knowledge that is adaptable to individual needs and problems in a day-to-day, real-life context.

The dynamic health course is one in which students actively engage in fact finding, discussion, and field experiences that lead to conceptualization and conclusions. Active participation is essential. Students are not merely passive recipients of information but are encouraged to react, to take part, to develop the ability to think critically, and to choose rationally among alternatives. Choices and decision making demand thinking, and the more thinking involved, the greater the contribution to the general education of the student.

The dynamic health course deals with today's problems. It might take advantage of a current drive for funds to fight cancer to make the subject of cancer prevention an organizing center for health instruction. It might focus on local traffic problems, or special health problems with which the local community is concerned currently. It will not focus alone upon the *facts* about drug abuse or the physical signs of venereal disease, but upon the human motivations and behaviors of which these problems are but the symptoms. It will not purport to speak of health while it studies only disease.

Whatever the topics or problems or concepts used to structure the dynamic course, the outcome should be a student who can generalize from the separate learning experiences he has encountered to the more powerful ideas that will be useful long after the facts have been forgotten or rendered obsolete.

Furthermore, a dynamic health course allows the students to share in its planning. What they need to know is only partially a decision to be made by teachers and society. Not only does student participation ensure that his own perceptions of his needs, which are inherently more valid, will influence selection of course emphasis areas, but it also promotes his interest and involvement in the learning.

– the scope of the curriculum

What is learned in health education is not entirely within the province of the school. Children at any age are learning something about health every day and from a wide variety of sources such as television commercials, advertising in the news media, observation of adult behavior, and hearsay from their peers. What is taught in the classroom has tended to be dependent upon the textbook or textbook series adopted by a school. In essence, therefore, the scope of health education has been determined less by school administrators and teachers than by authors and publishers. What has been taught has been whatever subjects or topics the textbook authors thought to be most worth while. The major administrative decision has been the choice among alternatives in textbook presentations. Teachers who fear that the so-called packaged learning systems emerging in many disciplines are mechanistic and threaten the central role of the teacher fail to recognize that packaging is nothing new. The difference is that the new packages are often more valid tools because they reflect the research and best work of many skillful educators rather than the philosophy and knowledge of one or two authors only. In fact, the writers of some textbooks are full-time staff members of publishers, whereas the credited author simply reviews and approves the result and lends his name and prestige to the resulting book.

When the separate course is taught is an administrative decision, and varies with the philosophy of the school or school district. There is no standard practice regarding either the content of health courses (what is taught) or the grades in which health education is provided (when it is taught). In elementary schools some health instruction is usually given each year in relation to the growth and developmental needs and characteristics of the children. If there is any pattern at the upper levels, it is that one course is offered during the middle or junior high school years and another course during the senior high years.

Many organizations, groups, and experts in school health education have made recommendations about direct health teaching. Most agree that elementary school children should be given a minimum of 20 minutes health instruction each day, that students in the middle grades should have a minimum of a class period once a week for a year but preferably a full semester of daily health instruction during this period, and that a one-semester daily course in health be provided senior high school students.

Curriculum decisions must be made locally with reference to the particular needs of the students, the problems of the community, the faculty, and the facilities available. If the administrative commitment is to give direct instruction, the program should be of high quality and taught by qualified health educators. Equal time, space, and essential equipment on a par with other subject areas must be provided for health education. No once-a-week sharing with physical education or rainy-day scheduling will suffice.

In the self-contained elementary classroom it is possible that health may be assigned its own special time slot in the day and taught directly as a separate subject. In most elementary schools one teacher works with the same group of students throughout the school year and is responsible for teaching about health as well as all the other subject areas. Unhappily, however, most elementary-education major programs neglect to require even a basic health content course for prospective teachers. Where a two-unit course in methods and materials in health and physical education is required, the focus is typically on physical education alone. The result is that health education may be perceived more narrowly than is desirable and may fail to receive the comprehensive treatment it should have. According to Cushman, "Emphasis in health education since the 1920's has been on the promotion of health habits, teachable moments, and correlated learning rather than on knowledge."[10]

In the secondary schools, administrators have often assigned physical educators or coaches to teach a health course because teacher preparation institutions have long awarded degrees in Health & Physical Education. Some of these programs may indeed have given equal emphasis to both areas, but they did not always produce teachers whose interests were so neatly halved. In most cases, health preparation is minimal at best and, more often, is largely an assumption based upon some commonalities among the required science courses basic to each field. Today the trend is toward the requirement that health education be considered separately as an area of study. At last report, colleges and universities in thirty-one states are offering a program of specialization in health education at one or more of three degree levels. A total of one hundred four institutions presently offer such degree programs, an increase of twenty-six in the years between 1967 and 1970, and more programs are reportedly in the process of development.[11] This growth mirrors the swiftly mounting demand for health teaching specialists for the already authorized specific health courses in many areas.

It can be demonstrated that children in every grade have problems in sufficient quantity and of sufficient importance to make direct teaching every year desirable. From the seventh grade on, a one-semester course each year can be justified. Some might believe that if so much health instruction is provided, the subject will be exhausted in the first two or three years and the rest would be repetitive and useless. The truth is exactly the reverse. There is not enough time to teach all that could be taught, even if health were taught every semester. Few schools are so organized as to permit this much teaching in health education, however. The next best allotment of time would be a semester course at the seventh, tenth, and twelfth grades, with the tenth omitted if need be. This arrangement would at least reach the students entering and leaving both the junior and the senior high schools.

The strength of the separate course rests upon several factors. Because it *is* the traditional pattern of teaching anything, it is the pattern that teachers have themselves experienced, and consequently they feel most comfortable and secure in it. The full class period, five days a week, for a semester at a time allows enough time for a comprehensive study of the subject. A separate course allows the teacher time to be more flexibly responsive to student needs or special local problems. Interest and motivation to learn are more easily sustained when a day-by-day program can be planned and carried out.

Where the course is assigned to a health educator on a full-time basis, the instructional strategies are more apt to be dynamic and relevant than where the instructor teaches primarily in other areas and gives his principal effort and interest to his own subject. The full-time instructor has time to focus all of his energies on new developments in the literature, to incorporate these fresh data in his teaching, and to evaluate the results for use in replanning and renewal of his own insights and understandings about health behavior and how it may be changed.

A weakness of the separate course is that it may tend to be compartmentalized as an approach to general education, and valuable integrating experiences with other subject areas may be neglected. In some schools, overdependence on the textbook may cause more attention to be given to covering the book than to emphasizing content areas that may be of greatest concern to the students. Because teachers tend to teach as they have themselves been taught, direct teaching may consist of dreary daily lectures, and these may more often be a set of warning restrictions than suggestions for positive health behavior and greater pleasure in life. "Don't smoke. You'll die of lung cancer!—Don't engage in premarital intercourse. You might get venereal disease!—You might become an unmarried mother . . . or father!"

Wherever the separate course is provided, in the absence of an effective health-coordinator, other subject area teachers often fail to provide reinforcing experiences. Health instruction is regarded as taken care of fully by the health course and is often forgotten by the rest of the faculty.

However, the specific course seems to many to be the best and most fruitful way to convey to youth the great lessons of science as they may be applied to the maintenance and promotion of the health of the human organism. The easiest and most sterile way to structure direct teaching is to divide the material by the great systems of the body, to lecture about the anatomy and physiology of the systems, and then to field any questions as time allows. But people need to *live* effectively, and cramming facts into their heads regarding the structure and function of the liver will do little to motivate them to make choices among behaviors that will not be detrimental to the structure of that vital organ. The material to be taught must be chosen in relation to living needs, and it must be sensitive to changes both in knowledge and human needs and interests.

A comprehensive, dynamic health course will not only enrich the lives of the students but will serve as an important reinforcement for other educational areas. If man's essential need is to learn who he is, and to discover meaning in his existence, then health education, *at its best,* can contribute in an important way to the success of that quest. The specific course taught by a qualified health educator is, potentially at least, health education at its best.

CORRELATION

Organization of health instruction in a correlation pattern is the planned inclusion of health information within a host subject or series of subjects. Host subjects are often physical education, home economics, and physiology, or broad fields of study such as biology, life science, or social science. Whatever the host course, or courses, natural relationships are sought between health concepts and concepts central to the primary disciplines.

Traditionally, the school curriculum has been composed of a number of more or less related subjects or disciplines, each with a body of knowledge structured upon certain fundamental ideas, and typified by special modes of inquiry by which related new knowledge is generated. So we have the basic subjects of reading, writing, and arithmetic and, built upon these, the more advanced subjects of history, mathematics, science, literature, music, art, and all the rest. Subjects have multiplied to the point where it is no longer possible to find time or space to teach them all. Choices must be made. For some, choices are made in relation to future career plans, for others, in terms of personal interests. In an effort to make sure that certain subject areas will be studied by all students, administrators have fused related courses into broader fields affording an overview of a wider area for nonspecialists and have employed correlation as a means of including other subjects by means of a curriculum-wide strategy.

But it is through a systematic study of the separate courses, however they may be organized for teaching, that one usually pursues one's education.

> Emphasis is thus placed on the subject as the organizing basis of the experience of the learner. Establishment of relationships between subjects is encouraged, but elimination of subject lines is held to destroy the foundation of education. Ability to meet common problems of living is the central purpose of the subject cur-

riculum, but the achievement of this purpose is held to be best realized through systematic study of the various subjects.[12]

In the college and university experience, degree requirements and scheduling pressures push the student even more into taking a cluster of courses whose interrelationships, even among those of a planned major program, may be less than well understood. The relevance of one course to another often depends upon the individual's ability to synthesize and generalize on his own. But, inescapably, there is some overlap among subjects. It is difficult not to learn some English and spelling while studying biology. Biology teaches one a great many facts relevant to health. In health education it is possible to learn something of politics through a discussion of needed public health facilities or programs. As a process, then, correlation exists naturally and inevitably both in and out of school. As a means of organizing the curriculum for health education, correlation is the planned, or in some cases the claimed, interweaving of health instruction throughout parts or all of the rest of the school curriculum.

– potential relationships to health education

Correlation has rich possibilities. There is such a close relationship between biological science and the science of living that correlation is unavoidable. In many modern science textbooks, human biology and health have been deliberately included for this reason.

Science has much to teach about the human organism. Science provides some answers to man's questions of "how." How are we born, how do we grow, how are the brain cells constructed, how does the brain work? What are the laws of genetics? What is DNA? What does it have to do with reproduction? Microbiology provides the fundamental facts about communicable disease and its control.

It would be foolish and wasteful if in teaching government all of the attention were given to the structure of the courts and their role in law enforcement and none to the causes of criminal behavior necessitating their existence, or if much thought were given to government structure and none to the responsibility of government to provide for the comprehensive health care of the people whose taxes support it.

In physiology, teaching can be centered around human health problems that are related to the physiological structures and functions rather than upon structure and function as isolates. The physical sciences have a great deal to contribute as well. Blood chemistry, immunity processes, hormone structure and function, blood pressure, osmosis, digestion, muscle action, and fatigue can be explained by the physical sciences and at the same time meaningfully related to human life.

In social studies we can teach something about the relationship of the appalling health conditions in the inner city ghettos to today's social problems and issues. History is filled with incidents that can be related to health problems and health behavior.

The study of literature is rich with potential for influencing health attitudes and practices. Human relationships, family structure and function, the extent to which mankind has been subjected to and has conquered disease, and personality problems that have shaped lives and history can be learned perhaps more effectively from reading literature than from a health textbook. The shifting perceptions of moral behavior held by young people today and the growing violence and bloodshed on high school and college campuses have been attributed by some to the constant exposure to violence on television, which these young people have watched since they were children.

There are countless opportunities to relate health material to the traditional subjects. And, of course, health instruction can draw upon all of the other disciplines in the curriculum as sources of the information required in the solution of health problems. Look at the *Reader's Guide* and the *Education Index.* It is possible to find writings that are directly and indirectly concerned with health in a wide range of professional and popular journals.

What is taught in the correlated health education curriculum, then, is a decision that must be made and adhered to by all of those whose responsibility it will be. Ideally, a curriculum committee under the leadership or with the assistance of a qualified health coordinator should plan the total program. Only with the effective cooperation of coordinator and host teachers can health instruction be given comprehensive treatment and reach all of the students. Planning of this kind considers not only what is to be taught, but also when and how.

SUGGESTIONS FOR CORRELATION

Below is a selection of suggestions developed from a few of the fields that are most likely to be rich in possibilities for correlation with health education.

With Physical Sciences

1 Ventilation and heating
2 Vision, refraction, optics
3 Disinfectants, germicides
4 Chemistry of food, nutritional needs
5 Weather, climate, and health and disease
6 Water and food preservation and sanitation, freeze drying

7 The use of X-ray in medicine, of radioactive substances in disease control
8 Health problems in space, space travel
9 Velocity in relation to safety in driving
10 Relationship of physics and chemistry to physiology
11 The control of sex in the embryo through physical means
12 The atom, fissionable material, and health
13 Fluoridation and chlorination of water

With Social Sciences

1 Health status compared internationally
2 Governmental health organizations here and abroad
3 Functions of government relating to health of people
4 Current issues of medical and health care
5 Studies of environment, home and community planning, city planning
6 School and community recreation
7 The family, domestic and comparative
8 Traffic control, automobile hazards, industrial safety, legal backgrounds
9 Poverty, sickness, economic status, race, depressions, and disease
10 Health in relation to rural and urban populations
11 Growth of superstitions, fallacies, rumors, prejudices
12 International relationships as they relate to health
13 The World Health Organization and kindred groups
14 The influences of health factors, e.g., the great plagues, on history
15 Health problems in specific world areas
16 Health problems and economic and industrial development

With Problems of Democracy

1 Official and voluntary agencies, and their function in public health, the public health service, local health department
2 Functions of health officers, health commissioners, coroners, inspectors, sanitation directors
3 Knowledge of available community health services
4 Consideration of health activities of clubs, labor organizations, and various other societies
5 Legal requirements for driving, use of firearms, installation of certain machines and apparatus
6 Analysis of the recreational facilities available in the community
7 Health status of the community and the nation
8 Study and discussion of current health legislation, fluoridation, socialized medicine

9 Discussion of family health problems, the advisibility of voluntary health insurance, cost of medical care

10 Health problems of the nation's elder citizens

11 Relation of slum areas to physical and mental health

12 Sociological aspects of disability and disease

13 Effect of city zoning in promotion of community health

14 Problems of community sanitation and efforts to control communicable disease, inspection, adequate waste and sewage disposal

15 Importance of food preservation in interstate and international commerce

16 Health regulations and inspections relative to international travel

With Physical Education

1 Cleanliness, infection, skin infections

2 First aid and care of injuries, protection against injury

3 Clothing and weather

4 Use of physical examinations, limitations and possibilities for activity, development of compensating activities

5 Experience in participation in developmental and individually prescribed activities

6 Experience in planning, decision-making, social conduct, and emotional control through competitive situations

7 Experience in choosing activities for current and later use and in evaluating results of participation

8 Relation between vigorous and restful activities

9 Fatigue, conditioning, "training," diet, and nutrition in relation to activity

10 Safety precautions in all activities

11 Experience in the development of a sense of achievement, in personal evaluation, and in self-direction

12 Individual differences in size, strength, endocrine factors, and ability in relation to performance

13 Sex differences in performance, organic and psychological development

14 Experience in the appreciation of play, fun, and recreation

15 Experience in acceptable boy-girl relationship through corecreation

With Driver Education

1 Importance of mind and muscle coordination

2 Effect of alcohol and narcotics on driving ability

3 Study of eyesight and the necessity of adequate vision

4 Safety rules for drivers, pedestrians, and bicycle riders

5 Need for stable emotions and logical thinking

6 Study of accident facts and statistics

7 Organization of safety patrols and safety councils

8 Relation of sleep and proper eating to personal energy and stamina

9 Emergency procedures to follow in case of an accident, first aid[13]

These topics are some that could be studied in correlation with health education. Now let us look at an actual correlation plan as it was worked out for a California school district.[14] The rationale for deciding what would be taught was that certain key topics were important and that these would be taught as a part of the existing course offering, which appeared to be the best vehicle for such study. The key organizing centers or health topics decided upon were the following:

1 Growth and Development (including family life education, mental health, and structure and functions of the human body)

2 Nutrition

3 Personal Health

4 Community Health

5 Stimulants and Depressants

6 Chronic and Communicable Diseases

7 Consumer Health Education

8 Safety and First Aid

It can be argued that these topics in fact reflect most of what is considered representative of the body of knowledge embraced by health education. Now let us look at how this is correlated in the school curriculum. The plan for the first and broadest area, growth and development, is given here as an example of the vertical sequence, which considers this topic every year from the seventh through the twelfth grades.

I. Growth and Development

A. Grade 7

1 *Home Economics* (First semester required of all girls)
Unit: Interpersonal Relationships—1 week
Unit: Child Development and Family Relationships—3 weeks

2 *Home Economics* (Second semester, elective)
Unit: Interpersonal relationships—1 week
Unit: Child Development and Family Relationships—4 weeks

3 *Physical Education* (Required)
Unit: The Process of Growing Up—2 weeks
Significance of the period of adolescence to boys and girls
Fundamental needs of growing boys and girls
Physical development during adolescence
Personality development and social development

B. Grade 8

1 *General Science* (1 year, required)

Unit: Body Chemistry and Health—3–5 weeks
Health and effective living—one of four sections included in this unit
The needs and interests of teen-agers—one of four areas considered in the section

C. Grade 9

1 *Home Economics* (First semester, elective)

Unit: Interpersonal Relationships—1 week

2 *Home Economics* (Second semester, elective)

Unit: Child Development—1 week
Unit: Family Relationships—2 weeks

3 *Physical Education* (Required)

Unit: Teen-age Health Problems—2 weeks
Structure and functions of the human body—one of two sections included in this unit

4 *Ninth Grade Advanced Science* (Introductory physiology, elected by small proportion of college-bound students)

Unit 1: Human Behavior—1 semester
Unit 2: Human Physiology—1 semester
Unit 3: Human Conservation—1 semester

5 *English,* Grade 9 (Required—three units to be chosen from a list of twelve)

Unit: Growing Up Socially
Factors that influence dating practices
Social skills that can be learned
Acceptable teen-age activities

Unit: Over Twenty-One
Emotional and physical needs that adults have in common with teen-agers
Responsibilities of adults to teen-agers
Responsibilities of teen-agers to adults
Factors that influence relationships between teen-agers and adults

Unit: Getting to Know Us
Groups to which teen-agers belong
Ways groups influence teen-agers
Decisions teen-agers have to make
Ways to make decisions wisely
Ways persons can contribute to others and gain self-satisfaction

D. Grade 10

1 *Home Economics* (Grades 10–12, elective)

Unit: Personality Development and Interpersonal Relationships—4 weeks

2 *Physical Education* (Required)

Unit: Growing into Maturity—2 weeks
The human machine
Boy-girl relationships
Developing sound attitudes

3 *Health Science* (Taken by approximately 75 percent of the noncollege bound students—elective. Students elect one of four areas of study in this course: Health Science; Life Science; Earth Science; Physical Science. Health Science, given here, is the most popular.)

Unit: Health and Personality—1 week
Unit: Structure of the Body—3 weeks
Unit: Vital Processes of the Body—5 weeks
Unit: Control of the Body—6 weeks

E. Grade 11

1 *Senior Home Economics* (Grades 11–12, required of all girls, 1 semester)

Unit: Child Growth and Development—4 weeks
Unit: Family Relationships and Personal Development—4 weeks

2 *Biology 1–2* (Grade 11 or 12, 1 year—taken by approximately 75 percent of college preparatory students. One of three parts of this course deals with the differences in structure and functions of animals including the human being.)

3 *Physiology and Hygiene 1–2* (Grade 11 or 12, 1 year—taken by approximately 5 percent of the college-bound students, elective)

Unit: Human Body: Structure and Function

F. Grade 12

1 *Senior Home Economics 2* (Grade 11 or 12, elective, 1 semester)

Unit: Personal Development—2 weeks

2 *Physical Education* (Required)

Unit: Reaching Maturity—2 weeks
"Preparation for Marriage," one of four parts of the unit, includes the following:

The reproductive process
Premarital preparation
Marriage
Parenthood

4 *Problems in American Life* (Required, 1 semester)
Includes consideration of the achievement of stability in marriage and family.

How many of the above courses are required of all students? Notice the heavy emphasis on structure and function. Two courses are mentioned more often than others—home economics, required only of girls and usually elective in any case, and physical education, which offers bits and pieces snatched from physical education class time.

What about the horizontal sequence, those studies correlated with health education in any one year? The plan for the seventh grade is given below.

Growth and Development	1 Home Economics (Required of girls) Unit: Interpersonal Relationships—1 week Unit: Child Development and Family Relationships—3 weeks

	2 Home Economics (Second semester, elective) Unit: Interpersonal Relationships—1 week Unit: Child Development and Family Relationships—4 weeks 3 Physical Education (Required) Unit: The Process of Growing Up—2 weeks Significance of the period of adolescence to boys and girls Fundamental needs of growing boys and girls Physical development during adolescence Personality development and social development
Nutrition	1 Home Economics (First semester, required of girls) Unit: Foods and Nutrition and Family Meals—4 weeks 2 Home Economics (Second semester, elective) Unit: Foods and Nutrition and Family Meals—5 weeks
Personal Health	1 Home Economics (First semester, required of girls) Unit: Personal Grooming and Health Habits—1 week 2 Home Economics (Second semester, elective) Unit: Personal Grooming and Health Habits—1 week
Community Health	(Starts in Grade 9)
Stimulants and Depressants	(Starts in Grade 8)
Chronic and Communicable Diseases	(Starts in Grade 9)
Consumer Health Education	(Starts in Grade 9)
Safety and First Aid	Home Economics (First semester, required of girls) Unit: Safety at Home and in the Classroom—1 week

In this plan, health education is correlated with only two courses, one of which is for girls only. The other, physical education, gives one 2 week unit to The Process of Growing Up. Although some of the other years are more fully developed, none of them is very inspiring. Only 4 weeks are actually required of all students in the ninth grade, for example, and all of it in physical education.

The strength of the correlation curriculum is considered to be its planned reinforcement of previous and parallel learning experiences in health education. The correlation curriculum should focus on the reality of the impact of health on every facet of life and make health teaching a dynamic of every other area of general education.

The weakness of correlation lies in its total dependence on the host teacher's ability to organize his teaching economically and effectively enough to achieve all of his own course objectives as well as those proposed for health. Not just his ability but his interest is critical to the success of correlation. A biology teacher is not as apt to spend time stressing the social and mental-emotional forces influencing health behavior as the physical. Nor is he as apt to view health as a behavioral science rather than a biological, even though human, science. Social science teachers may be more interested in examining the social aspects of health, and less concerned or knowledgeable about the physical and mental components of those aspects. It is apparent that attempts to provide health education only through correlation are likely to reach only certain students, to consider only certain topics, and to be unevenly effective, depending upon the teacher and the host area. Correlation plans are at best never perfect, and they never can cover the area of healthful living as it should be covered. The school district formerly using the plan above has shifted to the conceptual approach and requires separate health education courses of all seventh and tenth graders.

Correlation is probably best employed as a supplemental form of curriculum organization. What good would a social studies course be, for example, if it did not tackle the problem of health care, or comprehensive health planning, or relationships between consumers and providers of health products and services, and not just the economic aspects but the shared responsibilities involved? If no other pattern is possible, correlation is better than nothing. In such a case the following suggestions may help to stabilize and enrich the process.

1 The faculty must be receptive to the idea of correlation and ready to receive and use such recommendations as appear reasonable.

2 An individual or small committee must become sufficiently familiar with all areas of study and with the wide area of health education to recognize where each could enrich the other, and be prepared to make recommendations for the inclusion of health material in other areas.

3 A program of inservice training should be provided for the teachers involved to improve their ability to handle the acceptable health material.

4 Conferences should be held during the year as necessary for the exchange of ideas between teachers in the different areas, for example, between the social science teachers and the health group. Such conferences would be useful in checking facts, exchanging teaching materials and ideas, agreeing on purposes, and setting directions.

5 The health teacher or anyone close to problems and sources in the area of health education should make it a continuous practice to supply other teachers with ideas, resources, and teachable materials.

If these suggestions are followed, correlating health education with other subject areas becomes, if not the best way to teach health, at least a profitable one.

THE TEACHER'S ROLE IN CURRICULUM

Health education, being a study of human life and its processes, in broad outline would involve all related problems, interests, and needs. Indeed there is little that does *not* involve health in man's social, emotional, and physical life. Factors such as emotional stability, sexual and social maturity, physical development, adjustment to stress, illness, or disaster, and the problems associated with personality development—all these and many others influence a person's health. To define these problems, to examine and prepare to teach about them in a manner appropriate for each grade or level of achievement and ability, and then to arrange them logically and meaningfully in an organized curriculum plan is a task requiring great skill in curriculum construction.

Owing to its complexities, *curriculum* has emerged as a major field of study at the doctoral level. Perhaps the time is at hand when school administrators and teachers can begin to focus their own special skills where they can be most influential and effective and leave curriculum making to the specialists.

Sliepcevich differentiates between two levels of curriculum decision-making. The broader, more general view of curriculum development, entailing careful research and decisions applicable to any community because of the universality of certain needs and problems, she terms the "macroscopic view." The more specific curriculum problems at the classroom level, the "microscopic view" would be the teacher's special area of decision making, with the former problems left to the curriculum specialists. The teacher brings special competencies, talents, and insights to the problems of adapting, modifying, and implementing the materials developed for his use that no curriculum expert can ever provide. The teacher and the curriculum expert complement each other and make each other more effective in such a team approach. Sliepcevich recalls:

> Letters requesting assistance provide evidence of the overwhelming task which curriculum development presents to local communities. In essence, such letters usually state that a curriculum committee has been appointed and request that guides, outlines, bibliographies, materials, and anything else that may be available

> be sent. Such letters often end with a plea for any suggestions as to how to proceed with the task.
>
> Too often, what results from collecting guides and outlines developed by local, state, or nation-wide projects and then formulating another guide using excerpts from these is a conglomeration of content or other curriculum components that are unrelated.[15]

She pleads that teachers would not be less involved in curriculum decisions, were this division of labor to come about and were development of general curriculum materials to be entrusted to curriculum specialists, but *more* involved at a more significant and sophisticated level than in hacking out the usual cut and paste, grab-bag job of curriculum guide preparation. The unending series of such documents, decorated with nice sounding but ambiguous objectives and bolstered with fuzzily stated "suggested activities" demonstrate this compulsion to rediscover the wheel. Studies of the *uses* of these kinds of curriculum materials reveal that most of them sit dust-laden on the bookshelf or in desk drawers. Meantime, the available textbook continues to structure what is taught.

CURRENT CURRICULUM CHANGES

Whether the scope of the curriculum is determined with a macroscopic or a microscopic view, or both, it will most probably be described conceptually rather than topically in the 1970s and beyond. Availability and acceptance of instructional packages in connection with broadly conceived curriculum plans will quite probably increase in most disciplines.

The word for the 1970s will be "accountability," meaning that schools and colleges will be judged by how *they* perform, not how their students perform. Educators have long claimed most of the credit for the record of the successful student and at the same time smugly disavowed any responsibility for the one who fails. They may say, "He doesn't try" or "He lacks ability." In 1970 the Office of Economic Opportunity launched a multimillion dollar experiment employing a variety of packaged teaching programs under performance contracts with industry. According to the terms of the contract, reading and mathematic skills are to be taught to poor children at guaranteed levels of achievement, and payment will depend upon the success of the program, not on the number of packages used.

The role of the teacher is already changing from the traditional stage-center lecturer to the from-the-wings facilitator of learning. Learning is the product, not the activity. Facts become the means by which the student learns processes, or ways of enquiring and creating knowledge.

Individualization, based upon precise specification of educational objectives, is an outcome of the shift away from the lockstep of graded schools. The so-called egg-crate school building is being replaced with buildings whose rooms are flexibly adaptable to individual, small-group, and large-group activities. Tomorrow's schools may be schools without walls and year-round programs. It is predicted that ultimately an even more sophisticated notion of providing "adaptive" education will tailor a curriculum to meet the special requirements and abilities of each learner.

In fact, all of these changes can be found even now in some places. But change in appearance is not change in substance. And in the long run, what matters is the outcome of education as a means of meeting the needs of the learner and the society, and of transmitting the body of knowledge. Innovation may or may not become practice. The traditional curriculum patterns will perhaps continue to serve to structure health education however the content may be defined and the methodology change.

When the sources of the curriculum have been examined, the recommendations of state and national authorities are significant additional data to be considered in making a decision. A recent statement of administrative guidelines was an outcome of a 1969 conference of leaders in health education, school superintendents, principals, schoolboard members, and physicians in California. Their resulting guidelines appear to exemplify current thinking about the best health teaching at the secondary level.

Prefacing their recommendations with the explanation that the guidelines are stated in general terms inasmuch as specific administrative decisions are the prerogative of local districts, the following were their conclusions:

Programs

1 Health education should be identified as a separate subject in the school curriculum.

2 School districts have an obligation to make provisions for health education as an integral part of general education.

3 Health education should be a planned, sequential program in grades kindergarten through twelve; crash programs emphasizing special health topics should be avoided.

4 Adequate time and resources for health education should be provided.

5 Districts should be encouraged to explore innovative organizational patterns for instruction such as flexible scheduling in order to provide for effective health education.

6 Districts should also offer pre-school and adult health education programs, *if not otherwise available.*

Curriculum

1 Curriculum development should focus on student achievement of desired behavioral objectives.

2 Relevant health concepts should be included at the most appropriate developmental levels of children and youth.

3 Health education should be responsive to the needs of students and the demands of society, and should reflect current scientific knowledge.

4 The curriculum should focus on the positive aspects of health.

5 Students and the community should be involved in curriculum development to insure the inclusion of instruction based on health needs, interests and problems.

6 Districts should be encouraged to explore innovative and creative instructional methods which actively involve students in the achievement of established behavioral objectives such as small discussion groups, independent study and team teaching.

Time

1 Health education should receive equal consideration with other subject areas in the curriculum.

2 Adequate time should be provided to achieve the established behavioral goals and program objectives.

3 Specific time allotment should be given to the treatment of health education in depth as well as recognizing it as an inherent portion of several other disciplines.

4 Time allotment will vary depending on individual and community needs.

Teachers

1 Health education in schools should be taught by an adequately prepared teacher with a demonstrated interest and aptitude in health education. Wherever possible, the teacher should have a specific preparation in health education, preferably a major or minor.

2 Desirable teacher qualities should include: ability to interact meaningfully and honestly with students, to act capably as a resource for students, and to be sensitive to individual differences and needs.

3 Districts should provide continuing programs of in-service teacher preparation in health education that should also reflect current scientific information.

Coordination

1 Responsibility for the development, coordination, and implementation of health education in the school district should be assigned to a specific person.

2 Districts should be encouraged to seek and utilize consultant services from county schools office, from medical and other sources.

Community

1 School districts should be responsive to and involve the community in planning, developing and implementing programs in a

variety of ways, including the establishment of and/or the participation in school-community health councils.

2 Districts should never assume permanent acceptance of health education by the community but should constantly assess and revise the program in accordance with changing needs and attitudes.

3 Districts should enlist the help and support of community leaders.

4 Available community resources should be utilized to augment and enrich the instructional program.

Financing and Facilities

1 Sufficient financial support should be provided to insure adequate facilities, personnel and instructional materials to achieve the established objectives.

2 School districts should seek resources which may be available from a wide variety of community agencies and organizations.

Evaluation

1 The program should be periodically evaluated in terms of effectiveness based on realistic and measurable criteria.

2 Pupils, teachers, parents and others should be involved in the evaluation of the program at regular intervals in terms of relevance to pupils.[16]

SUMMARY

Organizing the health curriculum is a problem doubly perplexing in today's disturbing climate of social change, divisive international involvement, generation gaps, and the unprecedented rate of growth in technology and knowledge. As the schools struggle to meet the challenge posed by the needs reflected in this wide range of problems, comprehensive health education for the total man seems more an imperative than ever before. Three curriculum patterns, direct teaching, integration, and correlation can be used as a means of teaching about health from kindergarten through the twelfth grades.

Direct teaching, or the separate course, is the pattern chosen by most health education authorities. Most would also agree that direct teaching should be supported and complemented by planned correlation and integration throughout the entire curriculum of the school if health teaching is to be effective enough to counteract the powerful social and emotional forces that often promote the very behaviors health educators seek to change.

Curriculum decisions at any level must answer the basic questions: What will be taught? When or to whom will it be taught? and How will it be taught? Chapter 3 has presented some answers to these questions at the school or district level. Chapter 4 will address these questions at the level of the classroom and from the frame of reference of the teacher.

NOTES AND REFERENCES

1 Adapted from Nelson B. Henry (ed.), *The Integration of Educational Experiences,* Fifty-seventh Yearbook, National Society for the Study of Education, Part II, Chicago, University of Chicago Press, 1958, pp. 10–11.

2 Adapted from R. L. Willard, "Integrative Issues and Methods," *Main Currents in Modern Thought,* 20, 2 (November–December 1963), 41.

3 Philip H. Phenix, "Key Concepts and the Crisis of Learning," *Teacher's College Record,* December 1965, pp. 137–143.

4 Wesley P. Cushman, "An Overview of Approaches to Curricula and Course Instruction in Health Education," *Journal of School Health* (January 1969), pp. 14–21.

5 School Health Education Study, Inc., *Health Education: A Conceptual Approach,* St. Paul, 3M Education Press, 1967.

6 John Gardner, *Self Renewal,* New York, Harper & Row, 1965, p. 26.

7 John Goodlad, "Direction of Curriculum Change," *NEA Journal,* December 1966, pp. 33–37.

8 Jerome S. Bruner, *On Knowing,* Cambridge, Harvard University Press, 1963, pp. 121–122.

9 Florence B. Stratemeyer *et al., Developing a Curriculum for Modern Living,* 2nd ed., New York, Teachers College, Columbia University, 1957, p. 355.

10 Cushman, *op. cit.*

11 School Health Education Study, Inc., *Directory of Institutions Offering Programs of Specialization in Health Education,* Washington, D.C., School Health Education Study, Inc., 1970.

12 Hollis L. Caswell and Arthur W. Foshay, *Education in the Elementary School,* 3rd ed., New York, American Book, 1957, p. 258.

13 These five sections are adapted from Elena M. Sliepcevich and Charles R. Carroll, "The Correlation of Health with Other Areas of the High School Curriculum," *Journal of School Health,* 28, 9 (November 1958), 283.

14 Ina Lundh, Assistant Director, Curriculum and Instruction, Health and Safety, Long Beach Unified School District, Long Beach, Calif.

15 Elena Sliepcevich, "Curriculum Development: A Macroscopic or Microscopic View?" *The National Elementary Principal,* 48, 2 (November 1968), 19.

16 Harold J. Cornacchia, Chairman, Editing Committee, Asilomar Conference, "Administrative Guidelines for Health Education in California Secondary Schools," 1969.

SELECTED READINGS

American Association of School Administrators, *The Year-Round School,* Association for Supervision and Curriculum Development, "Projects, Packages, Programs," *Educational Leadership,* 27, 8 (May 1970). Washington, D.C., American Association of School Administrators, 1970.

Berman, Louise M., *New Priorities in Curriculum,* Columbus, Ohio, Merrill, 1968.

Beyrer, Mary K., Ann E. Nolte, and Marian K. Solleder, *A Directory of Selected References and Resources in Health Instruction.* 2nd ed., Minneapolis, Burgess, 1969.

Department of Elementary School Principals, "Health Education in the Elementary School," *National Elementary Principal,* 48, 2 (November 1968).

Dorothy McClure Fraser (ed.), *Social Studies Curriculum Development: Prospects and Problems,* 39th yearbook, Washington, D.C., National Council for the Social Studies, 1969.

Gardner, John, *Self Renewal: The Individual and the Innovative Society,* New York, Harper & Row, 1965.

Goodlad, John I., *Planning and Organizing for Teaching,* Project on the Instructional Program of the Public Schools, Washington, D.C., 1963.

Joint Committee on Health Problems in Education of the NEA and the AMA, *Health Education,* Washington, D.C., NEA, 1961.

Mitzel, Harold E., "The Impending Instruction Revolution," *Phi Delta Kappan,* Bloomington, Ind., Phi Delta Kappa, April 1970, pp. 434–439.

Morphet, Edgar L., and David L. Jesser, *Cooperative Planning for Education in 1980. Designing Education for the Future:* An Eight State Project, Denver, 1968.

Morphet, Edgar L., and Charles O. Ryan, *Planning and Effecting Needed Changes in Education. Designing Education for the Future.* An Eight State Project, Denver, 1967.

National Association of Secondary School Principals, "Curriculum Change in Health Education," *The Bulletin,* no. 326, Washington, D.C., National Association of Secondary School Principals, March 1968.

Peddiwell, J. Abner, *The Sabertooth Curriculum,* New York, McGraw-Hill, 1939.

Pollock, Marion B., "Curriculum Planning: A Gamesmanship Approach," *Journal of School Health,* (October 1969), 523–25.

Short, Edmund C., and George D. Marconnit, (eds.), *Contemporary Thought on Public School Curriculum,* Dubuque, Iowa, William C. Brown, 1968.

Tyler, Louise L., *A Selected Guide to Curriculum Literature. An Annotated Bibliography. Schools for the Seventies Series,* Center for the Study of Instruction, Washington, D.C., NEA, 1970.

Young, Marjorie A.C., "Review of Research and Studies Related to Health Education Practice (1961–1966) School Health Education," Health Education Monograph, No. 28, New York, Society of Public Health Educators, 1969.

CHAPTER 4 ORGANIZING FOR EFFECTIVE TEACHING

The crucial decisions at the instructional level of organization center about What? When? and How? questions just as at the administrative level. The difference is that in this case, the decisions are made by teachers as they make their plans within the larger organizational structure. Instead of being concerned with patterns of curriculum organization at school or district level, the focus is on a plan for teaching.

What to teach and when to teach it are more closely related problems at the classroom level than at the administrative level. Yet these decisions must be made within the framework and supportive to the vertical sequence planned by administration for kindergarten through the twelfth grade. Whatever plans are made by a teacher, or group of teachers, for a given class or group of classes must build upon expected learnings acquired at lower levels and must contribute to goals established as essential outcomes of the total public school experience in health education.

We have said that at the institutional level, decisions regarding what is to be taught determine whether health instruction will be a part of the total school curriculum or not. If it is agreed that health education will be a part of the curriculum, when and to whom it will be taught is the next problem. It may be decided that health will be taught every year, and if so, either in whole or in part; or it may be required only at certain grades or levels. How health is to be taught is an administrative decision that generally results in adoption of one or more of the three patterns of organization. These are integration, direct teaching or the separate course, and correlation, as described in Chapter 3.

Horizontal sequence, the planned series of units of instruction for a single course, requires no less consideration of the sources of the curriculum than any other curriculum decision area. Choices among alternatives cannot be validly based upon intuition, assumptions, or conventional wisdom at the classroom level any more than at the institutional level. Teachers, too, should utilize information about the special characteristics and needs of the learners in their classes, the community and society in which they are living, and the methods of inquiry unique to health education as well as the structure of its body of knowledge.

Goals and objectives derived from careful analysis of data obtained from study of these sources must be examined to assure that they are: (1) feasible for the students involved, both in terms of student readiness and the availability of the necessary resources; (2) a legitimate concern of the schools; and (3) consistent with the philosophy of health education and the stated policy of the school and the district.

At the classroom level, decisions about what is to be taught focus first upon the alternatives among several schemes for ordering the body of knowledge. The organizing element may be a content area such as dental health or communicable disease; a health problem such as obesity or quackery; concepts such as the ten that form the framework of the curriculum devised by the School Health Education Study; or another such classification system. Too often the practice has been to follow the path of least resistance and "teach" the textbook selected by the school or textbook committee. Which is to say, whatever the notion decided upon by the author of the book for ordering his chapters, so is the planning for teaching structured. Whichever scheme is adopted, however, the content is essentially the same, although it may be developed differently. The first step in organizing for teaching should be to decide which organizing elements among those comprising the system chosen are most significant and meaningful for a given group of students. This is a decision of scope, a horizontal view of curriculum. There is far more known about human health than can ever be placed in a school curriculum. The storehouse of information is overflowing with teachable material, only a fraction of which can be investigated during the school experience of a student. And new information is being discovered more rapidly than it can be communicated. The problem is to select the most relevant, the most meaningful, and the most useful material for the students who are to work with it.

When to teach the selected material is a problem of sequence. A textbook may well provide a logical sequence of subject matter with acceptable application to the students' needs. Then again, it may not. The point is to decide what *would* be the most meaningful sequence of topics, problems, or concepts for the group and then plan the instructional objectives and learning opportunities accordingly.

To select and order the subject matter for a course of study so that it coincides with every aspect of student readiness is a challenging task. Nor is it easy to develop the sure ability to distinguish between what is unnecessary repetition and what is desirable reinforcement. Some revisiting of subject matter is advisable. It is foolish to believe that essential information about nutrition, for example, can be so exhaustively studied and learned as a result of one unit in the sixth grade that no further study will be necessary. For one thing, students at higher stages of development are concerned with different and more complex nutrition problems. No student can learn all he needs to know about social and sex-role relationships in the tenth grade and be presumed to be equipped to meet all problems in those areas for the rest of his life. Health problems keep recurring, even if in different forms and with different intensities or meanings. Ways of solving health problems keep changing, too. Organizing for effective teaching includes looking back to see what the learner brings to the class from earlier experiences and looking ahead to see what he needs to be able to do in the future. Effective plans build upon the former and arrange for his grasp of the knowledge and skills needed for the latter. Any one class can only contribute in part to the long-range goals decided upon by the schools. It is nonsense to think that one health education course, however effective it might be, could prepare an individual to solve all of the problems he will encounter in a lifetime. Yet any given course *can* contribute importantly to the development of an effective, positive life style—one that tends to promote rather than to diminish the individual's health and tends to make him behave in ways that promote rather than diminish the health of his family and community.

A COURSE OF STUDY We have used the term "course" to speak of health instruction as it is offered in a block of time set apart in the curriculum, during which direct teaching occurs with sole attention to the promotion of healthful living. Such a class may be required or elective, but it is given equal time among other courses and receives equal academic credit toward graduation. The intent is to provide students with an opportunity to learn ways of solving those personal and community problems that are the most pressing of all. Without the energy and zest for life and achievement that are natural outcomes of good health, learnings in all other areas of the curriculum are diminished or impossible. Where there are community health problems, the effectiveness of the schools and every other social institution is lessened. Whether health instruction is offered by means of a separate course or as part of another course or broad field, however, the basic structure of organization is the unit.

UNITS

A unit has been defined as the teaching-learning activities and supporting materials planned for the development of one organizing element. An organizing element may be a topic, a problem, a content area, or a concept. In any case, a unit is a plan to be used by teachers in a specific classroom or in a typical classroom situation. Tyler describes a unit as a structural organization of learning experiences covering several weeks, focused upon problems or major student purposes, and employed at the classroom level. "Unit" is also used with the modifying term "resource" to describe a similarly structured but more broadly developed plan in which emphasis is placed upon related resources (films, filmstrips, books, journals, transparencies, charts, tapes, models, pamphlets, and other teaching materials). Both unit and resource unit include a statement of general and instructional objectives, an outline of the subject matter, and a number of suggested student activities including a culminating or summarizing experience. Finally, ways of evaluating the outcome of the unit's suggested activities are described. To each sort of unit are appended lists of resources to be used in teaching but far more extensively developed in all ways in the case of the resource unit.

– unit construction

Once the organizing elements have been selected for a course in health education for a given population of students, and the sequence of their study has been agreed upon, the next step is to determine how the course will be taught. How? is a question involving both structure and methodology. The development of a teaching unit or guide is a function of structure. Increasingly, the trend in all areas of the curriculum is toward acceptance and use of teaching-learning guides prepared for general use by state or national specialists, often through Office of Education grants, and published with the cooperation of textbook publishers. More in the nature of resource units, detailed teaching-learning guides provide a rich array of learning opportunities and evaluation activities based upon research and careful analysis of the sources of the curriculum. The teaching-learning guides leave individual teachers free to use their time more profitably in planning for teaching in their own classrooms. Generally speaking, a framework of long-range goals or general objectives with sequentially developed behavioral objectives derived from and designed to build toward their achievement provides structure and coherence to a curriculum that yet is flexibly adaptable to individual classroom needs and interests. But whether the teaching unit is packaged or homemade, it typically considers but one organizing element and includes most of the following components:

1 The title and overview of the problem

2 Long-range goals or general objectives, stated in cognitive, affective, and action terms

3 The behavioral or educational objectives of the unit

4 An outline of the content—generalizations or key ideas drawn from the relevant subject matter

5 A series of suggestions for learning opportunities capable of implementing the objectives

6 Related evaluation activities

7 A list of available resources and materials for developing the classroom activities

These will be described and examples of each given in the following pages.

1 The Title and Overview of the Problem / A good beginning is the selection and use of a provocative title for the problem, concept, or other organizing element to be considered in the unit. The title page should be appropriately set up, with the title centered in capital letters, the names of the authors and the date in the lower right corner of the page. Page 2 should be titled "Overview." This might include a brief discussion or description of the intent of the material to follow in relation to the education of the students for whom it is designed. Ideally the overview should include data justifying the inclusion of the material in this course. Justification might involve pertinent research, authoritative statements derived from individuals, educational organizations, national or state curriculum studies, and professional organizations; morbidity and mortality statistics if relevant; and needs and interests determined through study of the learner and the community. Consider, for example, the following statement:

> This unit is designed to help students realize that as part of any community they can affect health conditions. Moreover, they can effect change in those conditions if change is necessary and desirable. It is also designed to show community organization which already exists for the promotion of public health.
>
> Environmental is meant to include mental and social as well as physical factors. Actual exploration of a local community's organization, problems, and viewpoints makes this unit a meaningful one. Classroom reading and discussion alone make community health too remote for student interest.[1]

2 Goals / General objectives or goals should be stated in terms of cognitive (thinking), affective (attitudinal), and action terms. These kinds of statements should be developed by the district health curriculum committee as representing the desired outcomes of the total school health education program, kindergarten through the twelfth grade. These goals remain constant for all units at whatever level and provide a common reference point by which planning at all levels can be guided. If teaching is concerned with changing behavior, these goals represent the long-range outcomes that the schools seek to achieve in health behavior and are nearly impossible to evaluate in the classroom situation for this reason. The goals are broadly stated, therefore, both as to behavior and content. Examples in each area are:

Cognitive: The student knows that there are inescapable interrelationships among the physical, mental, and social aspects of growing and developing, and that a change in one affects the others.

Affective: The student respects himself and his fellows as individuals, alike in some ways yet possessing unique capabilities and able to make a special contribution to the well-being of the community.

Action: The student chooses alternatives in behavior that tend to promote rather than hinder growing and developing.

3 Behavioral Objectives / Whether planning for a total health education curriculum or for a specific health class, the central problem is always the definition and selection of appropriate objectives for learners at any given stage of development, not development in the physical sense alone, but in dynamic interaction with the individual's social and mental-emotional level of maturation as well. We have said earlier that objectives can be defined at varying levels of origin and that these are described by Goodlad as being societal, institutional, and instructional. Only those objectives written at the classroom level, he believes, should be termed behavioral or educational objectives. Long-range goals, or general objectives, might be said to be defined at the institutional level since they represent outcomes to which the total effort of the school is dedicated. The teacher is responsible for working out the specific classroom objectives, those most operational statements that provide structure and direction for the organization of effective teaching. To do this, the teacher might ask himself, "What do I want my students to be able to do as a result of the instruction?" rather than succumb to the temptation to think, "What shall I teach today?" or "What should I include in this unit?" A behavioral objective should describe a behavior in connection with a given amount of content in such a way that the objective is operational (it can be achieved) and measurable (the student can be expected to demonstrate achievement of the objective in the classroom). A behavioral objective

should also be specific and unambiguous enough to communicate its intent unmistakably.

An educational objective should be stated clearly enough that any teacher, reading it, could develop a learning opportunity appropriate to its accomplishment. Not necessarily the same learning opportunity as any other teacher's, but one capable of giving the student practice in working with that content, using that behavior. In general, objectives designed to structure a unit can be stated clearly enough to be communicative without being so specific as to be single-lesson limited. Enabling objectives (short-term instructional plans) that may be needed in individualization of instruction can be developed by a teacher as necessary to organize a day or several day's instruction but always as an implementing step toward achievement of his principal objective.

Examples of behavioral objectives along with some of the possible enabling objectives follow:

1 Analyzes the many factors that motivate social drinking behavior in the United States

a Identifies social factors that tend to promote or make moderate drinking behavior acceptable
b Describes reasons why adolescents and adults begin and continue to drink

2 Evaluates those dangerous drugs and narcotics whose misuse constitutes the greatest problem in this country

a Identifies physiological and psychological effects of barbiturates, amphetamines, marihuana, and heroin
b Recalls and states the four kinds of dangerous drugs and narcotics whose misuse presents our great drug-dependence problems
c Describes the synergistic effect of alcohol consumption with simultaneous use of certain drugs

3 Applies sound criteria in evaluating claims for and against cigarette smoking

a Given a claim for or against smoking, the student can apply accepted criteria in the analysis of its validity and identify any half-truths or distortions of fact that may be present
b Given a claim for or against smoking, the student can identify appeals to emotion rather than to logic
c The student can differentiate between authoritative and other sources of statements about effects of smoking

4 Distinguishes among the variety of influences that continually affect growing and developing

a Given a dietary pattern, the student can predict its effect upon the weight or growth of selected individuals
b Describes ways an individual grows and develops socially and emotionally as promoted by his physical growth

c Relates the hormonal changes of puberty to the growth spurt of adolescence

4 Content Outline / It is neither possible nor necessary to include all of the subject matter that could be discovered relative to an objective such as any of those described above. There should be enough data indicated to ensure the teacher's clear perception of the breadth and the boundaries of the coverage intended but without so much detail as to be wearisome or as to obscure the important ideas. The content should expand but not go *beyond* that described in the objective. The content might be developed in outline, either in short-sentence form or in paragraphs. In any case, efforts should be made to present powerful ideas or generalizations rather than trivia. In a Washington state health education unit the content relative to a desired student competency at the primary level is developed as a series of concepts as follows:

Competency: Understand environmental factors which affect health

Concepts: Water and air are important

Clean food is important

Clean and comfortable home conditions affect health

Noise and space affect how people feel and respond

Hazards in the environment can cause discomfort and problems

Many people keep water and air safe

Many people help protect our food

Individuals can improve their surroundings

Water and air are essential to life

Waste disposal is an increasing problem

Disease is transmitted in many ways

Our surroundings, group activities, and group organization affect us[2]

Another health teaching unit, *Dependence-Producing Substances,* for middle-grade students outlines the content under "Concepts and Understandings" in this way:

Some people attempt to find enjoyment or solve the problems of living by consuming things which may be harmful to their health.

The substances sometimes used inappropriately vary from coffee, tea, cakes, and candy to tobacco, alcohol, and dangerous drugs.

Many people begin smoking cigarettes in order to achieve status in their peer group, to appear grown-up, or because of curiosity, and then develop a habit which is often difficult to break.

The use of alcohol by elementary school pupils should be restricted to certain religious or medical purposes and carefully supervised by responsible adults.

Alcohol acts as a depressant of central nervous system functions; it slows down a person's ability to think clearly or to act efficiently.

Most drugs should be used only under a qualified health advisor's guidance.

The main effect of tobacco, alcohol, and dangerous drugs is upon the central nervous system, especially the brain.

Advertisements on television, radio, billboards, and in news media are designed to encourage people to use tobacco and alcoholic beverages regardless of any possible hazards.

Public concern about the harmful effects of dependence-producing substances is increasing as scientific data accumulates.[3]

5 Learning Opportunities / In a way, objectives, learning opportunities, and evaluation activities are just different ways of looking at the same thing. The objective stipulates a behavior that the student is expected to use in connection with specified subject matter. The learning opportunity should provide him several (as many as needed) experiences in practicing that behavior and in dealing with that information. When the teacher wishes to evaluate the success of these experiences in changing the student's ability to "can do it" from "couldn't do it," an evaluation activity is presented which quite simply asks him to show that he can. Learning opportunities must provide the learner with two kinds of experiences, those that provide him with whatever foundation facts he needs in order to achieve the objective and those that furnish many situations in which the behavior involved may be practiced. Those that can accomplish both at one time are best of course. Learning opportunities must be designed with both purposes clearly in mind and directly related to the objective in general and to some specifics of the expanded content. Not one or two, but a wide array of suggested learning activities is desirable so that the unit can be employed by many teachers to fit many situations.

Here are the learning experiences suggested in association with the previously cited content for the unit on dependence-producing substances.

Have students list things people eat or otherwise consume in order "to feel better," e.g., coffee, tea, milk, candy, drugs, tobacco.

Analyze whether the feelings of well-being are social, physical, mental, or a combination of these: construct a chart.

Discuss what the State Health Texts have to say about soft drinks, coffee, and tea.

In buzz groups of five or six pupils discuss: "Why do some people begin to smoke cigarettes and why do some of these find it difficult to stop even when they find it unpleasant?" Share the group discussion with the entire class by means of a panel made up of one reporter from each group.

Students read about tobacco in State Health Texts for Grades 5 and 6. Discuss the effects of tobacco on the system.

Invite "Smoky Sam" (Mannequin with tape recorded message) to discuss tobacco and show how nicotine and irritants (tars) are trapped in lungs.

Show film, *The Huffless, Puffless Dragon.*

Describe general action of alcohol in the human body; how it acts as a depressant once it enters the blood stream.

Develop vocabulary list—depressants, stimulants, etc.

Have students list ways drinking alcohol may lead to ill effects.

Discuss how some are encouraged to drink to achieve certain effects—intoxication; be "one of the gang"; appear adult.

Explain term "drug"—that it is a general term describing medical substances. Point out that many are used routinely by doctors.

Discuss value of antibiotics and other compounds. Have students explain why such medicines should be used only when prescribed for them by a medical doctor or another qualified person.

Use picture or chart of brain and nervous system; briefly describe how these compounds affect the body.

Point out risks associated with "mind changing" drugs such as glue sniffing and smoking marihuana.

Collect advertisements for these products and discuss how advertisers help one assume that smoking, drinking, or use of drugs is desirable, harmless, etc.

Note newspaper articles and television programs about alcohol control, drug use, smoking and health. Use news clips and tape recordings of recent action as a basis for class discussion or committee reports.[4]

6 Evaluation Activities / An effective evaluation is a learning opportunity in itself if it is valid. An evaluation activity should ideally be a carefully prepared problem or situation that is different from any former classroom activity but allows the student to apply his new ability and knowledge to its solution. To suggest, as often is the case, that a teacher give a test to find out if students have grasped the basic ideas of the lesson or that he appraise the students' written reports is to say that he should evaluate by evaluating and that is no help at all. Whatever the suggested evaluation activity, it should be as clearly explained as was the learning opportunity. Not memorization of facts should be measured but ability to apply new skills in solving problems or making decisions or plans that are everyday health-related concerns. Objective tests have their uses in evaluating achievement or behavior to be sure. But a test is an instrument, not an evaluation. Let us not confuse the cookbook with cooking. Just as with the learning opportunity, evaluation activities should clearly describe a procedure that could be

used to provide the learner with the chance to demonstrate his new ability. A criterion level of success might be suggested as well. Further discussion of this vital aspect of effective teaching will be found in Chapter 6.

7 Resources and Materials / This section of a unit should contain a list of textbooks, references, articles in both popular and professional journals, audiovisual aids, pamphlets, and other meaningful teaching materials. In a teaching unit, those included are usually limited to those used in developing the plan. In a resource unit the list should be more complete, allowing for differences in needs and interest as well as problems of availability. Probably the most comprehensive such listings ever compiled are contained in the resources books developed by the School Health Education Study in connection with each concept and its set of teaching-learning guides.

However extensive the list may be, the materials should be cataloged separately as teacher or student materials, classified by kind, and their sources identified. Bibliographical data should be complete and enough information provided that a teacher would know where to write for such materials. Films and filmstrips should be annotated. The following items illustrate how various materials should be listed.

Textbooks:

Bauer, W. W., Gladys G. Jenkins, Helen S. Schacter, and Elenore Pounds, *Health for All,* Chicago, Scott Foresman, 1965 (for junior high school students).

Periodicals:

Richardson, Charles E., "Education for Family Planning," *The Journal of School Health,* 39, 8 (October 1969), pp. 537–543.

Films:

Why Man Creates, 25 minutes, color, 1970. Pyramid Film Producers, Box 1048, Santa Monica, Calif., 90406. Series of entertaining yet thought-provoking vignettes discussing the natural urge toward creativity as it is promoted and inhibited by frustration and social pressures (animated and live action).

Filmstrips:

Preparing for the Jobs of the 70's (Part I, 76 frames, Part II, 69 frames), color, sound, 1967. Guidance Associates, P.O. Box 5, Pleasantville, N.Y., 10570. Illustrates the changing employment picture and describes job opportunities in health and medical fields.

Transparencies:

Interpretation of Health Information (catalog number 4982), 20 visuals, color, 1967. Charts, maps, graphs, other commonly used means of presenting data in visual form to be used in developing skill in interpreting graphic materials used in disseminating health-related data. 3 M Company, Visual Products Division, 3 M Center, St. Paul, Minn., 55101.

Tape Recordings:
"Let's Meet the Doctor," 10 minutes, 1968. Wollensak Teaching Tape, 3 M Company, 3 M Center, St. Paul, Minn., 55101. Discusses common procedures followed by physicians, differentiates between family physician and specialists, and explores the contribution of the medical profession to community health.

SHORTCOMINGS IN UNIT CONSTRUCTION

Curriculum development is an exacting task at any level. Creativity, writing skills, patient research, and meticulous attention to the logic and structure of curriculum development are required. Few units or curriculum guides presently satisfy all the criteria described above. Goodlad points out that schools commonly lack a comprehensive and reasonably consistent set of objectives to guide them in making curriculum decisions and that in general curriculum guides do not specify the organizing elements that are to tie together the suggested learning activities. Of learning opportunities, which he terms "organizing centers," he says that very little attention is given to identification of the precise outcomes desired and to description of learner activities appropriate to their attainment.[5] Examination of typical teaching guides reveals that instead of research a cut-and-paste technique appears more common. The result sometimes is a patchwork quilt of content, learning activities of a sort, and some evaluation activities that, understandably, lack consistency or perceptible plan. Any objectives are usually ambiguously stated and therefore not operational. Typically, there are no stated objectives at all. The relationship between the content or concepts and unit objectives accordingly is more assumption than design. What is presented under the title of content or teachable material is often a series of statements of a differing order—a sprinkling of generalizations, admonitions, questions, facts, topics. Learning opportunities or activities seldom say much more than that the teacher is to discuss some aspect of the content.

If a learning opportunity is to be described as a part of a unit intended for general or wide use, it must be stated so clearly that any teacher, whatever his skills, experience, intuitive teaching ability (or lack of it), and academic preparation, will grasp the procedures without difficulty or question. A learning activity cannot depend upon unstated assumptions for its implementation. The most often seen teaching suggestion begins with the word "discuss." "Discuss" is a word that means many things. Which one is meant? Further, discussion leading is a skill not uniformly possessed by all teachers. The less skilled may need more help, for too many teachers interpret the word "discuss" as "tell."

A learning opportunity is in fact a briefly stated lesson plan and should therefore list all of the activities intended in some detail and suggest pertinent questions and materials to be used. For example, suppose that the teacher desires to develop the students' skill in analysis and application of criteria determined in an earlier teaching strategy concerned with consumer health. The next procedure might involve the preparation of some fictional advertising copy promoting the purchase and use of a product purporting to cure the common cold. The learning opportunity should describe the method of presenting a situation in which the learner can apply the criteria (the advertising copy prepared in advance); give an example of such copy; suggest how it might be used in the class (for example, placed on the chalkboard, projected by overhead projector, duplicated for handout, and so on); and include the significant points that should be noted by the learner in his analysis of the claims.

The learning opportunity might also suggest ways that the class could be organized for the lesson. Is the material to be discussed in small-group buzz sessions, with the resulting conclusion reported back to the total class? Should each group be given a different piece of copy or should all groups study the same one? Should each student work alone? Should the activity be done in class or assigned as a homework project? Should the activity be done with the book open or closed? All of these points should be made clear, if only as suggested alternatives. The plan should be preceded by a statement that explains *why* the activity would be done. In this case, such a statement might be, "Using prepared advertising copy as exercises in evaluating claims promoting health products."

Finally, there should be a suggested culminating activity to help the teacher make sure that his students recognize the relationship of what has been accomplished to some larger purpose that has meaning for them in everyday life. In this case, the students might be required to search through magazines or newspapers for advertisements whose claims they find questionable and to bring these to class for discussion.

It may be that the reason few people complain about the lack of rigor with which many units are prepared is that nobody really uses them once they are completed. Yet such units take a lot of time to compile, and when the amount of time spent on such a document is multiplied by the number of groups across the country at school, district, county, state, and national levels (to say nothing of all the special health interest groups who also put together small units for school use) the amount of time spent in the past few years must be astronomical.

The following examples illustrate some of the shortcomings described by Goodlad and others.

Example 1 / A "curriculum guide" for sex education that cannot be faulted for the way its objectives have been stated, for it has none. Unevenly structured "teachable material" and "profitable activities" are followed by a list of concepts and attitudes that it is hoped will evolve through the interaction of the first two with each other and the intended students. No evaluation activities are provided, which is logical in the absence of objectives. It is difficult to find out how far you have come when you don't know where you are going. It's rather like the airline captain who announced to his passengers, "Folks, I'm very sorry to tell you that we're lost, but you'll be glad to know that we're making excellent time!"

Example 2 / A ninety-page book developed at the national level that details concepts, suggested learning experiences or activities, resources, and related evaluation. The book indicates no objectives but escapes criticism on this point inasmuch as its authors stipulate in advance that this is not a guide but a list of suggestions. In some ways it is more complete than similar documents which do claim to be guides. The problem here is that the preponderance of the suggestions involve telling rather than teaching. The teacher, not the learner, is most often involved in the activity. For example, it is suggested that the concept "Differences in time of maturing can be of great importance to the individual" can be communicated by the activity, "Discuss the reasons for individual differences in growth rates." The concept "Drug abuse by young people is a serious problem in today's society" is presumed to be understood when the teacher has done this: "Study and discuss the causes of drug abuse—social and psychological." Or is it the student who is supposed to do that? It is hard to tell. The one other suggestion for this concept is "Assign readings on these causes and discuss." Who is assigning and who is the discussant? The related evaluation suggestion is equally fuzzy—"Relate drug abuse to emotional illness."

Example 3 / A curriculum guide prepared under the guidance and financial support of a health agency in a New York State county and representing the work of over a hundred educators. The preface advises that it will present a general pattern of concepts, problems, activities, experiences, and resources with a bold present-day outlook utilizing the conceptual approach to learning. The boldness involved appears to depend upon the fact that the content has been developed in the form of a list of related conceptual statements. In the guide developed for the junior high school there follow four units, each including an overview that discusses the importance of the topic to be considered, a list of concepts, a list of activities (the relevance of which is not clear), and a list of resources. Neither objectives nor evaluation activities are provided. Again, most of the activities are teacher-oriented or are so ambiguously stated as to be nonsensical or at best confusing. For example, "Make a scrapbook of good food." The teacher, or the students? Why? And how does one make a scrapbook of good food? One gets an image of a book with a ham sandwich pasted in it, or a bit of desiccated pie! Or how about these? "Compile a chart of varying heights and weights." Who? What use is to be made of the chart? "Suggest that students discuss the behavior of teenagers with adults." How many adults? Why? Observation suggests that teen-agers are weary of the subject already, at least as discussed with adults who are their parents.

Example 4 / A curriculum guide adopted in 1970 by a large school district in California. Its subject is sex education and health education. Designed for kindergarten through the twelfth grade, it is the only guide reviewed here to present objectives. There are lists of general objectives for the elementary school, the junior high school, and the senior high school. Those for the elementary school are teacher objectives, describing the intent of the instruction. Those for the upper levels are stated in terms of the learner but specify vague or multiple behaviors such as "to review and to understand and interpret dynamic physical changes." The units are centered around a topic, with some related concepts, teaching suggestions, recommended texts, teacher references, and audiovisual materials. The learning activities are heavily oriented toward discussion and lecture. For example, to teach the concept "There is much more to being a parent than just having the biological ability to reproduce" here is a suggested activity. "Discussion in small groups and with entire class." Another is "Suggested guest lectures: a. Society for the Emotionally Handicapped; b. psychiatrist; c. psychologist; d. pediatrician; e. nurse." The assumptions in this suggestion are monumental. Only one more suggestion is given relative to the concept and that is "Assign special reports in areas of interest, Delacato's Theory, etc." How any of these suggestions relate to the concept, or why they would be worthwhile, or how to do them is left entirely to the teacher. Some multiple-choice tests and opinionaires are appended as resource materials, although not in relation to any one learning opportunity, concept, or unit. And although concepts are supposed to be the outcome, the tests are entirely fact and physiology concerned.

A trend toward greater precision in unit construction is increasingly evident in many disciplines, however. Along with acceptance and use of behaviorally stated objectives has come the realization that the corresponding elements of a teaching unit must also be clearly stated. Planning for effective teaching in the 1970s will very probably continue toward a more detailed and lucid description of all of the components of a unit of instruction.

At present, as has been illustrated, a typical unit suggests content as a series of loosely related generalizations or concepts and lists an array of very briefly described teaching suggestions. And perhaps it can be argued that teachers need nothing more than a suggestion in order to plan their lessons. Perhaps. But considerable evidence exists to show that not all teachers are skilled in a wide range of methods, nor are they uniformly familiar with many techniques. Success in communicating a plan for teaching, when that plan is given in shorthand, depends upon an assumption of equality among teachers in regard to their experience, interests, motivation, attitudes toward health education, beliefs about the concept of health, and a host of other variables. It is safe to say that such an assumption is not supported by the facts.

If a unit is prepared by a teacher, or a small group of teachers, for short-term use in a given situation, then less carefully described materials may suffice. If a unit is to be widely distributed and intended for teachers of all degrees of experience and ability, then considerably more care needs to be taken in its preparation.

Many of the Social Studies Projects have produced excellent teaching units and guides for national distribution and adaptation. The *Anthropology Curriculum Study Project,* University of Chicago, has developed a self-contained, ninety-two page unit with detailed teaching instructions. Evaluation activities parallel the behavorial objectives. Content is provided for the teacher and for the student in separate reading materials. The project *Development of Economics Curriculum Materials for Secondary Schools,* Ohio State University, has developed eighteen units for teaching high school economics. The developers view economics as a system of concepts and patterns of reasoning to be learned by progressive examination of the concepts. The teaching suggestions emphasize the unfolding structure of ideas, and suggestions for handling each teaching situation are provided. Potential teaching problems are explored along with specific suggestions for handling student activities and materials. Evaluation materials, including multiple-choice tests and written exercises to measure concept comprehension as well as grasp of their interrelationships, are provided as well as semantic differential instruments and questionaires to assess affective responses to the course. Another economics course for high school, *Econ 12,* San Jose State College, California, designed as a teaching system, provides behaviorally stated objectives, procedures to be used in pursuing the objectives, and measures to see if the objectives have been achieved. Flexibility is provided in that teachers are free to use or not use parts of the four units, depending on class ability and interest. The *Taba Curriculum Development Project* and the *High School Geography Project,* University of Colorado, are other examples that reflect a growing trend toward the construction of carefully planned units by national educational projects in nearly every discipline.[6]

The guides developed by the School Health Education Study writers are nearly impeccable in their attention to recommended curriculum procedures. Of these guides Tyler says:

> No other curriculum project that this reviewer knows has made its conceptual design as clear as this project has. Furthermore, the conceptual design has utilized most of the best that is known about curriculum planning. In addition, the entire conceptual structure has been evaluated for scientific accuracy by competent individuals in medicine, health, and health education.[7]

The chart beginning on page 125 represents a short sequence of content, learning opportunities, and evaluation activities for students in the primary grades along with the behavioral objectives they are designed to implement and evaluate.

Note that the column marked Teacher and Student Materials is purposely left blank so that the teacher can write in her own choice of materials after consulting the accompanying Resources Book with reference to local materials.

OTHER APPROACHES TO TEACHING

Once the content has been determined and a unit developed, yet another critical area of decision making confronts the teacher. What is the best approach or organizing principle for teaching the course? How is the class to be introduced to the unit? What is to be their first contact with the material? At the elementary level should one begin the study of nutrition by telling students about the functions of proteins and carbohydrates, or would it be better to talk about the kinds of foods that make up a good lunch? Should a teacher begin a unit on dental health for first-graders by describing the parts of a tooth? Should a second-grade teacher explain the germ theory of disease as a first step in promoting the use of disposable tissues in the control of respiratory disease? Would citing National Safety Council accident statistics spur third-graders to greater caution on the playground? At the college level, is study of patterns of mental illness any help in beginning to explore ways of promoting a balanced emotional and social life?

Several approaches have served as a rationale for ordering the study of course materials. Five of these approaches will be identified and discussed here.

– the anatomical-physiological approach

This approach to lesson planning is a favorite among the "give them the bones of the body to learn" bunch. The subject matter is comfortably concrete, it is reasonably free from controversy, and it is easy to construct tests to measure achievement. For many years, teachers and textbook authors have believed that health instruction should be introduced by teaching the structure and function of whatever part of the anatomy was of concern. Digestion could not be related to human behavior until the structure of the stomach and intestines was learned.

A chapter in a textbook using this approach would order its discussion of mental health as follows: (1) structure of neurons; (2) structure of the nervous system; (3) functions of the central nervous system; (4) functions of the autonomic nervous system; and (5) functions of the reflexes. Then, after the anatomy and physiology has been investigated, unrelated to anything but itself, the text may discuss emotions, adjustment and maladjustment, personality problems, and other important aspects of human interactions.

Students understandably lose interest in this kind of health teaching. Facts of anatomy and physiology are significant to health education only when they are used as a means to an end, not as an end in themselves. For instance, in order to investigate the effect of cigarette smoking on health, it is useful to explore the physiological effects of nicotine and tars upon the structure of the respiratory system or the function of the vascular system. Inevitably some facts about the anatomy of these structures must be involved, but not as the principal goal of instruction. Physiology is a course with its own importance, but it is not health education. The structure of the tooth is not health behavior. "Blood and bones" hygiene is as out of date as the bustle. Would that it were as little seen today. Health teaching should be concerned with the development of behaviors and skills with lifetime utility in the solution of real life problems. Facts in isolation are very easily forgotten.

– the chronological approach

Under this rationale, the unit, chapter, or lecture is always begun by tracing the history of the subject to be learned. The student begins his study of any given health problem by retracing the events that preceded present-day solutions. For example, the chronological approach used in a unit on personal health might be structured as follows: (1) bathing practices in ancient civilizations; (2) bathing and cleanliness problems during the Middle Ages; (3) bathing practices in early America; (4) changing concepts of the need for personal cleanliness. If the goal of such teaching is to change student behavior (assuming that it needs changing) it is doubtful whether the first three points will contribute very much to that change. The information might be amusing or mildly interesting, but it is unlikely to be motivating.

Another such revisiting of the past is to introduce the study of disease control by presenting in chronological order the several major theories that have evolved to explain the sources of disease. Interesting, probably, but not germane to daily problems of today's student.

– the etiological approach The etiological approach is more likely to be seen in small units or single-lesson constructions than in a total course of study. This approach involves the cause-effect pattern. It is likely to be used in studies of disease. For example, a series of lessons might be constructed to explore causes of communicable diseases (bacteria, viruses, metazoa, protozoa, rickettsia, fungi) and the effects of these disease agents as evidenced by the symptoms they produce. Or the course might be structured according to causes of transmission of diseases and effects on individual and community health. As a means of exploring these cause-effect relationships, factual descriptions of the disease agents, means of transmission, portals of entry, modes of escape, and characteristics of diseases caused by each agent are studied. The usefulness of all this detail depends upon the student's ability to make generalizations successfully as well as to detect their relevance to his own needs.

the psychological approach

There is less than total agreement on the distinction between *psychological* and what would appear to be its antithesis, *logical,* approach to teaching. Tyler perceives this difference as being between the way the relationships of curriculum elements are viewed by the expert in a field and the way they may appear to the learner. The latter arrangement, the psychological, is defined in terms of its meaningfulness to the learner himself.[8] Goodlad, on the other hand, believes that a scheme of organization can be either logical or illogical, but that it cannot be either logical or *psychological,* since what happens to the learner as a result of a teaching plan can be either psychologically bad or psychologically good. He argues that an approach that is defined in terms of the kinds of learning processes desired in the learner actually describes the desired *outcomes* of the plan and not the plan itself.[9]

In health teaching, the psychological approach has been perceived as one that begins with demonstrated or revealed student needs and interests rather than with some aspect of subject matter. This approach is contemporary, aiming more at the solution of immediate problems than at the accumulation of information for possible later use. It deals with the stuff of health instruction in relation to the need for it and not as background information that is intended for general education only. Whatever use is made of the facts derived from bacteriology, chemistry, anthropology, anatomy, physiology, or

Concept: Protection and Promotion of Health is an Individual, Community, and International Responsibility

Behavioral Objective and Content

A. *Defines the Meanings of Health and of Community.*

1 *Health* means different things to different people in different environments.

a Health to some may mean not being sick, not feeling bad, or not having a disease.

b Health can mean feeling well and being generally happy in one's surroundings, wherever one may be—at home, in school, at play, and in other situations.

c Health involves the ways a person thinks (mental), the ways he feels (physical), and ways he acts with others (social).

d An individual's understanding of the meaning of health may affect his actions (e.g., he may work toward feeling his best most of the time in all ways and in all environments; he may not be concerned about health until something happens to him, his family, friends, or others).

2 A *community* may be thought of in various ways—from the limited context of one's family, neighborhood, or school, to the broader scope of the world and universe. Basically a community is a grouping of people together—working, playing, living, and in many instances caring for or about others.

a A family is a community of people who are usually related and who may live together (e.g., families may include aunts, uncles, grandparents, brothers, sisters, parents, guardians, and some people not related to the family).

b A neighborhood is

Teacher and Student Materials

*Behavioral Objective and Learning Opportunities**

A. *Defines the Meanings of Health and of Community.*

Words to Understand

city
community
family
health
mental
nation
neighborhood
physical
planet
social
state
town
village

Using Tape Recorder To Explore Personal Meanings of Health (A–1)

Have children discuss what "health" means to them, mentioning as many things as possible that come into their minds. Suggest that they rephrase their ideas into short statements and tape them to summarize what they think about health.

After class members have recorded, a volunteer listening committee might use the tape to develop a list of all the things that students mentioned as being health. Others may wish to use a portable tape recorder to collect comments of older students, parents, friends, or neighbors, when asked, "What does 'health' mean to you?"

Have students work in small groups to classify these statements in some way (e.g., health is physical, mental, social; health is absence of disease; health is being comfortable and happy). After this, discuss with them how the statements differ.

Analyzing Pictures To Discover Meanings of Health (A–1)

Have children select (from magazines, posters, newspapers, books) pictures which illustrate, for them, some aspect of health. They may choose to put these in booklets, make a group or class bulletin board, or arrange them on feltboards. (Students should find pictures to show various aspects

Behavioral Objective and Evaluation Activities

A. *Defines the Meanings of Health and of Community.*

Have children select from a list of simple statements those that best describe the meaning of health. Sample descriptions might be:

1 Health means being able to run very fast.
2 Health means eating a lot and having strong muscles.
3 Health is being tall.
4 Health is being rich and important.
5 Health means that we feel ready to enjoy the day's activities when we wake in the morning.

or

Have children make up short sentences describing health as they see it. Have each child write his statement on a strip that can be placed on bulletin board or used to decorate the room. Students not yet able to write might dictate statements to the teacher.

Evaluate the activities and the extent of students' understanding of the overall concept of health by noting the development of student ability to express verbally the physical, social, and mental aspects of health.

Collect a set of pictures or transparencies which illustrate contrasting physical, social, or mental health conditions or situations. For example: well nourished, energetic appearing children and adults versus thin and listless or obese and lethargic individuals.

Present each pair of

Behavioral Objective and Content

a community of people living within a defined area (e.g. apartment complex, people on the same block, in the same within several blocks, in the same school zone).

c A village, city, or town is a community of people who have organized a government to help meet their needs. These communities vary in size from very small to very large.

d A state is a community of people who live within many cities, towns, and neighborhoods in a defined area. It is organized to help the communities within the state, but may also help other communities.

e A nation is a community of people who live in states (or territories). It is organized to help the people within that nation, but may also help other communities.

f The planet earth is a community of people who live in nations, states, cities, neighborhoods, and families.

g The universe may be thought of as a community, as space flights explore and expand boundaries.

3 A person is part of many kinds of communities at the same time, and is affecting and being affected by these communities.

Teacher and Student Materials

*Behavioral Objective and Learning Opportunities**

of individual, family, and community health.)

Short descriptive statements may be written or dictated to accompany certain pictures (e.g., "This mother with a new baby is . . ."). Have children work in small groups to decide who is healthy (e.g., individual, family, community) in the pictures.

Have the entire class discuss selected pictures and respond to questions such as, "If this person is healthy, what tells you that he is healthy?" Use a circle, square, or some other symbol the children select to indicate the part of the picture identified by class as a "clue" to health.

Using Audiovisuals To Identify Various Kinds of Communities (A–2)

Select appropriate films, filmstrips, tapes, transparencies, or other media which portray the variety of communities with which the student may or may not be familiar. Students may view these individually or work in small groups to identify the wide range and size of communities and their boundaries, likenesses, and differences.

Students may record their observations on a chart entitled "What to Look for in Communities." The chart could have columns with such headings as "Kind of Community," "Boundaries," "Like Others," or "Different from Others." Students may then come together and discuss types of communities, seeking to develop a list of many communities and characteristics as they can.

Using Local Study To Explore One's Own Communities (A–2)

There are many ways to explore one's own

Behavioral Objective and Evaluation Activities

visuals to the children to study as a basis for performing one or more of the following activities:

1 Ask each child to point to some aspect of a given picture and state whether its effect on health is physical, social, or mental. Have him give reasons for his selection and tell what effect it might have upon an individual's health.
2 Give each child a visual illustration of an adverse health condition or situation and have him draw his own picture of what would be a positive view (or remedy) for that situation or condition.
3 Ask children to pick a pair of contrasting pictures and write or dictate a short story explaining how a person might behave to become like one or the other.

Evaluate the activities in terms of the understanding students exhibit as they illustrate pictorially, or express verbally, the physical, mental and social aspects involved in the total concept of health.

Collect pictures or maps of as many kinds of community as possible, ranging from family, neighborhood, school, and town to metropolis, state, nation, and world. Show these one by one and have children decide if each one is a community and tell what kind of community it is. Ask questions such as:

1 What kind of community is this?
2 What makes it a community?
3 Might you be a member of a community like this?

Evaluate in terms of ability to differentiate among communities and identify the factors which make each community different from the others.

Construct and administer simple true-false test using statements such as:

T F 1 A family is a kind of community.
T F 2 Detroit is a city.

Behavioral Objective and Content	*Teacher and Student Materials*	*Behavioral Objective and Learning Opportunities**	*Behavioral Objective and Evaluation Activities*

communities. Possibilities to explore one's own for class, small group, and individual exploration include a walking tour of the school area: drawing a map of the local area (or using a street map which has already been prepared) and marking locations of familiar places on it; collecting clippings of local news and relating these incidents to places where various events happened, who was involved; writing or dictating stories about people and places in the community to illustrate how people in the community work together.

After this exploration, have the class develop a short descriptive story of the different communities they explored. These could be tape recorded for future use.

Making Documentary Records To Understand the Dynamic Nature of Community (A–2)

With the view of understanding that each of us lives in a variety of communities, have children keep a diary of the places they go for about a week. Have them record activities, note locations, kinds of buildings, people, and conditions. If possible, an 8mm film camera could be used to record short scenes throughout the communities (with an eye for health conditions and community problems).

After data gathering has been completed, have children map out their activities and movements on scale maps, using symbols to indicate their movements. Have them discuss these maps to show that a person's community is in constant change, and involves many people and places. From analyzing their maps, children may note some smaller communities within their range of movement (e.g., school, home, block, playground, shopping center). They may also note that some of their smaller communities overlap those of other classmates (e.g., same school, same block) or that some do not overlap (e.g., different locations for after school activities).

T F 3 A community is always a place on a map.

T F 4 A community is best described as town or city.

Develop a simple test and ask students to match the persons from Column I with the kind of community with which they might be most closely identified.

Person	Community
1 mother	a school
2 neighbor	b state
3 mayor	c neighborhood
4 governor	d city
5 aunt	e family
6 teacher	f nation
	g world

Duplicate a map of your state and parts of the adjoining states. Indicate locations of major cities and the community in which your school is located. If possible, add a second, more detailed map showing the local community by streets. Ask children to color in their state and circle their town or city on the first map. Use the street map to have them outline their neighborhood area (block, school, shopping area). Evaluate students' understanding of community areas by their ability to identify them on maps.

* The code after each Learning Opportunity relates to the specific Behavioral Objective and Content in Column 1.

Source: School Health Education Study.

other disciplines is made in explanation of a problem or its solution. The psychological approach focuses on process rather than on content. The emphasis is on skills and behaviors rather than on knowledge, although knowledge is prized as fundamental to rational decision-making. The psychological approach is designed to help students learn how to learn. It does not teach content so much as the effective application of content as a means of problem solving. Not based upon an arrangement of content as are the foregoing approaches, it is more flexibly responsive to individual or class needs.

– the conceptual approach

The current rush to focus upon concepts as a means of ordering the content of health education is an outcome, in part, of the so-called knowledge explosion. It is no longer possible to teach more than a fraction of what is already known in relation to human health problems, and the fund of knowledge keeps growing rapidly. As every discipline has struggled to cope with an overabundance of fresh data, the solution has been the same. Each group has been forced to identify its key concepts as a means of structuring its body of knowledge with some amount of economy and stability.

In health teaching, the conceptual approach has found wide, even enthusiastic, acceptance among many teachers while at the same time engendering feelings of hostility and threat among others. Changes in ways of doing things always seem to threaten some people. But conceptual learning is not new, rather it is the way people learn naturally, without (or perhaps in spite of) instruction. In order to discuss this approach it is necessary first to define some related terms.

One must first distinguish among "concept," "conceptualization," and "conceptual teaching" before thinking about the conceptual approach. Exact definition is difficult, especially in the case of "concept," because authorities do not all agree about what a concept is. In general, most will agree that concepts are the basic focusing ideas of a discipline and that they are mental constructs by which the individual orders related perceptions. However, when it comes to *stating* a concept, there is some difference of opinion. One man's concept is likely to be another's generalization, principle, or fact.

For purposes of this discussion, let us agree that the word or statement used to structure content (the concept) should be broad enough and abstract enough to allow the categorizing of a great number of related but less powerful ideas, facts, or experiences. Even preschool children have already formulated a great many concepts. The word "dog," for instance, is a concept. There is in fact no such thing as "dog," but only particular instances of dogs. But look at all the elements of "dogness" that we have learned and classified as identifying certain creatures as "dog" and not "tiger," "bear," "horse," or even "wolf." A multitude of experiences have given even small children perceptions of sizes, snout shapes, tooth arrangement, ear forms, leg lengths, textures and lengths of fur (or lack of it), colors, patterns of colors, barking sounds, breathing sounds, behavior patterns, and other data too numerous to mention. Concepts have affective components as well. One's concept of dog may be accompanied by emotions of fear or pleasure, depending on one's experience with dogs, especially as a child. Still, though certain specific data may differ among individuals, the concept of dog is relatively universal whatever it is termed. From infancy on, we all accumulate a constantly growing number of observations that we quickly sort out and classify in our data banks as "dogness" or "not dogness."

Internalization of a concept depends upon the ability to identify all things correctly which are members of that class (which is generalization) and also to identify all objects or ideas which however similar are yet *not* members of that class (which is discrimination). Total possession of a concept is probably too much to expect of anyone except the specialist in a given field, but the health educated person ought to be able to generalize and discriminate among the concepts involved with health education to the degree that he can function in society and make choices affecting health as a purposeful, rational human being.

Conceptualization, the process of mentally sorting out all of the perceptions that crowd in upon us as long as we live, occurs naturally and is internal, totally individual, and mediated by prior experiences. Two or more people often view or participate in the same experience without perceiving the same things at all because of prior learnings that each brings to the situation. One of the first acts of conceptualization a child performs is probably the formulation of the concept of food. At first, he reacts with pleasure due to the relief of the discomfort of hunger and associates that good feeling with the tactile sense of food on his lips and in his mouth. Then he begins to experience tastes, smells, and food textures, and associates some of them with this something that brings relief-of-hunger pleasure. He finds that some things can be placed in the mouth that are *not* foods, and he acquires preferences among the substances offered him as foods. Long before he can communicate by language a child communicates his grasp of the concept of food quite well. We know that he knows what is food and what is not, and we know how he feels about certain foods. Conceptualization is a process, and the difficulty is not in arranging for it, but in arranging for desirable kinds of perceptions leading to positive concepts.

However one sorts out the perceptions that crowd in upon him (and without which he cannot live) groupings inevitably begin to occur in the mind and increasingly abstract ideas begin to represent groups of groupings. Conceptual teaching, then, is the planned arrangement of experiences which afford the learner the kinds of perceptions that logically lead to the idea groupings, or concepts, selected as representative of the structure of a discipline. The concept itself cannot be taught, only the words. One does not teach concepts, one teaches *toward* concepts.

A conceptual approach to teaching is one that (1) employs concepts or powerful ideas to structure the body of knowledge concerned; (2) uses methodology that emphasizes the modes of inquiry by which new knowledge is discovered in that discipline; and (3) uses a planned sequence of learning opportunities derived from the concepts and employing the identified inquiry methods. Elements of the psychological approach are not precluded.

The conceptual approach differs from traditional patterns of categorizing content and from traditional teaching methodology. Not pontifications delivered by the stage-centered teller of facts about health, but creative situations designed to place the learner at center and the in-the-wings teacher as facilitator of that learning. Not passive listening but active participation in individual and group investigations and reasoning that lead to meaningful generalizations and conclusions rather than a cluster of meaningless facts. Not book learning but perceptions of many kinds relevant to health behavior, reflecting the functioning of the total organism, and judged criterial to the ultimate formulation of the most powerful ideas in health education. Conceptual learning goes on all the time, in and out of school. The conceptual approach merely arranges the best environment possible and allows it to happen.

SUMMARY

If we are to meet the needs of the twenty-first century and help the changed people who will live in those times, education must change as well. A new set of human values, as well as the new technology, demand new approaches to learning. Planning for effective teaching to meet this challenge will require attention to the special needs of every student. Learning must be focused upon the development of human capacities—capacities for effective interpersonal skills, creativity, love, and for *continuing* growth.

These critical changes must be implemented at the classroom level. Teachers need to be skilled in analyzing student needs and potentialities. They need to be able to define content with relevance to these needs and devise teaching strategies that help the learner to learn. If students do not learn, it is not they but the teachers and the schools that will be held accountable.

We have said that *how* to teach is a problem involving both structure and methodology. Unit or curriculum guide construction is concerned with the structure of teaching. A major problem here has always been a lack of time, energy, and resources with which to develop creative units that are designed to fit into a planned sequence. Today there is an increasing trend to purchase already developed curricula that are adaptable to local philosophies and needs, leaving the teacher free to spend his time on vital decisions at the classroom level. However, whether developing his own or adapting a packaged unit, ability to evaluate the excellence of curriculum materials is essential.

This chapter has explored unit construction and alternatives among instructional approaches. Chapter 5 will focus upon alternatives in methodology and techniques of teaching.

NOTES AND REFERENCES

1 State of Washington, Elementary Health Education, *Guide to Better Health* (working copy), Olympia, Wash., State Office of Public Instruction, p. 36.

2 *Ibid.,* pp. 38–45.

3 Alameda County School Department, *Dependency-Producing Substances,* A teaching unit, Grades One through Twelve, Hayward, Calif., Alameda County School Department, 1968, pp. 5–7.

4 *Ibid.,* pp. 5–7.

5 John I. Goodlad, *Planning and Organizing for Teaching,* Washington, D.C., NEA, 1963, chap. 2 *passim.*

6 Norris M. Sanders, and Marlin L. Tanck, "A Critical Appraisal of Twenty-Six National Social Studies Projects," *Social Education,* 34, 4 (April 1970), *passim.*

7 Louise L. Tyler, *A Selected Guide to Curriculum Literature: An Annotated Bibliography* (schools for the 70's), Washington, D.C., NEA, 1970, p. 99.

8 Ralph Tyler, *Basic Principles of Curriculum and Instruction,* Chicago, University of Chicago Press, 1969, p. 97.

9 Goodlad, *op. cit.,* p. 36.

SELECTED READINGS

Anderson, Robert H., *Teaching in a World of Change,* New York; Harcourt, Brace, and World, 1966.

Berman, Louis M., *From Thinking to Behaving,* New York; Teachers College Press, 1967.

Bruner, Jerome S., *The Process of Education.* Cambridge; Harvard University Press, 1963.

———, "The Skill of Relevance or the Relevance of Skills," *The Saturday Review,* April 1970, pp. 66–68; 78–79.

Goodlad, John I., *School Curriculum Reform in the United States,* Fund for the Advancement of Education, 1964.

———, *The Changing School Curriculum.* Fund for the Advancement of Education, 1966.

Morphet, Edgar L., Charles O. Ryan, and David F. Jesser, *Designing Education for the Future,* Vol. I, *Prospective Changes in Society by 1980,* New York, Citation Press, 1967.

NEA, *Rational Planning in Curriculum and Instruction,* Washington, D.C., NEA, 1967.

Oliver, G. L., "Toward Improved Rigor in the Design of Curricula," *Educational Technology,* April 1970, pp. 19–23.

Parker, J. Cecil, and Rubin, Louis J., *Process as Content: the Application of Knowledge,* Chicago; Rand McNally, 1966.

Pollock, Marion B., "What's So Good About Behavioral Objectives for Health Education?" *Journal of School Health,* 60; 4 (April 1970), 173–79; (May 1970), 274–275.

Popham, W. James, *The Teacher Empiricist,* Los Angeles, Tinnon and Brown, 1970.

Postman, Neil, and Weingartner, Charles, *Teaching as a Subversive Activity,* New York, Delacorte Press, 1969.

Taba, Hilda, *Curriculum Development Theory and Practice,* New York; Harcourt, Brace, and World, 1962.

Taylor, Calvin W., "Questioning and Creating: A Model for Curriculum Reform," *The Journal of Creative Behavior.* 1, 1 (Winter 1967), 22–32.

Tiemann, Philip W., "Analysis and the Derivation of Valid Objectives," *Journal of the National Society for Programmed Instruction,* 8 6 (1969),

Woodruff, Asahel D., "The Use of Concepts in Teaching and Learning," *The Journal of Teacher Education* (March 1964), pp. 81–99.

CHAPTER 5 SELECTING TEACHING-LEARNING STRATEGIES

Should teachers be concerned more with how well they perform certain techniques before a group of students than with what the students learn because of the techniques employed? Teaching and learning are not discrete but are connected events or transactions. In health teaching, perhaps *how* to teach is a more critical decision than *what* to teach. We are not really so intent upon communicating a certain amount of information, however meaningful. It is what is *done* with information that is of real concern.

Health behavior is essentially a decision-making process, and decision making involves intellectual skills. The belief that education should seek to train the mind is not new, of course, but the assumption has usually been that stuffing the students' minds with facts was the logical way of so doing. An encyclopedia is full of facts, so are the data banks of a computer, but neither of them is of any use without the trained intelligence of the human being. This constellation of skills and abilities has been defined as follows:

> A trained intelligence is one which can work operationally with ultimate efficiency, which functions in the individual's own idiosyncratic way, and which can at will engage in a variety of related mental performances. It has recourse to relevant information, whether in the

> memory or elsewhere. It can sort and arrange the facets of an idea into a functional order and bind them with what Cousins calls 'connective tissue.' It commands a portfolio of different intellectual techniques put together with a system of deciding when each ought to be used.[1]

Teaching-learning strategies must be selected thoughtfully and purposefully for their potential contribution to the development of intellectual skills or *processes* rather than solely for the transmission of information.

If concepts, topics, or problems give structure to a curriculum then processes, or intellectual skills, define its essential functions. Processes are the complex skills that are used to interpret or use data of all kinds in order to find solutions to problems. As such, they can be termed more simply "problem-solving skills." Problem solving is perhaps *the* method of health education. It is also fundamental to lifelong sensible decision making whatever one's situation. The necessity of emphasis on a process rather than an information-oriented curriculum is therefore overwhelmingly clear. Burns and Brooks argue that

> Today's living calls for problem solving skills, concept formation skills, data processing skills, the ability to make judgments and discriminate, the ability to relate causes to effects, the ability to analyze, the ability to summarize, and the ability to form valid conclusions. The cultivation of these general abilities is not and never will be the result of curricula which are solely information oriented. To develop behaviors associated with these abilities requires curricula which are specifically designed to achieve such ends. Curricula must be process-oriented if the learners are to develop processing behaviors.[2]

Curricula that are specifically designed to develop processing behaviors are built upon soundly derived and carefully specified behavioral objectives. The most important part of such objectives is the action word. Behaviors such as "identify," "describe," "differentiate," "synthesize," "compare," "interpret," and "demonstrate" are processes. Behavioral objectives not only provide direction in teaching toward process, but also let the learners know where they are going so that they can participate in the choices made among alternative ways of getting there.

An effective health educator seeks not to provide all of the answers in the form of structured, prescribed "content covering," but rather to provoke lifelong habits of questioning. The critical content of a learning experience should not be information, but the process through which the learning occurs, and that is to be a learned or sharpened part of the learner's repertoire of abilities. Edgar Dale points to this need for learning ways of *using* information rather than making information itself the goal:

> Much of our thoughtlessly memorized knowledge is inert, undynamic; it isn't going anywhere. A mental miracle will occur when we learn to restructure or rearrange what we already know in response to the solution of real problems. The chief emphasis will then be on *reconstruction* of knowledge, not on its *reproduction.*[3]

In the preceding chapters we have talked about excellence in curriculum design and unit construction. But the success of the best-planned curriculum in the world depends in the final analysis upon the skill of the individual teacher who is to implement it. However carefully curriculum plans are made, without equal care in designing or choosing teaching-learning strategies the purposes of the course are not likely to be attained. Most methods courses required of prospective teachers tend to describe specific techniques and ways of imparting information in the classroom, rather than strategies for teaching processes useful in real-life problem solving. Are "techniques" and "methods" terms that can be used interchangeably to describe the same thing or are they different things?

DEFINITION OF TERMS

"Teaching method" has been defined as the formal structure of the sequence of acts commonly denoted by instruction. The term covers both the strategy and tactics of teaching and involves the choice of what is to be taught at a given time, the means by which it is to be taught, and the order in which it is to be taught.[4] Richard K. Means views method just as broadly, defining it as a "process which involves a rational ordering or balancing of the elements which enter into the educative function—purposes, nature of the learner, materials of instruction, and the total learning situation."[5] If we accept this relatively global notion of the total instructional problem as "method," then the word cannot be used to refer to the techniques or procedures used by teachers in the classroom. Such activities as field trips, lectures, debates, role playing, and panel and buzz-group discussion are *techniques,* and they, along with materials and teaching devices, constitute the kit of tools from which the teacher chooses in designing teaching-learning strategies.

PLANNING—AND LEARNER CHARACTERISTICS

Just as a physician or surgeon first diagnoses a patient's illness and then chooses a procedure or treatment most likely to bring about his recovery, so the teacher diagnoses his students' present behavior and needs, then selects a teaching technique most likely to help them achieve a particular educational objective. However, designing a plan for teaching involves a great deal more than choosing among alternatives in technique. Teaching competence requires not only knowledge of the special inquiry processes and subject matter of a field, as well as mastery of a broad range of teaching tactics, but also a valid system of beliefs about the characteristics and abilities of the children to be taught.

The teacher must study the individuals in his class. Instruction must begin where the student *is* if it is to make much sense to the learner. Do all the students in this group already have the ability to employ the processes specified in the behavioral objectives defined in the unit, or only some of the students? Will there need to be some enabling activities provided first? What prior knowledge can be built upon in the investigation of the content identified as pertinent to the objective?

What are the cultural and socioeconomic characteristics of these students? Assumptions about background experiences whether in or out of school or value systems consistent with the typically middle-class orientation of teachers simply do not hold true for culturally disadvantaged children. The ghetto child tends to learn less from what he hears than from what he sees or touches. He learns more readily from induction than deduction.[6] More than usual attention may have to be given to the development of listening skills for the child who comes from an inner city environment where he has learned to shut out sound as a means of adjusting to it. Poor children, whose knowledge of hunger and want is painfully real, are understandably less interested in learning activities that are focused on the past or concerned with happenings too far in the future. For these children, teaching strategies may at first have to deal with the immediate and very concrete rather than the remote and abstract. Instruction will have to be planned as a series of very small developmental steps with immediate recall and reward. In the same group, more experienced and advantaged children may, on the other hand, make intuitive leaps forward, requiring the teacher to be flexibly responsive and ready to free them to range beyond the planned activities.

For all children, but among the poor particularly, low self-esteem makes them distrust their own judgment and conclusions; task setting during the first weeks of a class should be planned so that success is the inevitable outcome. Success is essential to self-esteem, and self-esteem breeds the kind of confidence that allows its possessor to risk failure, suggest hypotheses, try new ways. This kind of confidence flourishes also in a classroom environment where failure is viewed as a learning experience and risk taking as fun!

The middle or upper class child comes to school already convinced that education is a necessary and desirable long-range goal toward which he must work. The lower class or poor child is apt to view school as a dull and irrelevant routine that he must endure until he is old enough to leave it and get a job. When this time comes, the immediate gain represented by wages today may be more meaningful for him than some possible reward many years postponed by educational requirements, especially if his school experience *is* dull and irrelevant.

The time required to learn certain skills varies among individuals. Children learn and develop intellectually not only at their own rate but in their own style.

Still, the same teaching goals can be attained for most children. The differences among children do not change our goals so much as they change the teaching-learning strategies selected to achieve them. Learning is an individual happening resulting from the interaction between the student and the learning activity. The teacher's role is to provide a situation which will make a child's active participation in that interaction both likely and worthwhile. Subject matter should be a reasonable outcome of that activity rather than a list of arbitrarily selected and presented "eternal truths" or clusters of facts to be memorized.

Skill in diagnosing student needs is basic to the selection of appropriate learning opportunities. It is not enough to know *how* to carry out teaching techniques or follow specific procedures. The teacher must base his selection on reason rather than on whim or habit. *The question he must continually ask himself is: Why has this plan been chosen? The answer to that question must be as clear to his students as to himself!*

GENERAL PRINCIPLES OR CRITERIA

Some general principles or criteria for the selection of teaching-learning strategies are well established in theory if not always employed. Ralph Tyler suggests that there are five principles that should guide the teacher in this task.[7] Primarily, of course, a teaching plan should afford the learner an opportunity to practice the behavior specified in the objective. It should also give him an opportunity to deal with the kind of content implied in the same statement. It should be within the range of ability and experience and perceived as worthwhile by the students for whom it is intended. He points to the fact that since there are many particular learning experiences that might be used to attain the same objective, those should be chosen which appear to give promise of achieving more than a single outcome. For example, as an outcome of preparing a report about some health problem of interest, a student might also learn to use library and community resources, to read selectively and with comprehension, to generalize, conclude, and synthesize, and employ a host of other skills as well. Not all concomitant learnings are sure to be positive, however. The teacher must be alert to possible negative outcomes of learning opportunities. For example, as a consequence of many lessons on how to brush the teeth or uninspiring lectures on personal hygiene or the structure of the eyeball, many students automatically assume expressions of distaste or boredom at the very mention of the words "health" or "health education." Health instruction becomes associated with a series of prohibitions against things people like to do and with a dreary set of prescriptions about things people *do not* want to do. This kind of negative outcome is nearly inevitable when the emphasis is upon information rather than process. When process or problem solving is the focus of instruction, decisions to take or not take an action emanate from the learner himself as a result of the processes he has learned to use.

Goodlad refers to teaching-learning strategies as "organizing centers," which he describes as "instructional flesh on curricular bones." He lists eight criteria for selecting such organizing centers, some of which are similar to, while others go beyond, Tyler's principles. Goodlad says that the good organizing center (1) encourages the student to practice the behavior sought; (2) encourages the simultaneous practice of several behaviors; (3) supports learnings in other areas of instruction; (4) is planned with full awareness of preceding and forthcoming learnings for this particular group of students; (5) reaches to both the highest and lowest level of accomplishment in the group; (6) is sufficiently comprehensive to provide for a wide range of differences in student interests and learning styles; (7) has educational significance in its own right (that is, the materials selected for use in a given lesson are both valid and worth learning about); and (8) leads beyond itself to other times, other places, other ideas. Of this last criterion, he adds:

> Current curriculum revision seeks to provide this binding of time, place, and ideas through the identification of powerful concepts. The linking together of these concepts provides the structure of a field of inquiry. Instruction, then, is designed to help the student find and use a very few basic concepts . . . which become tools in dealing with data. Data are used to develop the concepts; the concepts in turn, help in the interpretation of new data. The student develops tools for independent inquiry.[8]

ACTIVE TEACHING TECHNIQUES

Any teaching technique or procedure must actively involve the learner if it is to be effective. Active participation can be either direct or vicarious. Direct participation exists where the student is himself physically involved in the activity; vicarious, where he is a viewer of an activity that is going on in another place or another time. Either way, the individual must be affected positively and provided perceptions and experiences contributing to the attainment of desirable long-range cognitive, affective, and action goals.

Direct teaching techniques may be group activities or individual activities. Group activities are those in which two or more people participate in the same learning situation, each taking a part and contributing to the whole. Committee work, discussions, dramas, field trips, panels, and role playing are examples. Individual activities are those in which each student interacts with some form of live communication in class or works alone on a project. Note taking during a lecture or while listening to a resource speaker, reading, performing his own experiment or observation in laboratory, interviewing, or developing a unique project are typical.

Vicarious teaching activities are usually media connected. The learner is viewing, or listening, to some presentation by means of television, film, videotape, transparency, sound slides, film strip, or tape recording. These also may be experienced either individually or as a member of a group.

It is important to remember, however, that techniques or procedures can be meaningless used as an end in themselves. It is not enough to have mastered an array of ways to present information. Both information and techniques must be means to an end—means whereby the learner is given an opportunity to develop ability to demonstrate the process defined in the instructional objective. These processes used in problem solving help the individual to discover new knowledge when he needs to, to become an independent, continuing learner.

A person gets better at what he practices. What better way to learn problem-solving processes than by solving problems? The most effective teaching-learning strategies focus upon problems the solutions of which are perceived by the student as rewarding and in his immediate self-interest. Selection of techniques should be guided by their potential contributions to one or more of the steps taken in solving a problem.

PROBLEM-SOLVING STEPS

A problem exists for an individual when his present background of experience and skills does not allow him to find a solution. Used in teaching, problem solving is an activity that follows certain logical steps which lead to the discovery of some new knowledge or behavior. In essence, a successful solution results in learning.

The steps in problem solving are generally agreed to be the following:

1. Recognizing the Problem / Health problems may be perceived by the individual as primarily physical (for example, overweight, acne, illness); or social (for example, boy-girl

relationships, shyness, aggressiveness); or emotional (for example, insecurity, frustration, anxiety). It is important that the teacher assist the student in identifying all components of any health problem. When the problem to be solved is recognized by the student as highly significant in his own life and a solution appears both possible and acceptable to him, he is far more motivated to work it out. It is a curious fact that this very obvious fact is so often forgotten in lesson planning.

2. Proposing a Tentative Solution / Some amount of thought must be given to a reasonable theory as a means of limiting the search for relevant data. Instruction at this point may be desirable in order to give the student criteria for the evaluation of an acceptable solution discovered later.

3. Collecting the Data / The necessary information may be already a part of the individual's experience or it may have to be discovered. In either case, a selecting process is applied in sorting out and classifying those facts, concepts, or principles needed to solve the problem or answer the question. The teacher may need to give instruction at this step to help the learner to recall or locate appropriate data.

In the process of collecting data the student might consult the *Reader's Guide* or the *Education Index* to identify relevant recent articles in professional and popular magazines and journals. Recently published textbooks can provide a starting point for investigation, and additional references are usually listed in connection with each chapter. Human resources who might be helpful include physicians, school nurses, psychologists, health educators, and other health specialists. The process of collecting information should be thorough and orderly rather than haphazard. The student should also assure himself that his sources are scientifically sound rather than biased or invalid in any way.

4. Formulating Trial Solutions / During this step, the learner combines the selected facts, concepts, and principles in various ways until he arrives at one best combination. Instruction at this point may be given in order to save time by eliminating the least likely combinations.

5. Matching Solutions / In the fifth step, the best hypothesis is matched against the criteria suggested by the solution tentatively proposed in step two. If the two appear to be similar, then the final step is to verify.

6. Verifying / Here the learner tries the solution by applying it to the problem. If it fails to work, then he generally returns to step four and selects another promising hypothesis for trial application. If the solution does work, he may wish to verify

it against several examples before concluding that the solution has indeed been validated.

Let us suppose, for example, that a teen-age girl is troubled by a 10-pound overweight problem. Her first step is to identify the problem, verbalizing it in terms that admit of its reality and the possibility of solution. Next, she might conceive a tentative solution to the problem such as to lower her calorie intake by skipping breakfast and lunch every day. Step three would be to recall or discover the data she needed to solve her weight problem most efficiently—data such as her present weight in relation to the desirable weight for her age and body build; her present calorie intake and calorie expenditure patterns; basic calories needed; nutritional requirements; health status as determined by medical examination, and any relevant rules or principles of weight control. Combining these bits of information, she might logically conclude that the best solution would be to choose a diet that supplied all of the necessary nutrients but substantially fewer calories. She might also figure that increased exercise, as an added factor, would help speed the process. Looking back to her preliminary plan she would find that in some ways the plan was similar but that her present hypothesis appeared to be sounder and more manageable. Not fewer calories through meal skipping but through better food choices is a wiser regimen. Adhering to the dietary plan over a period of time should verify the correctness of her solution. Raising her calorie expenditure through increasing her activities should verify that part of the solution as well.

What are the processes that have been learned or used in this series of steps? Analyzing, classifying, hypothesizing, conceptualizing, concluding, inferring, generalizing, theorizing, constructing, and interpreting to name only a few. Problem solving builds competence in intellectual skills. The teacher can select from a wide array of techniques and instructional media in designing teaching-learning strategies that contribute to or reinforce process development.

DIRECT TEACHING ACTIVITIES

– group procedures

Discussion / As a procedure contributing to finding solutions to problems, group discussions have undeniable value. Discussion helps students to practice and sharpen cognitive skills, formulate concepts and principles in their own words, and gain confidence in their own creative ability; discussion also shows them areas where further reading or study is needed. In addition, discussion provides the instructor with clues relative to the degree to which his objectives are being attained.

Considerable research exists to demonstrate the effect of the group environment upon the behavior of individuals. The effect can be either positive or negative, however. Changes in motivation and attitudes are far more easily effected by group discussions. People tend to be persuaded more readily as members of a group than as individuals. Group sanction or endorsement and public commitment to act are powerful aids in changing behavior. During World War II this was demonstrated by a great deal of research in relation to promoting acceptance of hitherto unpopular yet nutritious foodstuffs. It was shown that discussion *followed by group decision* was more effective than lecture or individual instruction in motivating women to adopt new food practices. On the negative side, when the group environment is not favorable to creative ways of looking at questions, an individual may find it easier or more comfortable to keep innovative ideas to himself rather than make what could have been a valuable contribution. The teacher must structure discussions in such a way that each student is allowed to present his suggestions or ideas in a climate of mutual respect both among students and between the teacher and students. At the same time, enough organization must exist to avoid wasteful expenditure of time on irrelevancies or trivia. If the goals of the discussion are clearly perceived by the teacher and the students, they can learn to differentiate between issues where it is appropriate to question and hypothesize—to try new ideas—and those where one's behavior is necessarily controlled by established routines.

Leading a discussion successfully is not a task for an amateur, nor is it a skill uniformly possessed by all teachers. The direction "discuss" so often seen in resource units is far more glibly said than done. The most difficult of all the discussion forms is that involving the total class. Discussion is not a series of answers to leading questions asked by the teacher, nor is it a bull session of opinion-airing or ignorance swapping. Rather it is a goal-seeking interchange of ideas leapfrogging upon the backs of other ideas, and this is difficult to achieve. Some teachers cannot seem to resist the urge to dominate the discussion and do most of the talking themselves. Any student participation in this situation is usually limited to questions that are answered by the teacher. Some teachers have difficulty in accepting the relatively unstructured classroom environment necessary if a pupil to pupil dialogue is to build to a vital discussion situation, and instead they maintain an individual pupil-teacher interaction only. Some students are talkers, whereas others are not, and it is difficult to keep the former from dominating the discussion even where pupil to pupil dialogue is encouraged.

Most of these difficulties are avoided when the class is divided into smaller groups, each with its own elected leader. But even in small groups, leadership that insures each member an opportunity to be heard with consideration is essential to the success of the activity. Maier showed that a minority member or members of a group (those with other than the majority opinion or idea) contributed reliably and significantly to better solutions of problems facing the group when leadership conditions favored their participation rather than rejection.[9] Another factor favoring the use of discussion techniques is the fact that apparently less able learners profit from participation and observation of the contributions of other group members.

There are a number of forms or structures in which discussions may be organized, six of which will be described.

1. *Brainstorming.* This can be teacher led in a total class situation or employed in small groups as a quick means of obtaining a large number of ideas for later analysis or evaluation. As an initiating procedure, the teacher or class identifies a problem or question that is to be the focus of the subsequent reactions and suggestions. An example might be "What are the effects of urbanization on health?" The teacher might simply ask the students to think of as many of the effects of urbanization as they can. Every suggestion or idea should be recorded without judgment as to its merit. The tenor of this activity should be receptivity and ideas. When no more effects can be suggested, each might be reconsidered for the purpose of further analysis and classified as either positive or negative. In a total class situation, the teacher acts as moderator and recorder. Use of chalkboard or transparency with overhead projector is an effective way of recording and summarizing class ideas. In small groups, each should be led by an appointed or elected leader and notes made by a group secretary. Each group brainstorms in the same way, and then reconsiders and categorizes its resulting pool of ideas as positive or negative in effect. Brainstorming is useful as a means of generating ideas to define problems of interest, to determine ways of locating data, or to theorize about possible solutions to problems.

2. *Buzz Sessions.* This is typically a small group, ordinarily about five or six in number, who are given a stipulated short period of time (for example, 6 to 10 minutes) to discuss some selected topic or problem and decide upon an approach or solution to a problem. The buzz session allows for the active participation of all the members. Such groups may be assigned the same topic or different topics. The culminating activity should be some means of conveying the group conclusions to the reassembled total class. This might be done by means of group leader reports or by forming an informal panel composed of group leaders who then discuss the broader issue to which these subgroup discussions are related. The other members of the class form the audience and are encouraged to ask questions or offer suggestions.

3. *Panel Discussions.* In the more formally organized panel discussions, the panel members spend some time in advance preparing for their contribution. As a teaching-learning strategy, panel discussion is often done in the nature of a project whose preparation is expected to take considerable advance

time, both in and out of the classroom. This kind of discussion is best carried out in a fairly structured manner. Each group should be provided an outline of its objectives and responsibilities along with suggested procedures. Time should be provided in class for each group to elect a chairman, prepare a tentative outline, allocate tasks, and set a timetable for their completion. The chairman should be responsible for submitting the outline in advance of the formal discussion, indicating the area for which each member is to be prepared in depth. When the panel makes its presentation, which is usually in the form of a conversational interaction among the group members, the chairman acts as discussion leader and summarizer. Panel discussions are especially successful in areas where there is controversy such as fluoridation, compulsory medical insurance, or standards of sex behavior.

4. *Forum.* This is a form of discussion that typically follows either a lecture by an authority or by a panel of experts speaking on the same subject but often with opposing views. Audience members are invited to ask questions, express disagreement, or add opinions and information. With large audiences the forum is frequently controlled by restricting the audience to handed up written statements or questions for comment and answer. The forum may also be structured by placing microphones at several points in an auditorium to which questioners must go in order to speak with the presenters.

5. *Symposium.* The symposium is usually a series of brief but formal presentations relevant to different aspects of a given problem. Following these, the audience participates either by means of questions or by joining in the discussion. The symposium usually involves a smaller and more intimate audience situation than the forum.

6. *Lecture-Discussion.* Many teachers, particularly at the high school or college levels, describe their mode of course conduct as "lecture-discussion." This means that the instructor presents some new and relevant material by lecture, after which the students are permitted and expected to ask questions, express views, and generally talk about the subject at hand. As a technique, the lecture-discussion allows the instructor to set the stage by giving the class a defined area of information in a short period of time, thus insuring a basic, common fund of data about which the discussion is centered. Its success depends upon the nature of the discussion matter and the skill of the instructor in leading discussions.

One of the best ways to initiate discussion is to present some common point of reference or experience through demonstration, film, transparency, or other teaching device. After the presentation, a question about the proceedings the class has just seen or heard makes discussion follow easily. Everyone has seen or heard the same things and can comment on those experiences on an equal footing. Another means of starting a discussion is to ask provocative questions. Question asking is not easy. The questions must be phrased in such a way that there is no pat answer, and they must be concerned with a problem that is meaningful to students. How many deaths from lung cancer are predicted within the next decade according to the film we have just seen? results in a factual answer with little promise of sparking further comment. A better question would be: Why is the death rate from lung cancer, formerly primarily a problem among men, now rising rapidly among women as well?

Whatever the form of discussion technique selected, the teacher should help the class to formulate summarizing conclusions or suggestions for action. These may not always be clearcut; they may be developed in the form of alternatives. In any case, the class should be urged to express itself in terms of a recommended action or point of view as a result of its talks.

Committee Projects / The cooperative participation of a small group of individual students in exploring some designated problem or topic is sometimes preliminary to other techniques. As described earlier, committee projects might be part of the procedures involved in planning a panel discussion. They might also precede other forms of presentation such as a drama or skit; a film or 2″ × 2″ slides with accompanying live or recorded narration; a debate; or a written report. Committee work can help students learn how to do research; to work effectively with others; to gather and organize data; and to synthesize data as a result of preparing a report. Careful structure is essential to the success of this technique however. Simply assigning a number of students to work as a committee in solving some problem or investigating some topic is not enough. We all have had experience with committee projects in which a few did most of the work and whose largely encyclopedia-derived factual reports were as boring to hear as they were meaningless as a learning experience.

One way to structure this kind of activity is to develop committee report forms relating to the various tasks implicit in committee projects. Such forms can be duplicated and given to each committee member or given to the committee chairmen when this is appropriate. In any case, a schedule giving the date by which the forms are to be completed and handed to the teacher should be posted and adhered to. One such form might require committee members to itemize library or other resources consulted as a preliminary step. Another might indicate purposes and results of committee meetings attended and planned for the future. A third might be a report detailing work completed and underway. And the last should be developed by the chairman and handed in a short time before the presentation. This final report should be carefully designed to include the title of the report; its specific purpose or planned contribution to the course; the responsibilities allocated to each member; a list of all sources of information consulted; the format to be used (dramatization, debate, panel discussion, media study, or other); any plans for class participation or evaluation; and so on.[10] Committee reports on major social problems such as pollution, the cost of medical care, or needed fringe health benefits in industry can be a successful method of examining the issues involved.

Role Playing. This technique is one that appeals to all ages. It is an ad lib, 3 to 5 minute acting out of a social situation in which the participants assume fictitious identities and then dramatize their parts. Role playing can portray a concept or dramatize a problem-solving situation. Two or more people may participate, and ordinarily a short amount of time is allowed for planning. The problem should be derived from the curriculum unit being studied and represent a real-life concern appropriate to the interests of the group involved. Although informality and even fun are associated with role playing, some instructional objective should be the obvious purpose of its selection as a teaching-learning strategy.

Role playing can be used to introduce an area of study through dramatizing a problem or to give students practice in using what they have learned by applying some principle to the solution of a problem. Role playing may also be used to illustrate the impact of tradition or values or social pressure on individual behavior. It might be used to provide an outlet for feelings or to put across ideas that, if approached more directly, might be awkward or uncomfortable for the students. Where it is possible to present a second dramatization without its players having seen the first, the fact that differing perceptions may result in different responses can be demonstrated by giving the same situations to two groups.

In general, the teacher should provide a well-structured explanation of the activity and its intent. Whatever the subject of the role playing, it should not have too direct personal meaning for any class member. The situation and resulting reactions should be those of people in general, not of specific participants or their friends. It may be wise, especially early in the course, to call for volunteers to take part in this activity.

Any nonparticipating members of the class should be instructed to observe the action carefully and watch for stipulated elements. One way to insure active observation is to allow the role players to choose and illustrate some principle, problem, or other health-related concept, which the class members are to interpret from the action. For example, teams of two or three might be given generalizations drawn from the subject matter, such as "Stress can be helpful or harmful in its effect on human behavior." Each team is given perhaps ten minutes to plan a way of presenting this idea through role playing. Role playing can also be used as a summarizing device, with the other students asking questions and commenting on the meaning of what they have seen.

Field Trips. A dynamic means of linking course purposes and individual concerns and responsibilities is a visit to a local community health resource, or an on-the-spot exploration of a health hazard or problem. As with any teaching-learning strategy, this technique should be chosen for its potential contribution to a desirable instructional objective and offer promise of being the best means of doing so. Although there is no reason why a field trip cannot be an individual experience, the term is usually used to describe a total class movement to some place other than the classroom. The place can be somewhere on campus or away from and at a considerable distance from the school.

Much preliminary planning is essential if the trip is to be off campus. Class discussion might be used to identify the exact place or resource to be visited, the kinds of information needed, and the perceived relationships between this information and the health concepts being studied. Depending on their age and ability, some or all of the actual arrangements may also be made by class members (arranging for the visit by letter or interview, setting the date and time for the visit, providing the hosts with necessary information about the class members and the purpose of their visit, *always following up with a letter of appreciation*). In this situation, the teacher acts as counselor throughout but stays in the background, allowing the students to practice the problem-solving skills they are acquiring.

The purpose of a field trip should not be to divert, although diversion it may be, but to provide a unique cluster of experiences contributing to the acquisition of some powerful idea related to health behavior. For example, on a field trip to a local health center, rather than focus upon what kinds of services are available as a survey, the students might be directed to look for evidence of *changing* services as they reflect new community needs. (The idea here is that community health programs must continually change and become more complex as the community itself changes and becomes more complex.) Not questions of fact so much as questions of Why? or, possibly, Why not? should structure a vital field experience.

All safety precautions for the care of the students making the trip should be planned for in accordance with school or district policy. Transportation, teacher aides, parental permission or assistance, and other logistic problems should be solved well in advance of the scheduled travel.

A post-field trip essential is a discussion of the data identified as relevant to the purpose of the trip. Cause and effect inferences should be drawn where possible and suggestions developed for improvement of the present situation or resource. Examination of present and future needs in the area could lead to some reasonable predictions relative to the changes necessary to meet them. Another profitable field trip activity is to encourage interested students to bring cameras and take pictures of the things they find significant. Following the trip, the pictures can be organized logically and an accompanying commentary written by other volunteers as a special project. The resulting presentation can be used in class as a stimulus for further discussion or review or shown to other school gatherings. It could also be used in succeeding years as a pre-field trip device to alert future classes to the purposes of the visit or to provide a base line for noting change.

To discover how different community groups live, the way they now meet or fail to meet their problems, the way the local community safeguards the health of its citizens, or to gain an on-the-ground insight into the larger social problems related to health provides a richer, more meaningful approach to an appreciation of personal and public health responsibilities. An enterprising teacher might work with his class as it seems appropriate to arrange a visit to one of the following:

1 A hospital or clinic to observe its programs

2 A commercial medical laboratory to observe methods of quality control and production

3 Recreational facilities in a given area to appraise their adequacy in relation to the needs of the people who live there

4 A food-packing plant to observe the care and handling of the food while it is being processed

5 A public swimming pool to study the sanitation and safety procedures followed

6 The kitchen of a large restaurant or series of restaurants in the company of the public health sanitarian to discover which factors are controlled by law

7 A large factory to study safety equipment and regulations provided to meet the special health and safety problems found there

8 A modern sewage or waste disposal facility to ascertain present means and their limitations

Other field experiences, such as public-opinion surveys concerning health needs or beliefs, analyzing building or zoning ordinances for their effectiveness in meeting present health needs, searching out traffic or fire hazards that need to be corrected, or investigating health quackery claims are just a few examples of less structured, individual or small-group projects that could be extraclassroom activities.

– individual procedures

Lectures / A lecture has been described as a long statement reflecting what one person perceives as the significant facts about some topic, resulting in a series of notes or impressions reflecting another person's perception of what he has just heard. The two perceptions may or may not be the same. Still, exposition is a highly satisfactory way to communicate certain kinds of information. Group work in every class meeting can be as boring as lecture or any other kind of teaching technique.

The lecture is particularly useful as a time-saving means of transmitting a great deal of information and can be as dynamic and interest-holding as any other well-executed teaching strategy. We have all experienced the sleep-inducing drone of a dull, meaningless lecture as well as the excitement generated by a meaningful lecture delivered by a dynamic speaker. The simple matter of maintaining eye contact with the audience rather than reading a prepared statement can make a big difference. It is important, also, that the speaker himself appear enthusiastic about his subject if his listeners are to be stirred.

If a teacher decides to provide some background information, or all of the material relevant to some health topic such as the arguments pro and con fluoridation of public water supplies, planned parenthood, noise pollution, or any other such issue, the following outline describes a desirable sequence to be followed in developing the lecture:

A Subject:	A topic chosen in relation to a present interest or logical progression of course content, rather than an isolated, unrelated bit of material.
A transition:	A sentence or two describing the relationship of this lecture to the preceding activities or lecture
An Introduction:	A brief presentation in which the problem to be discussed is looked at from the perspective of the learner and the society, and a quick sketching out of the content to be covered
The body:	All of the key points presented in logical order, with frequent illustrations chosen from human behavior and needs, and, where appropriate, with humor
The summary:	Main points brought together at the close of the lecture to aid the students in grasping the message of the total lecture
The transition:	A forecast of what is to follow in relation to what has just been said

As a means of actively involving the learner, it has been suggested that demonstrations or visual aids (transparencies, pictures, graphs, charts) be used to illustrate important points and to add a note of informality or change of pace to the presentation. Another effective device is to start with a meaningful problem, then present pertinent data organized in such a way that the students begin to perceive the solution before the instructor needs to point it out. Such a procedure might profitably be ended by asking the class to verbalize the solution either in discussion or in writing.

Value Sheets / Young people frequently detect a difference between their values and those of adults. Values have to do with the restless human need to know who we are. Many educators speak about the importance of teaching values and the relationship of values to human behavior, especially health behavior, but there is less talk about how to get at values in our teaching. Raths and others describe some very exciting ways of doing this that have special significance for teaching-learning strategies in health.[11] One such technique is the value sheet. This is essentially an individual procedure, although the results can be shared with others in small or large group discussions.

In its simplest form a value sheet consists of a thought-provoking statement or quotation and a series of related questions. The purpose of the statement is to pose an issue that the teacher believes has value implications. The purpose of the questions is to guide the student through a value-clarifying process in connection with that issue.

Value sheets may be based upon bipolar issues such as independence versus dependence; freedom versus license; love versus hate; upon provocative quotations; or upon concepts such as health, friendship, or love, supported by a series of short quotations amplifying that concept. The questions that follow ask the student to state his own position in regard to the issue and perhaps take a stand or make some commitment for action. An example of a value sheet is given below:

> *Directions:* Carefully read the material quoted below, underlining or otherwise noting those points that seem significant to you. Then write out answers to the questions that follow it. Later you will be given an opportunity to share your reactions with a small group of your classmates. You need not reveal your written statements to these students if you prefer not to do so.
>
> Some of a certain man's best friends are politicians. One of them has promised to produce legislation next fall requiring a type of vehicular device that just happens to be manufactured by one of this man's clients and associates. If the bill passes, it will be a small drop in the legislative well. If it passes, it will be a large boon to the manufacturer and his attorney. . . . I asked [him] whether such special interest legislation offended his liberal ethic. "No," he said, "that's the way the system works. Everybody does it!" . . . Then he went on to talk about his hopes for new leadership and how young people could make a real contribution to the electoral process. "The trouble is that most people don't care enough."
>
> The man's manners were impeccable. His personality was likeable. He didn't seem to have any qualms about wanting reforms and a little kickback at the same time. One was government. The other was business.[12]

1 Write your reaction to the statements attributed to this man relevant to government versus business as separate ethical problems.

2 Does the statement produce any strong feelings in you? What feelings does it produce?

3 Can you list other differences you see between the values people claim and their actual values as shown by their practices?

4 Under what circumstances do you believe it all right to accept a business-connected kickback?

- ☐ Only if it made no difference to anyone else's income
- ☐ Only if it could never cause me embarassment if it were to be discovered
- ☐ Under no circumstance of any kind.
- ☐ Only if my efforts had contributed significantly to the business success
- ☐ (Write any statement that better describes your position.)

5 If this is an issue that worries you, is there anything you can do about it personally? In association with friends? As a member of our society?

These kinds of questions get the student to take a position relative to the values involved. They call for critical thinking, self-analysis, and identification of his own values and require him to make some personal commitment to action if he finds that his values differ from those described. They may cause him to change his values if he finds they are the same as those above. They help him take one important step toward learning who he is.

Simulation and Case Study / Simulations can be described as operating models of physical or social situations, or as simplified representations of reality. An example of a physical model is the driver-training device that places the learner in a full-sized automobile seat in front of real controls, which he manipulates in response to filmed driving situations as they appear ahead of him in a realistic manner. The kind of social model used in school classrooms is similar to a game in which students assume the roles of decision makers in a simulated environment and compete for certain objectives according to specified procedures or rules.

The values of games are many. In the first place they are fun, so that students are highly motivated to take part. Play, after all, is the business of childhood and is not necessarily frivolous or useless. Real learning can come out of group situations far more effectively than from textbook or teacher-presented subject matter. Learning gained through simulation goes beyond the problem-solving task. As students assume and play real-life roles they also gain insight into the demands and rewards of adult leadership or social role activity.

One disadvantage in this technique is the amount of time it takes to carry out the game. Another is the amount of apparent disorganization that results in the classroom. Some teachers may not feel secure in permitting so much freedom. Few teachers have the time or the ability to devise simulation games.

However, an increasing number of very good prepared simulation games that could profitably be used in health teaching are available for purchase.[13] For example, "Generation Gap," a game for junior or senior high school students, simulates the interaction between a parent and a teen-age son or daughter with opposing views on certain issues. The purpose is to give some understanding of the structure of power and interdependence in the family and to formulate effective strategies for handling conflicts. "Pollution," a game for elementary school students, is concerned with the social, political, and economic problems involved in attempts to control pollution.

Among the kinds of learnings possible through use of simulation are (1) a better grasp of important generalizations; (2) improved decision-making skills; (3) an increased ability to work with others; (4) more positive attitudes toward the life roles involved; and (5) growth in ability to think critically.

A somewhat similar device is the case study, which is a prepared, fully described, social situation involving a real-life problem. It may be actual or fictitious. The students utilize the background information and relevant data about the individuals described as a basis for individual or small-group analysis and hypothesis formulating and other problem-solving skill applications.

Textbooks / American education is still very much textbook centered. Everybody—teachers, students, and parents—seems to be uneasy without textbooks in the belief, apparently, that if there is no textbook to study one cannot be learning anything worthwhile. A recent review made of classroom observational studies undertaken during the past fifty years found that no significant change in teaching behavior had occurred in that time. The work of the typical classroom has been and continues to be study and recitation of assigned textbook materials.[14] We recently witnessed a tenth-grade health class in which the instructor quite literally "taught the book." The students were required to open their books each day to the indicated chapter and read. When they finished, they routinely wrote out answers to the questions provided at the end of the chapter, and, if time permitted, these papers were exchanged, corrected, and handed in. Scoring was done by the students themselves in response to the teacher's reading of acceptable answers. Any chapter too long to be completed within the 45 minutes of class time was finished on the following day. The only other kind of participation was any questions that arose during the scoring of the written exercises. As too often has been the case, the teacher was not a health educator but an unwilling recruit from another discipline.

Effective teaching uses textbooks as a resource rather than a crutch. Many school systems prefer or are required by state law to adopt certain textbooks for each grade in each subject. There are a number of textbooks or series of textbooks written for health teaching purposes. Such books are not of equal worth. Some are almost entirely physiology-anatomy oriented; some are marred by scientific inaccuracies; some are old-fashioned and platitudinous; a few are very good. The first step in using any textbook is to determine whether, as organized, it fits into the sequence of objectives selected as relevant to the needs and interests of the students involved. The teacher need not be tied to the order provided but should assign reading out of sequence in the quest for solutions to problems. Where portions of a textbook may be out of date (and the latest edition is about two years old when it reaches the students' hands), fresh materials should be identified and used instead. In *any* case, discovery and use of supplementary current reading materials should be an ongoing teaching-learning priority.

In order to help the teacher judge the quality of a textbook proposed for adoption or use, the following criteria are suggested:

1 The contents of the book should be based upon the health needs and problems of the age group for which it is written and should be directed toward the same objectives as the course.

2 The major emphasis of the text should be upon problems crucial to the pupils and important to the community in which the book is being used.

3 The content material must be scientifically accurate throughout and in complete accord with the best available knowledge in science.

4 The first chapter of the book should provide a good springboard for the year's program in health instruction by appealing to the pupil's goals, such as interest in appearance, athletics, and vocational success, and by pointing out the relationship that exists between the achievement of these goals and the satisfactory solution of the health problems covered in the remaining chapters of the book.

5 The book should be written in an interesting and readable style, with the vocabulary on the comprehension level of the pupils who will use it.

6 The text should contain a glossary.

7 The text should cover suitable and purposeful activities, participation in which will help the pupils solve their problems related to growth, development, and adjustment.

8 At the end of each chapter there should be listed suitable references of books, pamphlets, films, filmstrips, and other audiovisual aids.

9 The charts, graphs, and tables contained in the book should be meaningful to the pupils.

10 All statistics should be accurate and up to date.

11 The illustrations should be attractive, accurate, and relevant.

12 The paper and print should be of a quality and size that will minimize eyestrain, and the cover should be attractive.

13 The authors should have sufficient training and experience to qualify them to write a satisfactory text.

Textbooks have their drawbacks, to be sure. They seldom make provision for increased reading ability from the beginning to the end of the book, and any single text will be too easy for some, too difficult for others. Nevertheless, a well-written text can be useful to the inexperienced teacher and an inquiring student.

Programmed Instruction / Some materials for teaching health are available in the form of programmed textbooks. Such a book is used by an individual student in class or as a kind of surrogate tutor for homework. The programmed textbook is usually written as a series of items, questions, or statements to which the student makes a response as he progresses through the book. His response may be to fill in a word left out, to answer a question, to select the correct answer among two or more alternatives, or to otherwise indicate a reaction to the material presented to him. As soon as he has responded, he is allowed to see the correct answer so that he knows at once whether he was right and does not proceed until he has mastered the step. The items are written so that the student is carried along, small steps at a time, making few errors, until he gets to the final responses, which represent the intended new knowledge. Programs such as these are based upon meticulously defined instructional objectives and are tried and revised repeatedly until their teaching efficacy is virtually perfect. A teacher could lead a student through the same kind of tutorial program just as effectively of course, but a programmed textbook is not limited to teaching one student at a time. Each student can work at his own pace, which relieves slower ones of pressure and brighter students of frustration and boredom. The programmed textbook is a means of transmitting factual information accurately and uniformly in a relatively short period of time.

Individual Projects / Special student interests or abilities can be capitalized upon by assigning or encouraging the development of individual projects. Use of creativity and practice in problem-solving skills are the chief goals. Collages portraying some aspect of health education such as consumerism, pollution control, or dental care; construction of a smoking machine, poster, or chart; experiments; oral or written research reports; surveys; and media studies such as photographs or motion pictures illustrating some health concept are some possibilities. The key is to allow the students freedom to identify the topic and the means by which it will be explored. Motivation is far greater when students are permitted to experiment and create a unique product than when they are required to crank out the usual report in a prescribed, uniformly structured manner.

VICARIOUS TEACHING ACTIVITIES

– televised instruction Although use of television in teaching is far from universal, there is no question that it works as an educational tool. Students *can* learn from television as well as they can learn from teachers, textbooks, or other educational media. The success of *Sesame Street,* begun in the early 1970s, attests to this fact. One problem has been lack of funds for equipment, another the lack of good quality programs. However, in schools where closed-circuit television equipment is available, the potential for more effective use of demonstrations and experiments is obvious. Increasing use of videotape makes it possible to record such experiences or presentations by specialists for future use as well. Each student has a far better view of the proceedings in this way than he might if he were witnessing the actual activity. Many school systems use scheduled ETV broadcasts as supplementary health instructional materials. A good source of current information can be found in commercial broadcasts of documentaries dealing with health-related issues such as environmental pollution, drug-abuse problems, or population control. Such programs are scheduled with considerable advance publicity and can be identified and used as homework or voluntary activities for later use in class discussion. Effective use can be made of the tape recorder in preserving the sound portion of television shows that seem useful to health instruction as well.

– overhead projection materials Professionally prepared transparencies are now available in relation to nearly every aspect of health instruction. Such prepared illustrations differ from photographs in that they are generally simplified linear abstractions with less confusing shading and detail. Research indicates that this kind of representation is excellent in promoting transfer of learning and total student understanding of the basic concepts involved.[15] These graphic illustrations can be used to stimulate discussion, to initiate new topics, to provide supplementary materials for independent study or group work, as a pre-field trip preparation, to illustrate lectures, and as an evaluation tool. The development of original transparencies by students is a worthwhile project that many like to undertake. A blank transparency can be used effectively as a chalkboard substitute by either teacher or students. The writing is more easily read in many cases and allows the user to face his audience so that he is more able to pick up suggestions or need for clarification.

– films, slides, and filmstrips

Through use of film media a kind of vicarious field trip, experiment, or demonstration can be experienced which otherwise might be difficult or impossible to arrange. Often a 15-minute film can cover an experience more effectively than an hour-long field trip or lecture. With a film all students are seeing the same thing, all can hear appropriate explanations, and certain details can be magnified so that every part is made clear. This is not to say that a motion picture always does the job better than an actual field trip, because in some instances learning is more effective when one sees the real thing.

The effectiveness of filmed presentations depends as much upon the way they are used as upon the skill with which they were developed. Few films are of any value if they are shown without comment or discussion. The instructor must preview and note the key points illustrated. He must be alert for any inaccurate or out-of-date material. The entertainment quality of some films may be such that the educational purposes may be obscured. It is doubly important with these that the students be told in advance to watch for certain points. As a means of further insuring the students' critical analysis of what is shown, it can be rewarding to ask for and use the students' evaluation of the effectiveness of the film in achieving its objective as a criterion for future use.

Although it may be too time consuming, research demonstrates that learning is greatly enhanced by a second showing of a film.

Slides and filmstrips lack the dynamic realism of motion picture presentations, but they have the advantage of greater versatility. Individual frames can more logically be viewed singly and for the length of time desired. Slide film presentations are the most flexible of all. New pictures can be added, old ones deleted, and the sequence altered at any time. Slides can also be easily and inexpensively created by the teacher or students. When combined with a taped commentary, a slide presentation rivals the dynamic quality of a film. There are many excellent films covering all phases of personal and community health. Some schools have film libraries of their own, and most school districts have a central audio-visual department with a wide range of materials. The teacher may refer to catalogs issued by commercial companies, state departments of public instruction, voluntary and public health agencies, or his own school district offices for available films.

– other resources

As long as the teacher relies only upon his own voice to communicate ideas to a class he is limited, indeed. He is denying the students opportunities to deepen their comprehension of the health material that is under discussion. Actually, there are few teachers who are so limited in their resourcefulness that they confine their teaching-learning strategies to a one-way communication system.

Teaching aids have increased enormously since the invention of the chalkboard. In addition to the techniques already discussed, the teacher has radio, libraries full of reference books, tape recordings, records, and individuals from the community willing to come to the classroom and present and discuss health-related topics. The class can also employ such visual devices as exhibits, scrapbooks, flannelboards, charts, posters, models, and specimens, all of which actively involve the learner in many sensory experiences.

Because learning is more likely to turn into positive behavior when the learning experiences involve the individual emotionally and as totally as possible, health educators need to employ as often as possible techniques that are as close as possible to a direct, vital experience. Models and mock-ups provide a scheme or situation (for example, the plastic head and torso for rescue-breathing practice). Forms of drama such as sociodrama, skits, and plays (putting oneself into the other person's shoes) also provide for possible *action* on the part of the learner that could in turn lead to the formation of desirable behaviors and attitudes. Exhibits of so-called health foods, quackery devices, or proprietary drugs, although taken out of their real setting, are nevertheless vital learning experiences. Extensive exhibits viewed in a health museum (found in cities such as Cleveland and Columbus, Ohio, Philadelphia, Pennsylvania, and Dallas, Texas) could contribute a great deal if the trip is planned and conducted by a skilled teacher.

The purely visual display via the pegboard, chalkboard, magnetic board, map, graph, cartoon, diagram, and others may lack movement and audio properties, but in many situations such a display can bring a lecture or discussion point into focus better than words.

Edgar Dale places these audio-visual techniques in a cone-shaped hierarchy, with a verbal symbol at the apex representing the most abstract of the techniques, and the direct, purposeful experience at the base representing the most concrete experience.[16] It would be difficult indeed to say that any one technique is always better than others; there are too many variables operating in the learning process. The teacher must be skilled in many techniques and must select the one that will do the best job that day for that topic for that particular group of students. Each technique has a contribution to make, perhaps in combination with another. Any technique *can* emotionally involve the learner when it is used wisely and well.

Finally, there are many useful resources and resource people within the school itself. Students should be given opportunities to know what the safety- and emergency-care policies of the school are and how they are arrived at, how the school lunch program operates, and what the disease-control procedures are. Teachers will find that school nurses, dental hygienists, physicians, psychologists, home economics teachers, dietitians, school custodians, school bus drivers, speech teachers, and guidance counselors all have a contribution to make to classes in health education and usually are willing to make it if invited.

REWARDS AND PRIZES A motivational device with considerable tradition behind it is what might be called the "gold star" ploy. Indeed, the newest instructional systems, the so-called contractual teaching programs, which guarantee learning results, reportedly are using such gifts as pencils, writing pads, radios, and even trading stamps to tempt the students to try harder. As a means of increasing learnings, rewards and prizes might justifiably be regarded as teaching techniques.

There are many rewards that may be associated with an activity either as an incentive or as recognition of good work. The most obvious are grades, which of course are also used to express disapproval. Self-satisfaction, approval from the group, fame, money, gold stars, trips, trophies, group acceptance, being captain—these are all available for use by the teacher.

Are they of equal value—equally sound as educational techniques? Obviously not. If the teacher is concerned only with the effects of the reward as a motivator, he will use a reward differently than if he believes that a reward should be a recognition of good work. "If you pass this test with a 90 percent score you will get an *A*" is the first approach. "*Because* you did well on the test you have earned an *A*" is the other. Rewards offered as an incentive may produce dishonesty, antagonism, and distort values. Used as earned rewards they may be productive of continued excellence and a clear understanding of sound values.

What criteria may be applied before a reward is fixed upon or before a system of rewards is established? These are suggested:

1 The reward should be inherent in the activity, not separate or unrelated to it.

2 The reward should lead the winner to further activity in the same line of endeavor.

3 The reward should have values no different from those of the activity itself.

4 The reward should produce no socially unacceptable consequences in the individual winner.

5 Above all, the incentive to excel should come from the satisfaction of engaging in the activity, not just from a desire to gain the reward.

In short, when rewards in health education help the student face reality and achieve, organize, and integrate values, then they are worthwhile. When they teach false or twisted values, distort ego, and dissipate energy, they are questionable.

SUMMARY

The tremendous capacity of the computer has made it obvious that intellectual power does not derive from ability to store data, but from the ability to handle them. Teaching, therefore, can no longer be confined to the simple act of transmitting information, but must focus upon process, the development of intellectual skills.

Disease is not avoided by memorizing the bones of the body, nor is a happy marriage relationship assured through ability to label the parts of the reproductive systems. The kinds of experiences believed to be valuable in health education are those requiring the learner to define and solve problems, make reasoned and scientifically acceptable choices, analyze and reflect upon perceptions, and, concomitantly, to learn to work alone or effectively cooperate with others.

The dynamic technological society in which we live today requires an educational system that is in touch with the real world. In such a world there is a powerful sense of urgency to strive for innovation. A wealth of techniques, procedures, and media are available to the innovative teacher. The question he must ask himself as he chooses among them is not "Would it be interesting?" or even "Would it be desirable?" but foremost "Is it *necessary* in order to understand the concept and does it give the learner a chance to practice intellectual skills?"

Teaching-learning strategies must be designed to meet the requirements of the behavioral objectives defined as significant to achievement of essential processes and powerful ideas and also to suit the learning styles and abilities of the particular learners involved. To be effective, the strategies must involve the learner actively, focus upon problems perceived by him as rewarding and in his immediate self-interest, and allow him to practice problem solving. Effective teaching activities can be direct or vicarious. Direct techniques include group procedures such as discussion, committee projects, role playing, and field experiences, and individual procedures such as lecture, textbook study, programmed instruction, use of value sheets, simulation, case study, and individual projects. Vicarious learning activities include the viewing of such media as television, transparencies, slides, films, and filmstrips. A host of other resources, both human and mechanical, are available for teaching.

NOTES AND REFERENCES

1 J. Cecil Parker and Louis J. Rubin, *Process as Content: Curriculum Design and the Application of Knowledge,* Chicago, Rand McNally, 1966, p. 18.

2 Richard W. Burns and Gary D. Brooks, "Processes, Problem Solving, and Curriculum Reform," *Educational Technology,* May 1970, pp. 11–12.

3 Edgar Dale, *The News Letter,* 35, 8 (May 1970), 3.

4 Harry S. Broudy, "Historic Exemplars of Teaching Method," in N. L. Gage (ed.), *Handbook of Research on Teaching,* Chicago, Rand McNally, 1963, p. 3.

5 Richard K. Means, *Methodology in Education,* Columbus, Ohio, Charles E. Merrill, 1968, p. 97.

6 Sol Adler, *The Health and Education of the Economically Deprived Child,* St. Louis, Warren H. Green, 1968.

7 Ralph Tyler, *Basic Principles of Curriculum and Instruction,* Chicago, University of Chicago Press, 1969, pp. 65–67.

8 John I. Goodlad, *Planning and Organizing for Teaching,* Washington, D.C., NEA, 1963, pp. 95–100.

9 Bryce B. Hudgins, *Problem Solving in the Classroom,* Macmillan, 1966, p. 33.

10 Phyllis Lieberman and Sydney Simon, "Vitalizing Student Reports," *Social Education,* January 1964, pp. 24–26.

11 Louis E. Raths, Merrill Harmin, and Sidney B. Simon, *Values and Teaching,* Columbus, Ohio, Charles E. Merrill, 1966.

12 Art Seidenbaum, *Los Angeles Times,* Part II, August 3, 1970, p. 1.

13 Richard Zieler, *Games for School Use: A Bibliography,* Center for Educational Services and Research, Board of Cooperative Educational Services, 845 Fox Meadow Road, Yorktown Heights, New York, March 1968.

14 James Hoetker, and William P. Ahlbrand, Jr., "The Persistence of the Recitation," *American Educational Research Journal,* March 1969, pp. 145–167.

15 Francis N. Dwyer, Jr., "Adapting Visual Illustrations for Effective Learning," *Harvard Educational Review,* Spring 1967, pp. 250–263.

16 Edgar Dale, *Audio-Visual Methods In Teaching,* rev. ed., New York, Dryden Press, 1969, pp. 42–56.

SELECTED READINGS

Allen, Rodney F., John V. Fleckenstein, and Peter M. Lyon, (eds.), *Inquiry in the Social Studies,* Washington, D.C., NEA, 1968.

Berman, Louise, *From Thinking to Behaving,* (*Practical Suggestions for Teaching*), New York, Teachers College Press, 1967.

Borton, Terry, "What's Left When School's Forgotten?" *Saturday Review,* April 18, 1970, pp. 69–72.

Brennan, Matthew J., "The Conceptual Field Trip," *Science and Children,* Vol. 7, Washington, D.C., National Science Teachers Association, March 1970, pp. 34–35.

Carin, Arthur A., "Techniques for Developing Discovery Questioning Skills," *Science and Children,* Washington, D.C., National Science Teachers Association, April 1970, pp. 13–15.

Carroll, John B., "Words, Meanings, and Concepts," *Harvard Educational Review,* Spring 1964, pp. 178–202.

Conte, Joseph M., and George H. Grimes, *Media and the Culturally Different Learner,* Washington, D.C., NEA, 1969.

Dubin, Robert, and Thomas C. Taveggia, *The Teaching-Learning Paradox,* Eugene, Oreg., Center for the Advanced Study of Educational Administration, 1968.

Edinger, Lois V., "Schools for the Seventies and Beyond," *Today's Education,* Washington, D.C., NEA, 1969 (reprint).

Edling, Jack V., "Programmed Instruction," *Innovations for Time To Teach,* Washington, D.C., NEA, 1966, pp. 69–75.

Gagne, Robert M., *The Conditions of Learning,* New York, Holt, Rinehart & Winston, 1965.

Glasser, William, *Schools Without Failure,* New York, Harper & Row, 1969.

Grimes, Peter, "Programmed Learning: Testing Its Use in School Health Education," *International Journal of Health Education,* July-September 1966, pp. 138–143.

Kapfer, Philip G., "Behavioral Objectives and the Curriculum Processes," *Educational Psychology,* May 1970, pp. 14–17.

Likert, Rensis, "Diagnose Your Teaching Role," *The Instructor,* September, 1968.

Markle, Susan, and Philip W. Tiemann, " 'Behavioral' Analysis of 'Cognitive' Content," *Educational Technology,* January 1970, pp. 41–45.

Moore, George N., and G. Willard Woodruff, "Materials from a Decade of Ferment/a Legacy of Choices, *Grade Teacher,* January 1970, pp. 114–116.

Murphy, Judith, and Ronald Gross, *Learning by Television,* New York, The Fund for the Advancement of Education, 1966.

Nesbitt, William, "Simulation Games for the Social Studies," *New Dimensions,* New York, The Foreign Policy Association, 1968.

Rogers, Virginia, and Marcelle Lysilka, "Simulation Games . . . What and Why," *Instructor,* March 1970.

Schramm, Wilbur, *Programmed Instruction: Today and Tomorrow* (reprinted *Programmed Instruction*), New York, Fund for the Advancement of Education, 1964, pp. 98–115.

Skinner, B. F., *The Technology of Teaching,* New York, Appleton-Century-Crofts, 1968.

Smith, B. Othanel, *Teachers for the Real World,* Washington, D.C., The American Association of Colleges for Teacher Education, 1969.

Taylor, Calvin, and Frank E. Williams, (eds.), *Instructional Media and Creativity,* New York, John Wiley, 1966.

Time To Teach Project, *Innovations for Time To Teach,* Washington, D.C., NEA, 1966.

Turner, Thomas N., "Individualization Through Inquiry," *Social Education,* January 1970, pp. 72–73.

Von Stoephasius, Renata, *Learning by Television,* New York, The Fund for the Advancement of Education, 1966.

CHAPTER 6 EVALUATION OF INSTRUCTION

Evaluation has always been a process fundamental to education, but current demands upon the schools for accountability in terms of the educational product make planning and implementing such procedures a more critical problem for the 1970s and beyond than ever before. Recognition of this need for increased rigor in evaluating is reflected in the nationally developing trend toward adoption of PPBS (planning, programming, budgeting systems) by school administrators. Central to a systems approach is the specification of performance objectives and related evaluation procedures capable of revealing success or failure in achieving them. Evaluation in this context is not perceived as measurement of student success alone, but also of teaching effectiveness and effectiveness of resource utilization. Evaluation of this nature is essential at any level, classroom, course, or schoolwide.

THE NATURE OF EVALUATION

In general, evaluation is a process of reaching decisions. The basic activity involved is that of collecting information. Observed outcomes are tested against objectives, expectations, or goals to determine the degree of success that has been obtained. Data may be gathered by formal procedures such as performance and written tests, or informal means as through casual observations, self-reports, or interviews. Judgment is a part as well as an outcome of the process in that value judgments are involved in deciding *what* to measure as well as in interpreting the results of that measurement.

The goal of measurement is always the same, whatever the object of its scrutiny; to appraise something according to a set of values. But it is important to differentiate between the *goals* of evaluation and the *roles* of evaluation. The *goals* of evaluation are always the same. Whatever is being evaluated, the sought for outcome is some index of its success or worth. The *role* of evaluation can vary according to its function. The role depends on *what* is being evaluated and whose standards are being applied to the criterion. For example, a great many different kinds of evaluation are possible in any particular educational setting. Evaluation can be part of a teacher preparation program, in which case the performance of the student teacher is being appraised, and the standards prescribed by the faculty directing his preparation are those applied. Evaluation should be a vital component of curriculum development, where the success or failure of every aspect of the curriculum is constantly being evaluated and the results used as a basis for decisions concerning modifications or changes where necessary. Whatever the educational activity, whether research, lesson planning, or selecting teaching materials, evaluation has a role unique to that activity. The goal in every role, however, is to appraise the outcome of that activity.

For every role there can be several specific goals. For example, a role of evaluation might be the ongoing improvement of a course. (Michael Scriven aptly terms this role "formative" inasmuch as it helps shape or *form* the course.)[1] The goals of evaluation in this role might be (1) to determine the feasibility of the proposed objectives for the age group involved, (2) to appraise the effectiveness of the learning opportunities selected to implement those objectives, and (3) to evaluate the contribution of particular learning outcomes, irrespective of their effectiveness in themselves, to the stated goals of the course.

There are many roles that evaluation plays in health education. These include the appraisal of student achievement, the total school health program, the evaluation process itself, and more.

Evaluation should not be perceived solely as a terminal procedure used to appraise the final outcome of a program or the final grade of a student, but as an ongoing (formative) process that begins before instruction (pretesting) and continues throughout the course. A final evaluation activity is, of course, inescapable, but it is usually of a different order. End-of-course evaluation procedures are often termed "summative" because they are designed to make an appraisal of the end product, the total growth or sucess of whatever is being measured. Formative evaluation may be the more worthwhile as a means of promoting desired behavioral changes inasmuch as it gives students information about their progress at a time when this information can be employed positively. When carried out fairly and meaningfully, evaluation contributes significantly to student satisfaction in learning and provides motivation to persevere.

EVALUATION AND MEASUREMENT

Is there a difference between evaluation and measurement? Most would agree that whereas good evaluation always includes some sort of measurement, measurement is itself but a part of evaluation. Measurement is descriptive only—a means of quantifying some amount of information or status. The resulting data are used as one sort of evidence in making evaluations. In teaching, measurement is also a means of ordering, or ranking, individuals based upon their responses to test situations associated with learning.

Evaluation is a dual process that includes description and judgment—the collection and use of data from many sources, both objective and subjective, as a basis for educational decision-making. A teacher may ask questions on a written test about nutrition to see how much students know about the material that has just been studied—that is measurement; but it is only a part of his long-term evaluation plan to see just how ability to make nutritionally sound food choices has been influenced or changed by the whole unit on nutrition and by prior learnings in the course. Measurement usually focuses on specific behaviors and content and is objective; evaluation is long range, broader in scope, and tends to be subjective.

PURPOSES OF EVALUATION

Simply stated, evaluation in health education seeks to find out if we are succeeding in favorably influencing health behavior.

Ideally, the purposes of evaluation in health instruction are the following:

1 To determine present health knowledge, beliefs, and practices as a basis for developing instructional objectives

2 To identify and diagnose sources of learning difficulties

3 To assess the effectiveness of teaching materials and strategies

4 To appraise the total health curriculum

5 To provide continuing information about student achievement as a basis for motivation or grading

6 To improve counseling effectiveness

7 To ensure the relevance of evaluation procedures employed to the specified course objectives

8 To serve as a basis for constructive revision or modification of all aspects of the curriculum

In essence, we must decide which things are essential to measure if the results are to be useful. The set of activities we are willing to accept as evidence of the students' achievement of an objective becomes an operational definition of what in fact we wanted them to learn, whatever the asserted objectives of the teaching.

– what is evaluated? The problem of evaluation in health instruction is more difficult than in many subject areas because its desired outcomes are not as easily measured as many other areas. We can give tests of many kinds that provide information about student success or failure to learn health facts. But information *about* health behavior is not health behavior itself. Most of us do not need to read the results of recent research to know that there is a great difference between what an individual knows and what he does in making choices that affect his health. Witness the number of teachers, physicians, and other presumably informed people who smoke, often drink to excess, and exhibit other less than exemplary practices.

The health teaching-learning process is hamstrung by shortcomings in the techniques and instruments used in evaluation. In health education, evaluation has many roles, but those principally concerned with students usually fall into one of four categories: health behavior, health status, health knowledge, and health attitudes. What are some techniques used in the measurement of these aspects of desirable change?

EVALUATING HEALTH BEHAVIOR

Health behavior describes those actions customarily taken by an individual which have to do with and affect his health and that of his family and other social communities. The goal of health instruction is to influence that behavior favorably. It is important to distinguish behavioral changes in this context from those sought as an outcome of achievement of a behavioral objective. In the latter case, the word "behavior" refers to the intellectual skill or process being learned or reinforced, such as "interprets," "defines," or "analyzes." It is the difference between *ends* (health behavior) and *means* (behavioral objectives)."Health practice" is used interchangeably with "health behavior," and for some it may be helpful to use the first instead, as a means of differentiating between the two ideas.

Evaluating health behavior is far from easy. Behavior can only be assessed at any one point in time at best, however valid the instrument employed, and generalizations based on one observation are notoriously unreliable. To add to the problem, there is the difficulty involved in observing or determining actual health practice. If the only feasible means of ascertaining what an individual actually does about one or more aspects of his health depends upon self-report as elicited in questionaires, interviews, or behavior inventories, the data may be strongly biased by unconscious or conscious "bending" of the truth. The respondent may report his behavior in terms of what he has learned he *ought* to do (or as he does when he does what he ought to do); or in terms of what he thinks you would *like* him to say that he does. Conversely, he may take a certain delight in saying he does certain things for the shock value or as braggadocio (smokes marihuana, for example) although it may not be true.

Certain informal procedures can be used to gather information supplementing that gathered through such structured means, of course. Casual observations of student behavior in the classroom or about the school, on the playground or athletic field, or in the cafeteria or lavatory may yield information about individuals that might be identified as critical incidents or that might be used in anecdotal records. Such notations are facilitated by using a prepared check list or form for recording significant data.

Students should be encouraged to bring issues they find interesting to the attention of the teacher and the class, thus giving tangible evidence of their interests or concerns. Whenever possible, the teacher should talk informally with students and their parents on an individual basis, or with other school personnel who might have differing perceptions of behavior reflecting the success or failure of health instruction. Continuing insights into real needs and understandings will always be evident to the teacher sensitive to the outcomes of his teaching strategies. All of these kinds of findings add to the data used in evaluation, not only of the students, but of the teacher and the course.

A weakness inherent in some techniques for measuring behavior is their dependence on verbal descriptions of selected practices. Words do not mean the same things to all people. For example, self-report instruments often require the respondent to judge the frequency of given behaviors as a part of the analysis. The individual might be asked to indicate whether he smokes cigarettes (1) always, (2) usually, (3) sometimes, (4) seldom, or (5) never. One can place considerable faith in the validity of the first and last alternatives, given that the answer is truthful, but the remaining three are heavily dependent on one's interpretation of their meaning. One individual's "usually" may mean that he smokes only four to five cigarettes, another's that he smokes a pack or more every day. One person's "seldom" may mean that he too smokes four to five cigarettes every day, another's that he smokes only once or twice a month. Unless the directions for each query are carefully designed to ensure uniformity of meaning for each option, the results are of dubious value. Yet to design such a fail-proof instrument is nearly impossible if it is to be reasonably comprehensive and still economical in the time required for its administration.

Another frequent problem is the irrelevance of what is measured to health behavior. It is not unusual to find that a true-false test of facts about vitamins, other nutrients, and their functions has been used to appraise achievement of an objective such as "to know how to plan a nutritious diet." Information of the sort tested is essential to achievement of the objective; but in the absence of evaluation procedures designed to assess ability to use those facts in planning a diet, there is no assurance that the student knows how to plan a nutritious diet. Success in teaching facts can just as easily promote unthinking, rote behavior as sound health practices. To the dismay of her teachers, it was recently found that a former student was spending one fourth of her weekly food budget on breakfast bacon! The reason given was that she had been taught that breakfast was a very important meal and that a "good" breakfast consisted of bacon and eggs, orange juice, and cereal.[2] She had learned certain facts well and even incorporated them into her behavior, but she had not learned problem solving. She could recite the ingredients of a specific good breakfast, but she had not learned to identify any other breakfast foods that would be just as nutritious but within her means. Such an outcome is to be expected when teaching is content rather than process oriented. Overemphasis on content is reflected in the measurement techniques used in most classrooms. Analysis of typical teacher-made tests indicate that eight out of ten measure knowledge of specifics only.[3]

Finally, because health behavior does not begin or end in the classroom, and because some behaviors cannot be evaluated during school years, the outcome of some instruction may not show up for many years or may never be measured in any way. Attitudes and practices in regard to cigarette smoking may only change twenty years later, when a warning twinge of chest pain reminds the adult smoker of some things he learned about the effects of smoking while in school but which seemed too remote a problem at the time to be of concern. The influence of the study of concepts of marriage and family privileges and responsibilities upon behavior cannot be evaluated until the individual marries, and then only in part. These values are deferred and they are in many ways unique to health education in comparison with other disciplines. No classroom evaluation procedures can reveal such long-rage outcomes of health instruction. All one can do in evaluating the health behavior of students is to try to assess immediate results. Even so, it is difficult to know what outcomes result from the course and what from other influences such as peer-group pressures, advertising campaigns, and other community forces.

EVALUATING HEALTH STATUS

Most tests of student health status are the responsibility of physicians, psychologists, nurses, or other trained specialists. Only a very few simple screening tests for acuity of vision and hearing or measurements of height and weight are ever appropriate or expected of teachers. Procedures for making these kinds of tests are described in Chapter 12. However, every teacher should be alert to signs of ill health or disability affecting the performance and motivation of a student. Not only should signs such as a pallid or flushed appearance, marked weight loss or gain, or obvious distress be noted, but straining to see or hear, and inattention that might be traced to those problems. Abrupt negative personality or emotional changes, and changes in achievement and study patterns provide clues to health status as well. Teachers who work with the same students every day are, next to parents, those most able to observe such signs and report them to the school nurse or other person indicated by school policy.

EVALUATING HEALTH KNOWLEDGE

Health knowledge is that aspect of health instruction that the teacher can be most effective in evaluating. That all outcomes and expectations for health instruction cannot be measured precisely does not mean that the measurements which *can* be made are not useful and meaningful. And, although we have argued that information alone does not assure that the individual will choose wisely among health influencing behaviors, neither can it be denied that information is basic to a reasoned choice. If a person does not *know* that a vaccine is available for measles, he may never become immunized or see that his children are immunized. If he does not *know* what fluoridation is and what it can mean to dental health, he is ill equipped to vote intelligently for or against fluoridation measures proposed for his community.

– procedures in planning evaluation of instruction We have said that specification of instructional objectives in behavioral terms not only facilitates but assures the validity of related evaluation procedures. Validity, of course, means that the test measures what it is supposed to measure. If instructional objectives are ambiguously stated, or perceived only as introductory embroidery for a unit or lesson plan to be forgotten thereafter, then they might just as well not be stated at all. But when they are thoughtfully defined, based upon data derived from examination of the sources of curriculum decision-making, objectives provide a blueprint for what is to be evaluated and how it might be done.

Described simply, an evaluation activity, as a part of the instructional process, represents one side of a theoretical triangle, the other two being a given instructional objective and the teaching strategy or strategies designed to implement it. These three aspects of instruction might be expressed as three related questions: (1) Where are we going? (the objectives), (2) How can we get there? (the learning opportunities), and (3) Did we get there? (the evaluation procedures). Specification of objectives, then, is a necessary first step in planning the kind of instruction in which evalution is not only the means of appraising success or failure but also a contributing factor in instruction. Indeed it is difficult to separate objectives and evaluation, for implicit in an objective should be the activity acceptable as evidence of its achievement. In fact, some instructors find it easier to decide first what skills and knowledge they wish students to be able to demonstrate as a result of instruction and then to write behavioral objectives that describe the abilities and knowledge. Teaching strategies are the means by which the instructor builds a bridge between the desired behavior and the behavioral objectives.

Again, the objective specifies a behavior and a content to be learned. The teaching strategies are designed to give all of the students enough opportunities to practice the behavior in connection with the content as to make it possible for the learners to achieve the objective. Evaluation activities should be procedures designed to give the student a chance *to demonstrate that he can in fact now display a particular skill in dealing with a particular area of health information*—and not something else entirely. That is to say, if the objective were to stipulate that he should be able to infer causal relationships between specific social problems and drug-abuse behavior, then he might be given a description of people in given social situations and asked to infer what drug-abuse problems might result. Or he might be given a description of a drug-abuse problem and asked to infer what social conditions might have contributed to it. Such an objective is *not* evaluated by giving a student a test designed to measure his ability to describe the chemical components of heroin, marihuana, or barbiturates, the effects of such substances on the human body, or the legal complications attending their use.

TESTS AND MEASUREMENTS

The stated objectives of any educational program are generally concerned with effecting a change, whether it is in attitude, perception, skill level, or amount of knowledge. The measurement of change is usually based upon the difference between some preinstruction scores or observations (pretests) and those obtained subsequent to instruction (posttests). Without the use of pretests it is impossible to know either how much change has occurred or if any or all of the final test scores could have been made due to prior learnings without any instruction at all.

It should be remembered that a test cannot measure all that is encompassed in a course. A test is only a sample of an individual's achievement and as such can only give an estimate of what he knows about the material. Many things can affect his showing: the emotional climate of the classroom, his health status at the moment, social plans of his family or of the school that day or week, and even the kind of breakfast eaten by the student that morning. The most significant effect upon a test score, however, is made by the kind of questions the test asks.

Formal measurement techniques are usually more structured than informal measures and may be either performance or written tests. Performance tests of achievement are designed to provide an objective estimate of a student's proficiency in performing some motor ability. Their use is relatively limited in health instruction, but, for example, where first aid is included in their scope, such tests can be used effectively to measure ability to employ emergency techniques such as bandaging or rescue breathing. And, of course, there is always the toothbrushing technique demonstration.

Written tests in health instruction can be either standardized or teacher made. Standardized tests are important when the reference group must be larger than a class, for example, when we wish to know how the learning that has taken place in a particular classroom compares with that of other individuals in all schools in a community or state. Standardized tests are carefully planned and refined to ensure maximum validity and reliability Such tests are usually supplemented with norms established through extensive administrations. Teacher-made tests cannot be so painstakingly constructed, but both depend upon careful planning, creativity, knowledge of the subject material, and skill in item construction.

The validity of tests developed by teachers is often less than desirable. Common faults include ambiguity, lack of precision, and triviality of the content measured. Examples of some of these faults, along with suggestions for improving test items will be provided, although it is beyond the scope of this discussion to give comprehensive instruction in test construction. Some very excellent texts on measurement presently available are listed in the additional readings at the end of the chapter. One of the best is the third edition of Thorndike and Hagen's *Measurement and Evaluation in Psychology and Education.*[4] In addition to the fact that their descriptions of test construction techniques are carefully developed and easily understood, most of the examples given are directly concerned with health instruction.

Teacher-made tests are usefully categorized by Thorndike and Hagen as either free response or structured response.[5] A free-answer test is defined as one in which the student uses his own words, organizes his own answers, and responds in his own writing to a relatively small number of questions. The merit of the results is judged more or less subjectively; but the test requiring the most subjective judgment is the least structured of the tests, the essay test. Tests with structured responses are those in which the student can only select his answer to an item from a limited number of alternatives provided by the test writer: the student responds to as many of a large number of items as he can within the alloted time and receives a score for each correct answer according to a standard key.

Free-response tests require recall of information in order to prepare an answer, whereas structured responses appear to depend only upon a student's ability to recognize the correct answer among those offered. When skillfully constructed, however, both kinds of tests demand recall and reasoning. Whether a given response represents rote recall or reasoning depends also upon how the student has been taught, not solely upon how the question is asked. When facts are the focus of instruction, facts will be the end product as well. This is perpetuated in evaluation by course-specific questions. Statements are often lifted from the textbook, especially in the case of completion and true-false items, so that only the person who has been specifically taught to recognize what is being asked can answer the question. An example of such a question is: "Cold vaccines are ———." The answer to that could be a great many things, but chances are its author accepted only one, the one in the book or the one identified in class as correct. In what forms may tests be constructed within these two categories? Brief discussions of those most often used follows.

FREE RESPONSE TESTS

– the essay test

Essay tests take less time to prepare than do objective tests, but they require much more time to score. However, good essay questions are not easily written. First, they should ask the student to exhibit the cognitive skill or process stipulated in the instructional objective. If it was "compare" then the question should ask him to compare—not list or describe or discuss. The question should be written in such a way that he is not asked simply to parrot information, but instead must use it in a novel situation to solve the problem posed by the question.

A poorly constructed essay item is more apt to measure a student's ability to figure out its meaning than his knowledge about it. A question such as "Discuss the importance of various locations of accidents" is not only impossibly global but baffling as well. Does it mean to itemize locations and describe their importance as a factor in the occurrence of accidents? For that matter, what does "importance" mean in this context? Should the student evaluate the incidence of accidents at given locations? Should he rank all locations with respect to the probability of an accident? How many is "various"? Is there a location where an accident could *not* occur? What is meant by discuss? The question, quoted from the teacher's manual of a college health textbook is so ambiguous and its meaning so obscure that suggestions for its improvement are difficult to offer short of discarding it and writing another.

A good way to ensure that every student will perceive the task similarly is to pose a problem situation and ask a series of questions based upon that situation. For example:

> Automobile accidents claim more lives than all other accidental causes combined. Of these deaths five of six occur among males, most of them between the ages of 15 and 24. Describe, in a short paragraph or two for each factor, how the following might contribute to those statistics: (1) age; (2) fatigue; (3) emotional state; (4) drug abuse, including alcohol; (5) environment (weather, vehicle design or fault, street lighting, etc.); (6) social forces.

An essay question so structured is more easily scored, because the possibility of misunderstanding the question is diminished, and the range of possible answers is reasonably delimited. Yet the student is given freedom in composing his answers, and the requirement that he apply knowledge about these factors to the explanation of accident occurrence among the age group for whom the complexity of the question would be appropriate makes it meaningful and relevant to the needs and interests of young adults.

Examples of more simply developed yet clearly posed essay questions are:

> There are five times as many deaths per mile due to motorcycle than to automobile accidents. Explain why this great difference exists. Describe ways the potential for accidents could be lessened for motorcycle riders.
>
> A married couple and their three small children have just moved to a large city in another state where they have no relatives or friends. They wish to locate a family physician and pediatrician. Suggest four sources of sound information about competent physicians that could be contacted. Describe ways or criteria by which physicians might be evaluated in making a selection among those recommended.

The essay test is notoriously difficult to score fairly and consistently. Many biasing factors, some of them entirely unrelated to the quality of the answers, influence the judgment process—whether a given paper is read before or after a poor or an excellent one; whether the handwriting is legible, the spelling correct, the paper neat; how fatigued the reader is when he reviews it; the skills of composition possessed by the writer; how the reader himself perceives the question; and how much he knows about the writer's personality and previous performance—all of these can bias the scoring of a paper. Some students are so skilled at putting down words that *sound* good that they are sometimes able to disguise how little they know by their eloquence. Judges tend to vary in their evaluation of the same papers from one time to another. Research shows that the same paper can be given every grade from *A* to *F* by different judges. And, besides the fact that it is such a laborious, time-consuming task to read a great number of essay tests, so few questions can be asked that the sample of student achievement obtained may not fairly represent an individual's grasp of the material.

The advantages of essay questions are that they give the student an opportunity to show his ability to analyze a problem and prepare a solution in his own words and more or less at his own pace. Some students do not perform at their best under pressure to read and answer a great many questions, nor do they enjoy being restricted to only a few prestated options in choosing their answer.

Scoring is facilitated when the item is constructed so that a set of criteria for its evaluation can be predetermined. Papers should be read without noting who has written each to avoid a subjective "set" on the part of the reader. All the answers to each question can be read at the same time and evaluated and graded for themselves alone. Another technique is to read through all the papers once quickly, sort them roughly into piles of excellent, good, fair, and poor work, and then to reread each in terms of that grouping, more carefully this time, making shifts between sorting where necessary. This helps to ensure that each paper is judged with those of comparable worth to see that its quality is really equal to, less than, or better than the others in that particular category.

– short-answer and completion tests

The short-answer test item is a more restricted form of the free-answer test. It may be composed of very specific questions that can be answered with one word or a short sentence such as:

> Amino acids are components of which class of nutrients? ———
> Give an example of a voluntary health organization. ———

Completion items are similar to the short-answer question but are usually written as incomplete statements rather than questions. The student supplies the missing words. The following is an example of this kind of item.

> When a person is very afraid or angry, the adrenal glands, which are located above the (kidneys), produce a special hormone called (adrenalin) or (epinephrine).

The advantages of short-answer and completion tests compared to the essay test are that they are more easily and quickly scored and that a great many more questions can be asked, providing a better sample of the student's knowledge, yet the respondent is still preparing his own answer and must recall the information needed to do so. Because these kinds of tests must be so specific, they are best used in testing factual material such as dates, definitions, and terminology, and are not useful in appraising problem-solving skills. How accurately the answers can be evaluated depends upon the way the items are written. Teachers sometimes unwittingly reward rote recall and penalize thinking when only one answer is considered correct—the one associated with the statement in the book—when actually several other responses might be equally correct, as illustrated earlier. Some other weaknesses to be guarded against in constructing items include overemphasis on trivial information (for example, "The first year that manufacturers made seat belts available to new car buyers was (1949)." or omission of inconsequential words for example, "The first teeth to (erupt) usually are lower incisors.") Items written so that the desired answer is factually incorrect, such as "Insulin is a hormone manufactured by the (pancreas)," should, of course, be avoided. A better item would be "Insulin is a hormone manufactured by the islands of Langerhans, which are located in the (pancreas)". No item should omit so many words that what is left of the statement is incomprehensible as a question. For example, "The disease that causes ——— and is characterized by increased ——— within the ——— is called ———. The missing words are "blindness," "pressure," "eye," and "glaucoma," but as it stands, the item is more of a guessing game than a test of knowledge. A better statement would be, "The leading cause of blindness among adults in the United States is a disease called ———."

Scoring of the short-answer or completion test should not be done solely by key, but by a person competent to judge when alternative answers may be equally appropriate or correct.

– structured response tests

Tests that require the student to choose among already prepared alternative answers to questions are usually termed "objective," although only the scoring procedures are objective. Actually, subjective judgment is involved in devising these tests, influencing selection of the material considered important to be measured as well as the choice of the "best" answer. The most commonly used objectively scored tests are the true-false tests, the multiple-choice tests, and the matching-items tests, all of which are discussed below.

True-False Tests / The true-false item is simply a statement that the student is to read and judge one way or the other. It could be described as a two-response multiple-choice item, although the opposing alternative is unstated. Such an item may be written in a slightly different form so that the correct answer would be "yes" or "no" or "right" or "wrong." Another variation is to require the respondent to say *why* an item marked false is so or to correct any items judged false. This is an effective means of cutting down the effects of guessing but of course increases the scoring time.

True-false items are probably those most often encountered. They appear to be the easiest to write but are actually very difficult to construct so that they are unequivocally true or false, unambiguous, and yet concisely stated. Their best use is in testing a single fact, especially when this is so clear-cut that a multiple-choice with four or five plausible distractors is virtually impossible to devise.

There are the usual pitfalls into which the careless or inexperienced test writer can fall. Too often, statements from the textbook are used as is or doctored with a negative word to make them false. If it can be safely assumed that every statement in the book is correct, this is probably one way to be sure that the test items also are correct. However, dependence on such a procedure places undue emphasis on rote recall or recognition, and the items may be overconcerned with trivia as well. Words such as "all," "never," "always," and "only" are often employed as a means of making a statement false, and testwise students are comfortably aware of this fact. Another tip-off is the effort to qualify a true statement so carefully that the result is a markedly longer statement, which advises that this one is probably true. Another device is to use qualifying words such as "the best way to," "the most successful method of," "the chief reason," which forces the student to make a judgment when he has no way of knowing what other alternatives were considered. The most aggravating fault in true-false construction from the student's point of view is the attempt to *trick* the respondent into missing the item. A test should be for the purpose of measuring what students know, not a contest in which the goal is to outwit them with obscure or trick items. For example, how many would mark this item false? "A new born infant is judged stillborn when no heartbeat can be detected, there is no indication that he is breathing, and there is no visibile muscular movement." If the student said "true," he would be wrong according to the instructor who wrote and used this item. "I never catch nurses on this one," he chortled. "They know that if any *one* of them is true, the child is stillborn. It's false because you don't need all three signs." Not only did he intend to trick, but he was wrong. A statement is not false because it is even more fully supported by data than need be.

Ambiguity is a frequent fault. An item such as this is puzzling: "The best way to help a drowning person is to jump into the water and save him." Most certainly the best way to help a drowning person is to save him—but is that "best way" only associated with the part about jumping into the water? The student must decide and can only hope that he has guessed right. Another favorite gimmick is to make the correct answer dependent on knowledge of some unessential word, as in the statement "Xerophthalmia results from lack of Vitamin D." This item is not really testing anything but the student's familiarity with the first word. And what has that to do with health behavior except in the most trivial sense?

These are but a few of the pitfalls to be avoided in writing true-false items. Many of them are also true of all structured response tests, whether multiple choice or matching items, which are a variation of the latter. The alternatives in multiple-choice tests are actually a cluster of true-false statements relative to a given premise or "stem."

Multiple-Choice Tests / A multiple-choice question consists of a posed idea or problem called the stem and usually four or five possible responses or distracters, from which the respondents choose one best or correct answer. The stem may be written either as a statement or as a question. When a statement is used, the responses are ordinarily written so that they fit into and complete the sentence, as for example:

> Results of current medical research provide strong evidence to show that: (1) cigarettes made from pipe tobacco are milder and less harmful; (2) filter tips decrease tars to a harmless amount; (3) the longer the cigarettes the less harmful the smoke; (4) cigarette smoking is a principal cause of lung cancer; (5) mentholated cigarettes are less harmful than others.

An advantage of the multiple-choice items is that the desired one does not have to be the one true answer, although it does have to be defensibly the best among the alternatives provided. It can be constructed in such a way as to elicit problem-solving skills such as interpretation, analysis, application, and other cognitive processes as well as recall of knowledge. Construction of this kind of test is perhaps the most demanding of time. In a sense, each item represents four or five questions depending on the number of alternatives. A fifty-item multiple-choice test is the equivalent of a two hundred fifty question true-false test if there are five distracters used. This factor adds to the reliability. The more choices offered by an item the greater the reliability of its results as evidence of whatever is being measured. Of course, reading time is also increased, which can lead the student to make errors when he may actually have known the answer. When more than one alternative may be true, as in the case of the best-answer item, students often choose the first good answer without reading on to find the best one.

The most challenging task is to construct four or five distracters that are so plausible that only the individual who really knows the answer can choose among them sensibly. A distracter so unreasonable that not even someone guessing would choose it is termed "nonfunctioning." If the test writer is not careful, so many distracters may be nonfunctioning that the remaining choices dwindle to but two or three. For example: "Between 1940 and 1961, automobile accidents (1) were due to drinking drivers; (2) caused a million deaths every year; (3) decreased; (4) increased; (5) were greater on four-lane than on three-lane highways."

The first, second, and fifth options are clearly illogical, which brings us down to but two choices. Other faults illustrated are that the five options are not logically interrelated, so the two that do function are set apart at once from the others, and that the stem does not define the problem clearly enough for the respondent to know what to look for. The stem must include enough of the statement so that a problem is posed and the alternatives are readably short.

Matching-Item Tests / This type of test is really a variation of a multiple-choice test in which for each item in a list of terms, topics, or other elements a choice is made from another list of words that describe, define or otherwise relate to the items in the first list. Usually a list of terms is placed to the left and a list of alternatives to their right. The alternatives list should be longer than the other to prevent an automatic right answer to the last item for those who answer the other items correctly. The second list should not be longer than fifteen or so items so as to complicate and unnecessarily lengthen the search for the matching answer. In order to maximize the need for exact knowledge as a basis for discriminating among items, all of the words or statements in the first list should be homogeneous rather than an assortment of unrelated words or ideas. Finally, the directions should clearly explain what is to be done. An example of a matching test follows:

Number each item in column I to correspond to the item in column II with which it is most closely associated.

I	**II**
___Syphilis	1. Vision
___Glaucoma	2. Tumor
___Diabetes	3. Heart
	4. Spirochete
___Coronary	5. Insulin
___Sarcoma	6. Virus

Matching tests are best used to measure factual information such as definitions, terminology, or parts of something as in labeling parts of the heart or locations of glands.

– evaluating tests Textbooks on measurement can provide many more good suggestions for constructing well-designed tests, but no test is so good that it need not be evaluated and constantly revised for improvement. A practical way to do this is to study the results of its administration. Analysis of the responses to a multiple-choice test quickly reveals which distracters are not functioning, and these should be rewritten or replaced before the test is used again. Another valuable kind of information can be gained by looking at the results to see which items have been missed and which wrong answers have been chosen by many students. The first tells the teacher a great deal about misunderstanding when the items are used as a pretest; and the second tells a lot about the success of his teaching when the items are used as a posttest. In addition, the errors on pretest administration can be used for a basis of lesson planning. Two other valuable ways of evaluating a test are to try it out first on other teachers to check for ambiguities or errors and to go over each item with the students who have just taken it. The second not only serves as a valuable learning opportunity for the students, but it reveals weaknesses in the test. The outcome may be momentarily shattering to the teacher's ego, but the information gained can be effectively used to improve the items. Above all, when reviewing the test with students, the teacher should not be reluctant to listen to honest complaints about items and, if necessary, adjust test scores where they have been affected by ambiguities or errors.

In speaking of the classroom teacher and the teacher-made test, Diederich says:

> Teachers should not be in a position merely to declare that students are improving or not improving. They ought to contrive situations in which they will be trying to find out whether improvement occurs, and how much. In other words, they should approach the task of evaluation not with the arrogance of a judge but with the humility of an inquirer. The proper frame of mind for evaluation is fear and trembling. Then, if everything turns out all right, the relief of the teachers should be even more stupendous than that of the students.[6]

EVALUATING HEALTH ATTITUDES

Attitudes are harder to evaluate than other things. There are several sources of information about a person's attitudes, but all of them are subject to errors of perception and interpretation. First, the teacher can ask the individual himself what his attitudes are about certain subjects. However, although no one knows better than he what they may be, self-report is not always a reliable source. The person may wish to conceal some negative attitudes, and he may view some of his beliefs not as attitudes so much as truths. Second, the teacher can get opinions about a student's attitudes from his peers and parents and other adults who know him, but parents are understandably biased and so may others be. Another clue to attitudes is to observe an individual's reactions to certain issues or people. How one feels about something has a lot to do with the way he behaves. Again, however, the implications of observations, like beauty, depend upon the eye of the beholder.

There are some standardized written and projective tests that appear useful. Few, if any, of the written tests are presently available in published form, and use of projective tests such as the Rorschach and the Thematic Apperception Tests require the specialized training of a psychometrist or a psychologist with extensive experience in using these instruments. Some use has been made of semantic differential testing techniques in studies of attitudes.[7] In the main, written health-attitude tests ask the respondent to indicate his opinions or feelings relative to certain health behaviors or issues. Most written tests have been constructed in the form of the unstructured completion test or the structured multiple-choice. The first might be expected to be more evocative of attitudes than one in which some few alternative attitudes are offered from which the student picks one that may or may not accurately reflect his actual beliefs.

EFFECTS OF EVALUATION

Evaluation can have both positive and negative effects. A good evaluation activity should be as much a learning opportunity as it is a test. It enables the learner to discover his own areas of strength and weakness and, if he is provided quick knowledge of results, gives him satisfaction in his strengths while adding to his knowledge in weaker areas of study. Motivation for learning is increased when evaluation is treated as a tool for estimating present progress with mastery as the goal or for gauging total progress as an outcome of many such steps put together.

When evaluation procedures are used as a threat, they can have negative results not only on learning but on the students themselves as well as their perception of the course and the learning process. The pressure of examinations, especially when they are used to establish positions on an arbitrarily set grading curve (which assumes in advance that so many *A*s will be balanced inevitably by a like number of *F*s) can be motivating for a few. For too many others, the result is frustration, dependence on cramming, concentration on "psyching out" the teacher rather than on the joy of learning, and examination-taking tricks, cheating, or defeat and apathy. Examination procedures, whether for quizzes or finals, should be carefully planned so that their effect will be in all ways positive. The results of evaluation should not only be increased learning and desire to learn, but a feeling of reward and satisfaction in the activity for both teacher and students.

Bloom suggests that there are several necessary conditions if this is to happen.[8] First, the examinations must be concerned with those aspects of the learning which both teacher and students believe to be important and worthwhile, as well as directly related to the desired learning. Second, the evaluation must be objective, in that the results are not biased by the feelings of the scorer, and valid in that the range of things tested is comprehensive enough to permit the student to give a representative sample of his achievement. You cannot validly appraise an individual's knowledge in any one area of health instruction on the basis of two or three objective items such as true-false, multiple-choice, or completion sentences. It is always entirely possible, whatever the outcome, that two or three other items which might also have been used could have yielded quite the opposite results. Third, the results should be defined in terms of each student's achievement relative to the objectives rather than according to everybody else's performance on the test. After all, it is entirely possible, and desirable as well, that every student attain mastery of any objective judged appropriate to his needs and abilities. Bloom adds another consideration to these three:

> In addition to these elements, a well-designed examination with adequate previous indications to the student of what is to be expected of him can leave the student with a feeling that his preparation for it was eminently worthwhile. Such an examination can make the preparation for the examination an important learning experience if it requires him to bring the parts of the subject together in new ways—that is, if the examination causes him to interrelate and integrate the elements of the subject so that he finally perceives them in ways different from the ways he experienced them as he learned the parts or elements separately.[9]

EVALUATING TEACHING RESOURCES

– written materials A wealth of written materials, produced by voluntary health groups, industrial organizations, public health agencies, and other such interested associations are available for use in the classroom. The problem is not to find enough current pamphlets, booklets, and other supplementary printed matter for health instruction, but how to select those most relevant and acceptable among them. Very often a school or district will have an established policy that teachers must follow in choosing these materials for use in the classroom. Where no clear-cut guidelines have been established, the accompanying evaluation of health education material developed by the School Health Activities Committee of the Tuberculosis and Respiratory Disease Association of Los Angeles County could be adopted and applied with confidence.[10]

Evaluation of Health Education Material

Sample Policy

The Board of Education (Trustees) has found that there are many free and inexpensive materials available for school use for health education purposes.

The Board has further found that such materials need to be reviewed and evaluated in terms of their appropriateness and their potentials for helping children and youth achieve the understandings, attitudes, information and skills necessary to promote and maintain health.

Therefore, the Board recommends that the Superintendent of District appoint an evaluation committee which would periodically review new materials and re-evaluate materials in current use which might be outdated.

Members of this committee should include (1) an administrator; (2) a curriculum consultant; (3) an instructional aid specialist; (4) a teacher; and (5) representatives from the medical and dental professions to check for accuracy.

Health Education materials are appropriate when they meet the following objectives:

1 They are scientifically accurate and are free from bias.

2 They contribute to the development of critical thinking and use logical rather than emotional or propaganda techniques.

3 They are directed toward positive health practices.

4 They stimulate interest in the topic or lesson and provoke desirable pupil activity.

5 They reinforce other materials and the time involved in their use is justified.

For more effective evaluation, the following check list form has been devised as an objective appraisal instrument.

Sample Criteria

A. *Suitable Material Meets All of These Criteria*	*Yes*	*No*
1. Is appropriate to the course of study	_____	_____
2. Is a reinforcement of other materials	_____	_____
3. Is significantly different	_____	_____
4. Is impartial, factual, and accurate	_____	_____
5. Is up-to-date	_____	_____
6. Is non-sectarian, non-partisan, and unbiased	_____	_____
7. Is free from undesirable propaganda	_____	_____
8. Is free from excessive or objectionable advertising	_____	_____
9. Is free or inexpensive and readily available	_____	_____

B. *Pamphlets*	*Excellent*	*Good*	*Fair*	*Poor*
1. Readability of type	_____	_____	_____	_____
2. Appropriateness of illustrations	_____	_____	_____	_____
3. Organization of content	_____	_____	_____	_____
4. Logical sequence of concepts	_____	_____	_____	_____
5. Important aspects of topic stand out	_____	_____	_____	_____
6. Material directed to one specific group such as teachers, pupils or parents	_____	_____	_____	_____
7. Reading level appropriate for intended group	_____	_____	_____	_____
8. Based on interests and needs of intended group	_____	_____	_____	_____
9. Positively directed in words, descriptions and actions	_____	_____	_____	_____
10. Directed toward desirable health practices	_____	_____	_____	_____
11. Minimal resort of fear techniques and morbid concepts	_____	_____	_____	_____
12. In good taste, avoids vulgarity, stereotypes and ridicule	_____	_____	_____	_____
Total Rating	=====	=====	=====	=====

C. *Posters*				
1. Realistic and within experience level	_____	_____	_____	_____
2. Appeals to interest	_____	_____	_____	_____
3. Emphasizes positive behavior and attitudes	_____	_____	_____	_____
4. Message clear at a glance	_____	_____	_____	_____
5. Little or no conflicting detail	_____	_____	_____	_____
6. In good taste	_____	_____	_____	_____
7. Attractive and in pleasing colors	_____	_____	_____	_____
Total Rating	=====	=====	=====	=====

D. *Recommended for Use*

1. For use by:
   a. pupils ☐ b. teachers ☐ c. parents ☐ d. adults ☐

2. Appropriate grade level:
   a. primary ☐ b. elementary ☐ c. junior high school ☐ d. secondary ☐
   e. college ☐ f. adult ☐

E. *Not Recommended For Use*

Why Not? ______________________________

Date: ______________________ Evaluated by: ______________________

– audio-visual media Films, filmstrips, slides, transparencies, records, and tape recordings should be previewed by the teacher before their use in a classroom. Factors or qualities essential to note include the length of time required for effective use of the medium involved; its appropriateness for the students for whom it is intended (vocabulary, subject matter, relationship to the needs and interests of this age group, and so forth); its relevance and potential contribution to the behavioral objective; its scientific accuracy; and the major points demonstrated or emphasized in its message.

EVALUATING TEACHING EFFECTIVENESS

Possibly the most reliable gauge of teaching effectiveness is the amount of change that can be measured in the students' performance. Theoretically, most students should be brought to the point of mastery of every instructional objective identified by teacher and students as worth studying. Bloom believes that for most students, aptitudes are predictive of rate of learning rather than achievement and that given enough time and appropriate types of help, the grade of *A* could be achieved by about 95 percent of our students.[11] Bloom also suggests that teaching effectiveness needs to be evaluated on the basis of ability to present, explain, and order the elements of the learning task for the individual student in such a way that he can master it rather than, as at present, in terms of degrees of mastery symbolized by grades of *A* through *F*.

Such an outcome may not yet be a reality in most classrooms (and such is our conditioning to the grading system that a teacher who awarded 95 percent of his students an *A* would be regarded with consternation), but it is surely an ideal toward which a teacher should strive. Vopni suggests the following self-evaluative questions to be used by teachers as an ongoing means of measuring teaching effectiveness.

Were the objectives achieved?

Were the goals realistic?

Did I interpret the feedback?

Was I willing to modify the goals?

Did pupils become progressively more self-directing?

Were the objectives comprehensive? Did they include the less tangibles? Did I find ways to evaluate some of the long-range goals?

Did I change my plans and procedures because of the feedback from the evaluation?

How did I modify the goals, the content and resource materials, the space-time environment and constraints, or the opportunities for social interaction?

Did I make the objectives clear? Did I permit the students to contribute to the formulation of new goals?

Where did I seek help in improving instruction?[12]

These are only some of the questions, she admits, and suggests that teachers can think of many others that could be asked of themselves.

EVALUATING THE PROGRAM OF INSTRUCTION

It may safely be assumed that any progressive, well-taught, and scientifically sound course of study will be productive of results in the lives of students. There is evidence that both the integrated and the correlated plans have done well in broadening the base of student knowledge about health matters, just as there is ample reason to believe that a well-taught course in health education is a useful and productive experience. Not all courses of study, however, are equally good. They need evaluation. As stated earlier, the process of evaluation is essentially the same whether we are evaluating a student's progress, a lesson, a unit, a course, or an entire curriculum. The only real difference depends upon *what* is being evaluated and whose values determine the criteria applied. All of the techniques heretofore described can yield data to be used in formative evaluation of organized programs of instruction, whatever their level of remoteness from the learner. Indeed, formative evaluation is probably the only valid form of evaluation of actual instruction. Most courses have many goals that are not fixed but dynamic over time. Summative evaluation is therefore nearly impossible. Nor is it possible to evaluate a program of instruction without at the same time considering the teacher who is carrying it out and the student who is learning it.

Being of necessity structured and relatively static, formal documents or written plans for courses, units, or lessons are easily evaluated. Payne suggests the following guideline questions for the evaluation of plans or curriculum guides:

1 Does the plan provide the outline for organization and sequence of the course or curriculum area?

2 How specific is the treatment of subject matter? (unit topics, daily topics, specific examples, etc.)

3 Does the plan include specific activities for students? If so, are the activities described in sufficient detail to suggest what the student is actually to do and the related cognitive process? What is the general emphasis in types of activities described?

4 Does the plan give specific activities or methods for teachers? What is the general emphasis in types of activities?

5 Does the plan specify the materials to be used in instruction? Are there descriptions of what is to be done with the materials?

6 Are there any explicit statements about the nature of learning and the conditions under which it occurs? (e.g., statements about motivation, learning environment, maturation and capacity, cognitive processes)

7 Are there any explicit views on the structure of the subject matter? Are the criteria for selecting and organizing subject matter and materials given?

8 Is there a statement of objectives or desired results of instruction? To what degree of specificity have these been developed? (course, unit, or activity)

9 What are the suggested purposes for evaluating students? What evaluation methods are recommended? Are the specific procedures given? Is there a proposed schedule for evaluation? What suggestions are provided for the analysis and the use of the results of evaluation?[13]

Payne adds that two evaluative criteria are inescapable in analyzing curriculum plans—clarity of meaning and internal consistency. One important check on internal consistency is to compare the stated objectives with the learning opportunities and evaluation procedures suggested for their implementation. Clarity depends upon the care with which terms used to describe these aspects of the document have been defined. And where this important quality is neglected, it is not possible to judge the validity of any curriculum decisions at all.

A BIBLIOGRAPHY OF TESTS

To evaluate the end products of instruction, or to establish a base line for planning future instruction at a higher level, one must either construct and validate one's own test or use one of those already standardized by others. There are a number of carefully developed instruments available currently, some of which are listed below.[14]

Elementary School

1 Adams, Georgia S., and Sexton, John A., *California Tests in Social and Related Sciences,* Part III, Related Sciences, Test 5, Health and Safety, Monterey, Calif., California Test Bureau, 1953.

For grades 4 through 8, this 75-item test is composed of true-false and multiple-choice items designed to measure knowledge in the health and safety areas. Norms and a manual of directions are available. This test is one of a battery of subject matter tests in the sciences for the upper elementary grades.

2 Crow, Lester D., and Ryan, Loretta C., *Health and Safety Education Tests,* revised, Brookport, Ill.; Psychometric Affiliates, 1960.

For grades 3 through 6, this 90-item multiple-choice test was constructed to measure a student's knowledge, application of rules, understanding of cause and effect, and ability to select the best habits in health and safety areas. Norms and teacher's directions are available.

3 Dzenowagis, Joseph G., *Self-Quiz of Safety Knowledge,* Chicago; National Safety Council, School and College Department, 1956.

This test, consisting of 40 safety misconceptions, is designed to measure safety preparedness at the fifth and sixth grade levels. See "What's Your Safety I.Q.?" *Safety Education,* 36; 6–7 (November 1956), for a description of the test.

4 Klein, Walter C., *A Health Knowledge and Understanding Test for Fifth Grade Pupils,* La Crosse, Wis.; Northern Engr. and Mfg. Co., 1960.

This test has two forms and is composed of 60 best-answer type items. Norms and T-scores are developed. Refer to: Klein, Walter C., "Development of a Health Knowledge and Understanding Test for 5th Grade Pupils," *Research Quarterly,* 32; 530–537 (December 1961).

5 National Safety Council, *Bicycle Safety Information Test,* Chicago; National Safety Council (n.d.).

This is a 20-item true-false test suitable for use at the elementary level.

6 Speer, Robert K., and Smith, Samuel, *Health Test,* Brookport, Ill.; Psychometric Affiliates, Form A revised 1960, Form B revised 1957.

This test, for grades 3 through 8, has two forms and was designed to test the student's judgment, understanding, and knowledge of health facts. Multiple choice and problem-type questions are used. Norms and teacher's directions are available.

7 Yellen, Sylvia (Edward B. Johns, Consulting Ed.), *Health Behavior Inventory: Elementary,* Monterey, Calif., California Test Bureau, 1962.

This 40-item picture-question inventory is designed for grades 3, 4, 5, and 6. Personal health habits, nutrition, safety, rest and relaxation, dental health, cleanliness, and disease prevention are some of the areas included.

Junior High School

8 Adams and Sexton, *California Tests in Social and Related Sciences,* See entry 1.

9 Colebank, Albert D. (Edward B. Johns, Consulting Ed.), *Health Behavior Inventory: Junior High,* Monterey, Calif., California Test Bureau, 1962.

This 100-item test for grades 7, 8, and 9 evaluates health behaviors (25 items), attitudes (25 items), and knowledge (50 multiple-choice items).

10 Kilander, H. Frederick, *Information Test on The Biological Aspects of Human Reproduction,* 3rd ed. (mimeographed), Staten Island, N.Y., Dr. Glenn Leach, Wagner College, 1968.

This 33-question multiple-choice test is for junior high school through college levels. Norms are available. Single copies may be obtained free from Dr. Glenn Leach. The test is included in the Teacher's Manual for *School Health Education,* 2nd ed., New York, Macmillan, 1968.

11 ———, *Information Test on Drugs and Drug Abuse,* 3rd ed., Staten Island, N.Y.; Dr. Glenn Leach, Wagner College, 1968.

This 25-question multiple-choice test is for junior high school through college levels. Norms are available. Single copies may be obtained free from Dr. Glenn Leach.

12 ———, *Information Test on Smoking and Health* (mimeographed), Staten Island, N.Y., Dr. Glenn Leach, Wagner College, 1964.

This 25-item multiple-choice test is for junior high school through college levels. The questions are based on the Surgeon General's Report on *Smoking and Health.* Norms are available. Single copies may be obtained free from Dr. Glenn Leach.

13 ———, *Nutrition Information Test,* 5th ed. (mimeographed), Staten Island, N.Y., Wagner College, 1968.

This 33-question multiple-choice test is for junior high school through college levels. Norms are available. Single copies may be obtained free from Dr. Glenn Leach. The test is included in the Teacher's Manual for *School Health Education,* 2nd ed., by the author, New York, Macmillan, 1968.

14 Lawrence, Trudys, *Getting Along: Grades 7, 8, 9,* Temple City, Calif., 6117 North Rosemead Boulevard, 1964.

This instrument, for the evaluation of emotional health, consists of 45 situation-response items with multiple-choice answers. Original line drawings are used to illustrate the two forms of the test. Norms (3,114 pupils) and other information are available in an accompanying Teacher's Manual.

15 Schwartz, William F., *Achievement Test on Syphilis and Gonorrhea,* Durham, N.C.; Family Life Publications, 1965.

This is a 25-item multiple-choice test, reprinted from Schwartz's *Teacher's Handbook on Venereal Disease Education,* which is published by the American Association for Health, Physical Education, and Recreation.

16 ———, *Teaching Test on Syphilis and Gonorrhea,* Durham, N. C.; Family Life Publications, 1965.

This is a 50-item multiple-choice test, reprinted from Schwartz's *Teacher's Handbook on Venereal Disease Education,* which is published by the American Association for Health, Physical Education, and Recreation.

17 Shaw, John H., and Troyer, Maurice E., *Health Education Test: Knowledge and Application,* Brookport, Ill.; Psychometric Affiliates, Form A revised 1956; Form B revised, 1957.

For grades 7 through 12 and college freshmen, this 100-item test has two forms consisting of multiple-choice and true-false items. Knowledge and the application of knowledge are tested. Some physical education items are also included. Norms (based on over 6,000 students in various sections of the United States) and a manual of directions are available.

18 Speer and Smith, *Health Test.* See entry 6.

19 Thompson, Clem W, *Thompson Smoking and Tobacco Knowledge Test,* Mancato, Minn., Mancato State College, 1963.

This 25-item multiple-choice test was constructed from the concepts that had previously been established by experts as the most important facts in the physiological, psychological, and socio-economic areas of smoking and tobacco. The word difficulty of the test was established and found suitable at or above the seventh grade level. Refer to Thompson, Clem W., "Thompson Smoking and Tobacco Knowledge Test," *Research Quarterly,* 35; 60–68 (March 1964).

20 Veenker, C. Harold, *A Health Knowledge Test for the Seventh Grade,* Lafayette, Ind., the author, Purdue University, 1960.

Two test forms, each consisting of 70 multiple-choice items, were constructed. Printed forms and a test manual are available from the author. Refer to Veenker, C. Harold, "A Health Knowledge Test for the Seventh Grade," *Research Quarterly,* 30; 338–348 (October 1959).

Senior High School

21 Dearborn, *College Health Knowledge Test.* See entry 38.

22 Kilander, H. Frederick, *Information Test on the Biological Aspects of Human Reproduction.* See entry 10.

23 ———, *Information Test on Drugs and Drug Abuse.* See entry 11.

24 ———, *Information Test on Smoking and Health.* See entry 12.

25 *Kilander Health Knowledge Test,* 6th ed., Staten Island, N.Y.; Wagner College, 1966.

This instrument, designed for high school and college students and adults consists of 100 multiple-choice items representing nine areas of health knowledge. Norms are available.

26 ———, *Nutrition Information Test.* See entry 13.

27 LeMaistre, E., Harold, and Pollock, Marion B. (Edward B. Johns, Consulting Ed.), *Health Behavior Inventory: Senior High,* Monterey, Calif., California Test Bureau, 1962.

A multiple-choice instrument for senior high school students, consisting of 75 health behavior situation items focused upon problems met by students of this age.

28 McHugh, Gelolo, *Sex Knowledge Inventory,* Form Y, Durham, N. C., Family Life Publications, 1959.

Form Y of this inventory measures understanding of the human reproduction system and vocabulary relating to sex. It is suggested that this form could be used at high school, college, and adult levels. An instructor's manual and norms are available.

29 ———, *A Venereal Disease Knowledge Inventory,* Durham N. C., Family Life Publications, 1966.

This is a 52-item multiple-choice test. High school and college norms are available and a teacher's guide is being prepared.

30 New York State Council on Health and Safety Education, *Health Knowledge Examination for the Secondary Level,* developed by a committee of the council, 1962.

This test consists of 80 multiple-choice items. Sample test copies may be obtained from John S. Sinacore, State University College, Cortland, N.Y.

31 Schwartz, William F., *Achievement Test on Syphilis and Gonorrhea.* See entry 15.

32 ———, *Teaching Test on Syphilis and Gonorrhea,* See entry 16.

33 Shaw and Troyer, *Health Education Test: Knowledge and Application*. See entry 17.

34 *Test Your A. Q.* (*Alcohol Quotient*), Chicago; American Medical Association, Committee on Medicolegal Problems (n.d.).
This is a 20-question true-false test that provides a basis for a good discussion at the senior high and college levels.

35 Thompson, *Thompson Smoking and Tobacco Knowledge Test.* See entry 19.

College

36 Bridges, A. Frank, *Health Knowledge Test for College Freshmen,* Brookport, Ill.; Psychometric Affiliates, 1956.

This 100-item multiple-choice test measures knowledge in thirteen health areas. Norms (based on over 3,000 college freshmen from seventeen states) and a manual of directions are available.

37 Crawford, Marilyn, *Madison Health Knowledge Test,* Harrisonburg, Va., the author, Madison College, 1964.

This 100-item multiple-choice test was designed to measure knowledge in 11 health areas. T-scores and percentiles, based on 1,600 test scores, are available. The college population upon which norms are based was largely freshmen, female, and from the state of Virginia.

38 Dearborn, Terry H., *College Health Knowledge Test,* revised, Stanford, Calif., Stanford Uinversity Press, 1959.

One hundred multiple-choice items test knowledge in 11 health areas. Norms and a manual of directions are available. Although designed for the college level, this test is said to be suitable for senior high schools offering a full semester course in personal hygiene.

39 Gaines, Josephine. *Student Self-Appraisal Inventory of Interests and Estimated Knowledge in Major Health Education Areas,* mimeographed by the author, Department of Health and Physical Education, Staten Island Community College, New York, N.Y.

Although useful primarily in planning content in the college health education course, the knowledge portion of this inventory could be used in evaluating the change in extent of knowledge following teaching in specific health areas.

40 Leonard, Margaret L., and Horton, Clark W., *An Inventory of Certain Practices on Health,* Sacramento, California State Department of Education, 1949.

This inventory was developed for use at the college level by the California Community Health Education Project. Its 88 statements can be used to study actual health behaviors from the standpoint of the student's practices and also from the standpoint of the extent to which certain illnesses or health problems become a part of the pattern of behavior. An instructional manual is available.

41 ———, *An Inventory of Points of View Related to Health,* Sacramento; California State Department of Education, 1949.

This inventory, developed for college students by the California Community Health Education Project, consists of 109 statements that provide an opportunity for determining student attitudes on individual and public health.

42 ———, *Reactions to Certain Situations Related to the Health of Elementary School Children,* Sacramento; California State Department of Education, 1949.

This situation-response type inventory was designed to be used with preservice or inservice teachers at the elementary level. Consisting of 102 items, it explores opinions concerning the role of the teacher in the school health program. An instructional manual is available.

43 McHugh, *Sex Knowledge Inventory.* See entry 28.

44 ———, *A Venereal Disease Knowledge Inventory.* See entry 29.

45 Meise, William C, *A Scale for the Measurement of Attitudes Toward Healthful Living,* the author; Slippery Rock, Penn., Slippery Rock State College, 1962.

This Likert-type scale consists of 100 items and was constructed to evaluate opinions in twelve health areas. An instructor's manual is available. Consult the author about quantity purchases.

46 Reid, Carmen Patricia (Edward B. Johns, Consulting Ed.) *Health Behavior Inventory: College Level,* Monterey, Calif., California Test Bureau, 1966.

This test consists of descriptions of a number of health problems on which 100 multiple-choice test items are based.

47 Shaw and Troyer, *Health Education Test: Knowledge and Application.* See entry 17.

48 Southworth, Warren H., *An Inventory for Study of What College and University Students Know and Do About Health Services and Facilities,* Evanston, Ill., The American College Health Association, 1966.

This three-part inventory consists of 156 multiple-choice items. Student use of services and facilities is investigated in Part I by means of 76 items, whereas the 56 items in Part II relate to student information about services and facilities. Part III consists of 24 personal data items. Copies of the inventory may be purchased from ACHA. Refer to Southworth, Warren H., "An Inventory for Study . . . ," *Journal of the ACHA,* 15; 33–49 (October 1966).

49 *Test Your A.Q.* (*Alcohol Quotient*). See entry 34.

50 Thompson, *Thompson Smoking and Tobacco Knowledge Test.* See entry 19.

SUMMARY

Evaluation is a process of reaching decisions and involves description and judgment as opposed to measurement, which is descriptive only. Evaluation should not be just a terminal or summative activity, but a continuing procedure contributing to curriculum improvement as well as to student learning and motivation. The roles of evaluation are diverse, but those concerned most closely with students are health behavior, health status, health knowledge, and health attitudes. Other areas of concern within the scope of instruction are evaluation of health materials, audio-visual media, teaching effectiveness, and the total program. In this chapter techniques and procedures for the evaluation of changes in the learner were discussed and criteria for the appraisal of teaching materials, teacher effectiveness, and curriculum plans were provided.

NOTES AND REFERENCES

1 Michael Scriven, "The Methodology of Evaluation" *Perspectives of Curriculum Evaluation,* Chicago, Rand McNally, 1967, pp. 40–41.

2 James H. Myren, "It's Happening Now," Report of the Health Education Parent Participation Project, Tucson, Ariz. 1970.

3 Richard Burns, "Objectives and Content Validity of Tests," *Educational Technology,* December 15, 1968, p. 18.

4 Robert L. Thorndike and Elizabeth Hagen, *Measurement and Evaluation in Psychology and Education,* 3rd ed., New York, John Wiley, 1969.

5 *Ibid.,* p. 50.

6 Paul B. Diederich, "The Classroom Teacher and the Teacher-Made Test," *Educational Horizons,* Washington, D.C., Pi Lambda Theta, 1964, p. 20.

7 Charles E. Osgood, George J. Suci, and Percy H. Tannenbaum, *The Measurement of Meaning,* Urbana, University of Illinois Press, 1957.

8 Benjamin S. Bloom, "Some Theoretical Issues Relating to Educational Evaluation," *Educational Evaluation: New Roles, New Means,* Chicago, The National Society for the Study of Education, 1969, p. 46.

9 *Ibid.,* p. 47.

10 Barbara M. Osborn and Wilfred Sutton, "Evaluation of Health Education Materials, *Journal of School Health,* 34, 2 (February 1964), 72–73.

11 Benjamin S. Bloom, "Learning for Mastery," *Evaluation Comment,* Los Angeles, University of California, Center for the Study of Evaluation, 1968.

12 Sylvia Vopni, "What is Evaluation?" *Educational Horizons,* Phi Lambda Theta, Winter 1968–1969, p. 80.

13 Arlene Payne, *The Study of Curriculum Plans,* Washington, D.C., NEA, 1969, pp. 10–13.

14 Adapted from Marian K. Solleder, *Evaluation Instruments in Health Education,* Washington, D.C., American Association for Health, Physical Education, and Recreation, 1969.

SELECTED READINGS

Ahmann, J. S., and M. D. Glock, *Evaluation of Pupil Growth,* 2nd ed., Boston, Allyn & Bacon, 1963.

Ahmann, J. S., Glock, M. D., and Wardeberg, Helen L., *Evaluating Elementary School Pupils,* Boston, Allyn & Bacon, 1960.

Beatty, Walcott H. (ed.), *Improving Educational Assessment* and *An Inventory of Measures of Affective Behavior,* Washington, D.C., Association for Supervision and Curriculum Development, 1969.

Buros, Oscar (ed.), *The Sixth Mental Measurements Yearbook,* Highland Park, N.J., Gryphon Press, 1965.

———, *Tests in Print,* Highland Park, N.J., Gryphon Press, 1961.

Curriculum Innovations and Evaluation, Proceedings of the Association for Supervision and Curriculum Development, Pre-Conference Seminar, Princeton, New Jersey, Educational Testing Service, 1968.

Davis, Frederick B., *Educational Measurements and Their Interpretation,* Belmont, Calif., Wadsworth, 1964.

Ebel, R. L., *Measuring Educational Achievement,* Englewood Cliffs, N.J., Prentice-Hall, 1965.

Educational Testing Service, *Multiple Choice Questions: A Close Look,* Princeton, N.J. Educational Testing Service, 1963.

Garrett, H. E., *Testing for Teachers,* 2nd ed., New York, American Book Co. 1965

Hunkins, Frances P., "Bloom's Taxonomy as a Test Construction Guide," *Ideas Educational,* Kent, Ohio, Kent State University, 1966.

Lindquist, E. F. (ed.), *Educational Measurement,* Washington, D.C., American Council on Education, 1963.

Marshall, Jon C., and Powers, Jerry M., "Writing Neatness, Composition Errors and Essay Grades," *Journal of Educational Measurement,* Summer 1969, pp. 97–101.

McLaughlin, Kenneth F., *Interpretation of Test Results,* Bulletin no. 7, Washington, D.C., U.S. Department of Health, Education and Welfare, 1964.

National Society for the Study of Education, *Educational Evaluation: New Roles, New Means,* Chicago, University of Chicago Press, 1969.

Rosenshine, Barak, "Evaluation of Instruction," *Review of Educational Research,* 40; 2 (April 1970), 279–300.

Thorndike, Robert L., and Hagen, Elizabeth, *Measurement and Evaluation in Psychology and Education,* 3rd ed., New York; John Wiley, 1969.

Tyler, Leona E., *Tests and Measurements,* Englewood Cliffs, N.J.; Prentice-Hall, 1963.

Tyler, Ralph, Robert Gagne, and Michael Scriven, *Perspectives of Curriculum Evaluation,* Chicago, Rand McNally, 1967.

Veenker, Harold C., "Evaluating Health Practice and Understanding," *Journal of Health, Physical Education, and Recreation,* May 1966, pp. 30–32.

Webb, Eugene J., Donald T. Campbell, Richard D. Schwarz, and Lee Sechrest, *Unobtrusive Measures: Nonreactive Research in the Social Sciences,* Chicago; Rand McNally, 1966.

Wilhelms, Fred T. (ed.), *Evaluation as Feedback and Guide,* Washington, D.C.; Association for Supervision and Curriculum Development, 1967.

Wood, Dorothy Adkin, *Test Construction,* Columbus, Ohio; Charles E. Merrill, 1961.

CHAPTER 7 PROFESSIONAL PREPARATION AND RESPONSIBILITIES

As educators, all teachers share concern and some responsibility for the health education of their students. Health education in this context includes the instructional aspect that is the focus of the foregoing chapters in Part One of this book and health services and healthful school environment, which are discussed in the chapters comprising Part Two. A teacher cannot safely or effectively undertake responsibility for these three aspects of the total school health program without professional preparation.

We have said that learning depends upon the health of the learner. All teachers need to be sensitive to environmental and health care problems and able to solve or assist a student to find solutions for any that appear to diminish his chances for success and enjoyment in learning. All teachers need to be aware also that experiences with health problems and issues are learning experiences—and that health practices or attitudes exhibited by teachers can sometimes be more instructive, whether in a positive or a negative sense, than the words they utter. Whether one is an elementary school teacher, school nurse, school health educator, administrator, physical education instructor, or teacher of any subject whatever, there are certain areas of competence and knowledge that should be common to the professional preparation of all.

CORE AREAS OF COMPETENCE

Generally speaking, *all* teacher preparation programs should include experiences that equip prospective teachers and school administrators with competencies in the following apsects of health education.

1 Application of generally accepted concepts of educational principles, techniques, and evaluative procedures to specific health education objectives

2 Thorough analysis and understanding of the physical, social, and emotional growth and development characteristics of children and adolescents, including those special to exceptional or handicapped children

3 Development of a sound foundation of information and basic principles of healthful living as well as practice in identifying new scientific data relating to personal and community health as they are developed or discovered

4 Familiarity with the role and functions of the separate aspects of the total school health program as each relates to the others and to the total educational process and purposes

5 Knowledge of basic techniques of counseling and guidance as they pertain to health problems of children and youth

Although we have said that every teacher is responsible for the health education of his students, this is not the same as saying that any teacher can serve effectively as a professional health educator. No one suggests that a well qualified health teacher would be just as interested in or competent to teach physical education, yet the reverse assumption is very nearly universal among school administrators and even among parents and other teachers. This is an outcome of the long association of the words "health" and "physical education" and the reluctance of some teacher preparation institutions to recognize that the two disciplines have for a long time been distinct in their preparation, subject matter, methodology, and requirements. Sliepcevich points compellingly to the fact that although a physical education major might wish to make health science his minor field of specialization (or vice versa) such a choice should not be forced upon him. She urges that both physical education and health education majors should be free to decide which other subject areas they wish to emphasize:

> In our professional preparation programs where realistically a second field of competency is an asset for the beginning teacher, the student should not have to buy the "health and physical education" package. He should select one or the other for his specialized field of concentration and then be free to choose a second field in which he has interest, for which he has enthusiasm, and in which he has a chance of succeeding. The second field may well be the other area of our concern, but a choice has been made, rather than an ultimatum issued. The profession of physical education should recognize the fact that physical educators have

> been the scapegoats for many of the inadequacies in health education and poor health instruction and consequently their public image has not been helped. Far too many physical educators have been expected to become health teachers because they had no choice in the matter. Confronted with heavy and energy-consuming teaching assignments in physical education, burdened with additional responsibilities in coaching and intramurals, they have had the additional pressures of teaching and preparing for a subject which requires time to prepare and time to teach; a willingness to read extensively and continually; and which demands a strong conviction about the values of health education for all students.[1]

A nationwide survey of present practice in assigning responsibility for health teaching at the secondary level in school districts of all sizes in 1964 revealed that an individual with a combined health and physical education major was designated as health teacher in 65 to 80 percent of all junior high schools, and in 60 to 90 percent of all senior high schools. In the remaining proportion of secondary schools investigated, most health instruction was assigned to individuals who were physical education majors only.[2] Yet college catalogs detailing requirements for a major in physical education, or for a combined major where this is the only alternative, clearly reveal the paucity of course work in health science required of persons enrolled in these programs.

Until recently, unfortunately, personnel in health education have *had* to be drawn from other fields, mostly from physical education as we have shown, and from nursing, home economics, and the biological sciences. This has been due to a self-perpetuating circumstance linked to supply and demand. Because school administrators have tended in the past to view health instruction as a "frill," they have given it low priority in curriculum and staffing decisions. Owing to this lack of demand for teachers with major specialization in health teaching, many teacher preparation institutions have neglected to offer separate programs or any adequate preparation for health teaching at all.

Now, however, the demand for competent health teaching specialists is mounting rapidly. New legislation in New York State, for example, called in 1970 for thousands of fully qualified health educators. Other states, sparked perhaps by growing drug-abuse problems, the increased visibility given health education by national health curriculum projects, and cries for relevancy in curriculum planning emanating from the students themselves, are giving new attention to the effectiveness of present health education provisions and staffing practices. This increased need for qualified health teachers has led in turn to the establishment of numbers of new programs in colleges and universities across the country. As of 1970 there were one hundred four different institutions in thirty-one states offering either undergraduate, graduate, or both programs in health education.[3] These figures reflected an increase of twenty-eight institutions in a period of but three years and five more states reported one or more programs under development or pending approval. Just fourteen states (Alaska, Delaware, Hawaii, Idaho, Kansas, Maine, Mississippi, Montana, New Hampshire, North Dakota, Oklahoma, Rhode Island, South Dakota, Wyoming, and the District of Columbia) reported no programs at any level offering specialization in health education.

In addition, twenty-six institutions in fifteen states offer programs in community health education, with still others currently preparing innovative curriculums that will ready students to be comprehensive health educators able to function on a joint appointment basis between school and community agencies or capable of serving in either capacity as desired.[4]

HEALTH EDUCATION RESPONSIBILITIES

Those persons with the most specific responsibilities for school health education include elementary teachers, secondary teachers, health educators, school nurses, school physicians, and school administrators. Each of these requires special preparation for his role, not only as a planned outcome of his preservice professional preparation but as an essential continuing process. The dichotomy previously existing between preservice and inservice educational programs has given way to the newer concept of continuing education as a way of life, not just for teachers but for all adults.

Colleges and universities must prepare teachers who are not only committed to their need for continuing education but have learned the skills needed to do so. It is often said that teachers teach as they have been taught. Teachers of teachers must be innovative and also must focus upon process rather than memorization of facts if they are to turn out innovative teachers who are skilled in teaching rather than telling. Such an emphasis on process should be fundamental to any teacher preparation program, whatever the subject matter.

THE ELEMENTARY TEACHER

Because most elementary schoolteachers have direct responsibility for the health instruction in their classroom, and because these are the years when health attitudes and practices are most easily shaped, teachers at this level need to be especially well prepared. Unhappily, many students enrolled in elementary teacher preparation programs are not provided even a basic course in personal health. Recent studies show that prospective elementary schoolteachers hold a wide range of health misconceptions.[5] Elementary schoolchildren also have many health misconceptions,[6] and it may be that these have been learned in school. As Jesse Helen Haag says, "Most certainly if they were learned elsewhere, the misinformed teacher is not equipped to correct them."[7]

Experience has shown that most undergraduate curriculums for the preparation of elementary teachers do not give adequate preparation for health teaching. At a minimum, elementary teachers need a solid background of knowledge about personal and community health science and problems; methods of teaching health; growth and development characteristics of the young child; and the role of the school health program in promoting the total educational effort. Some of this background may be provided as an outcome of the general undergraduate program designed to fulfill specific state certification requirements. Too often, however, there is little consistency between certification requirements and teaching responsibilities. For example, most states have mandated the teaching of the harmful effects of alcohol, tobacco, and dangerous drugs in every grade, yet few states, if any, require that teachers must be prepared to give such instruction.

The interested teacher (and elementary teachers are typically vitally concerned with their students needs and interests) can broaden his grasp of the subject matter and methodology of health teaching by continuing to study on his own, or by participating in workshops, seminars, and other such structured experiences that may be available to him. Many colleges and universities, official, voluntary, and professional agencies, and health-concerned industrial organizations such as the National Dairy Council, Metropolitan Life Insurance Company, National Livestock and Meat Institute, and others provide educational materials and opportunities for teachers. Another source of continuing education is the vast amount of free literature available to interested teachers. Requesting that one's name be placed on mailing lists of printed material distributed by various health organizations, seeking the service and assistance offered by the health education section of the local or state departments of health or education, and consulting with nearby secondary school health educators or college health education faculty are other possible ways of meeting professional interests and needs of teachers.

THE SECONDARY TEACHER

Other than health education and physical education majors, few secondary schoolteachers receive any professional preparation relative to their responsibilities to the school health program. All secondary teachers have legal and professional responsibilities for the health and health instruction of their students, but few recognize this fact.

A survey of the health knowledge of over 200 teachers in all grades routinely charged with first aid and formal and incidental health teaching in New York State disclosed that a majority of this group, too, held a wide range of misconceptions about health. The conclusion was that teacher-training institutions should assume a major role in correcting this deficiency in future graduates. "If preparation in first aid and health education for the classroom teacher is viewed as a trivial or unnecessary burden by these institutions, then the level of expectation or proficiency may be insufficient to meet the daily needs of the educational setting," said the investigators in their report.[8]

Secondary teachers need to know and accept their role as members of the chain of communication in referring remediable health problems hindering the progress of students in their classes and as health teachers when some immediate interest makes health-related investigations or discussions particularly meaningful. Opportunities for guidance come to all school personnel, not just to health educators or nurses, for there is no aspect of life to which health is not central. Few young people get through the adolescent years without moments of stress adversely affecting their health and school achievement. For example, the boy whose overinvolvement in extracurricular activities causes his grades to slump and who is having troubles at home for a variety of reasons needs understanding and help if he is not to wind up so emotionally disturbed that he fails—or worse. And the girl whose premarital pregnancy causes great distress at school and at home will need help if she is to be able to handle any of her problems effectively. Less dramatic, perhaps, but nevertheless significant pressures affecting health and learning ability are common among students. Whatever the conflict or problem that makes a student seek the help of a respected teacher, that teacher is far better equipped to offer effective counsel and guidance if he is aware of the importance of his role in this aspect of the school health program and given some preparation to assume it. Every teacher needs to be alert to changes in patterns of behavior, appearance, or attitude in any of his students. Each student is his own norm, in a sense. A teacher needs to make observation a continuing process for this reason, not so much as a mechanical routine but as a sort of special sensitivity to change. For some individuals this sort of sensitivity seems to be God-given. For most of us it must be learned.

Hence, all secondary teachers need learning experiences enabling them to develop the core areas of competence described earlier. Such competencies are not easily acquired or to be casually accepted. They are central to the development of an understanding of the ramifications and interrelationships of the total educational program and process. The responsible secondary schoolteacher cannot afford to be without such competencies if he hopes to obtain the best results from his teaching and from his relationships with his students.

THE HEALTH EDUCATOR

Because health science is a multidisciplinary field, a health education specialist needs a general education program that provides experience in many fields including the social sciences and the physical and biological sciences. The basic general recommendation is that all teachers of health in the secondary school should be certified in health education as a separate subject. The following are specific certification standards for teacher preparation in health education recommended by the National Conference on Teacher Preparation in Health Education of the American Association for Health, Physical Education, and Recreation.

> The preparation of the health teacher should include courses in the biological sciences (such as human biology, anatomy, physiology, and bacteriology), the physical sciences (especially chemistry), and the behavioral sciences (such as psychology, sociology, and cultural anthropology).
> Minimum professional preparation requirements for certification in health education should include appropriate study in the following specific areas.
>
> 1 The school health program, including the areas of healthful school environment, health services, and health instruction.
>
> 2 Mental, emotional, and social health; alcohol, drugs, and tobacco.
>
> 3 Dental health, vision, hearing.
>
> 4 Emergency care including first aid.
>
> 5 Safety education, including occupational, home, and recreational safety; man-made and natural disasters.
>
> 6 Community health, including such aspects of environmental health as air pollution, water pollution, and radiation; fluoridation; agencies promoting community health; official, voluntary, and professional health agencies and organizations.
>
> 7 Nutrition in respect to health education, including knowledge of basic food nutrients, wise selection and use of foods; obesity and weight control; food faddism, food fallacies and controversial food topics.
>
> 8 Disease prevention and control, including the communicable and the degenerative diseases, and chronic health disorders.
>
> 9 Family life education, including human sexuality, and the psychosocial and cultural factors promoting successful marriage and family relations.
>
> 10 Consumer health, including intelligent selection of health products and health services, agencies for consumer protection,

misconceptions and superstitions concerning health, and health insurance plans and health careers.

11 Study in methods and materials for health instruction.

12 Student teaching in health education.[9]

Minimum standards for professional preparation were also defined by the members of this conference but preceded by the cautionary statement that specifics, competencies, and task responsibilities must always be viewed as an ever changing and emerging configuration resulting from the dynamic interaction among current social forces, values, and technological advances.

Some of these standards are the following:

There must be professional preparation in the specialized areas of:

1 Biological and behavioral sciences and their relation to health, for an understanding of the human organism from the biological standpoint and an understanding of man's ecology—man's interaction to society.

2 Health affairs, issues, and problems of the individual in society, with consequent identification of leading health problems and understanding and knowledge in this area.

3 Human growth and development and its relationship to health, with an understanding of the principles of growth and development and utilizing and relating these knowledges to the health instruction program.

4 Modification and reinforcement of behavior in understanding the principles of behavior modification and reinforcement, and applying learning opportunities that may favorably affect behavior.

5 The teaching process in health education, in the (a) formulation and utilization of specific instructional objectives, (b) organization of health content, (c) development and utilization of effective learning opportunities (methods, materials, techniques), and (d) evaluation of all aspects of the teaching-learning process with special concern for expected outcomes.

6 Modern concepts of health and health education for an understanding and development of these concepts, an understanding of the structure and functions of school-community health programs, and formulation of affective points of view in harmony with modern concepts of health and health education.

7 Health information and resources in order to evaluate the reliability and validity of health information and resources and identify the significance of emerging health problems and issues.

Specifically, the health teacher should have the ability to utilize understandings and to assist in solving emerging ecological health problems, including:

1 Factors which promote optimum health.

2 Health economics or consumer health.

3 Utilization of the services of voluntary, professional, and official health agencies and organizations in the community.

4 Interpretation of health information through biostatistics.

5 Human sexuality and social adjustment.

6 Bases of disease control, including problems such as air, water, and soil pollution, radiation, and immunology.

7 Dynamics of health behavior and an appreciation of its complexity.

8 Health counseling.[10]

Other recommendations for those preparing for health education careers have included experiences in physical education, recreation, and accident prevention and also professional laboratory experiences, including systematic observation, initial limited participation, full participation, student teaching, and field work in community health agencies.

THE NURSE

Because school nursing requires knowledge and skills in both the field of nursing and of education, graduation from an accredited nursing school as well as possession of a baccalaureate degree with a school health education major might be the best preparation. Tipple suggests that nursing preparation should be at the baccalaureate level and that school nurses should be qualified beyond that through appropriately planned master's degree programs.[11] The specific area of specialization at the graduate level would be expected to provide necessary understanding of school nursing principles and practice so that the nurse might apply her basic nursing skills effectively in the school situation.

Guidelines were proposed by the National League for Nursing as standards for the preparation of school nurses as follows:

> The role of the nurse in the school is to utilize, in collaboration with others, her knowledge and competence in nursing so that it contributes significantly to the achievement of the full health and educational potential of each student. Her ability to serve most adequately within the school setting is dependent upon basic preparation for professional nursing . . . and additional preparation that will enable her to:
>
> 1 Utilize concepts of human growth, development, and behavior in the milieu of the school health program.
>
> 2 Recognize development and health needs of students, especially in relation to prevention, detection, and treatment, which must influence educational programming.
>
> 3 Utilize existing community services for children and youth and spearhead the development of additional services when indicated by the needs of the school health program.
>
> 4 Comprehend the nature of the educational setting in which the school nurse works.
>
> 5 Select and use processes appropriate to the roles assumed by the school nurse.[12]

The role of the school nurse is changing, however. Ford believes that instead of being illness-oriented, school nurses should be wellness clinicians and that their basic preparation should stress growth and development concepts, counseling and guidance, behavioral and social sciences, advanced nursing practice, the educational processes, and much more. She suggests that three concurrent specific directions are needed in the future preparation for and practice of nursing in school settings: the development of a practitioner of nursing who (1) works intensively with pupils and their families to assess levels of wellness, using highly sophisticated conceptual, human, and when necessary, technical skills to do so; (2) applies epidemiological and demographic methodologies to achieve goals of preventive nursing; and (3) has the sort of statesmanlike stature and skill in public policy arenas needed to guide and influence the direction of the field.[13] Coleman, too, urges renewed emphasis on preventive nursing rather than on the concept of a nurse who waits passively for sudden illness or injury demanding her services . . . or the occasional service as a resource person for health educators.[14] More detailed discussion of the functions and roles of the school nurse will be found in Part Two, Chapter 11.

THE PHYSICIAN

An adequate knowledge of the goals and processes of education is highly desirable for the school physician. He must, of course, possess a valid state license to practice medicine, but it is to be hoped that he has in addition some understanding of the school health program and his role as a member of the school health team, as well as the total school curriculum and its requirements. As a school physician his role is primarily that of a practitioner, but he serves importantly as a consultant, counselor, and advisor as well. Special training in public health, pediatrics, and child psychology are particularly valuable. Above all, a school physician should have a deep interest in children and a desire to help them gain as much from their school experience as possible.

Whether school physicians are employed full time, part time, or serve on a volunteer basis, the qualifications for this kind of service are, in a sense, unique. Medical schools are beginning to appreciate the necessity for orienting medical students to the problems and practices involved in school health programs in order to prepare them for future advisory relationships. In addition, the role of the physician as a health educator is being given increased attention as a part of the medical training of all physicians.

A recently completed study of school physician behavior showed that despite a wide variation in professional characteristics, their activities in the school are remarkably similar because they appear to comply closely to central administrative directions. Perhaps the most critical factor influencing the effectiveness of the school physician, then, is the quality of personnel in leadership positions in health service programs. It would seem that the additional training of these latter key individuals is most essential to the success of the functioning of school physicians. The function and roles of the school physicians will be explored in detail in Part Two, Chapter 11.

THE ADMINISTRATOR The attitudes of the principal of a school, the district superintendent, and even of key administrators at state and national levels are crucial to the kind and amount of health education provided the students whose education is affected by their decisions. Mayshark's study of six large city and county school systems showed quite clearly that the quality of school health programs is related to the nature of administration involved. It was demonstrated that the perception of the extent of the health problems, the administrative action needed to solve these problems, and the amount of money spent for health education are all directly related to the strength of leadership given by the top administrators. Mayshark recommended that a course in the administration of school health programs should be included among the requirements for a school superintendency.[15] Such a requirement should be made a part of any administrative credential or training program.

An understanding of the purposes of the school health program and acceptance of leadership in its functioning are surely requisites for the responsible school administrator. Increasing recognition of this fact is demonstrated by a spate of recent significant publications, statements, and recommendations supporting school health education coming from state school administrators, and important organizations such as the prestigious American Association of School Administrators and the National School Board Association. The following is a recent statement published by the permanent Joint Committee of the above two groups:

> The Committee recommends a coordinated attack on all health problems with a comprehensive health education program extending from K through 12 and encompassing the total scope of such a program.
>
> Such a program places a responsibility on local school boards and administrators, state departments of education, and teacher training institutions to provide qualified teachers, adequate time for instruction, authoritative and up-to-date materials, and supervisory assistance for health education commensurate with other curriculum offerings.[16]

The competencies of any school administrator need to include those recommended at the beginning of this chapter for all educators, plus a keen awareness of the significance of the optimal health of each teacher to the success of the teaching-learning process. Few colleges or universities as yet offer courses designed to prepare administrators to assume this area of their responsibility, but acceptance of the need for such courses is unmistakable in the literature of the field of administration.

THE NEED FOR CONTINUING EDUCATION

Regardless of the nature or extent of one's specific responsibilities, a fundamental problem is keeping up to date with accurate, meaningful health information. The need for lifelong learning is by no means unique to health education, owing to the dynamic nature of knowledge, but nowhere is it more critical. Armer expands the Peter Principle (which holds that every employee in a hierarchy tends to be promoted until he reaches his level of incompetence) to include the Paul Principle, which avers that "individuals often become, over time, uneducated and therefore incompetent at a level at which they once performed quite adequately." The dilemma thus described becomes every year more crucial as the amount of available information becomes even greater.

Gardner insists that continuing education is essential to the kind of self-renewing society fit for free men, which is the American dream. He says:

> Education can lay a broad and firm base for a lifetime of learning and growth. The individual who begins with such a broad base will always have some capacity to function as a generalist, no matter how deeply he chooses to specialize. Education at its best will develop the individual's inner resources to the point where he can learn (and will *want* to learn) on his own. It will equip him to cope with unforeseen challenges and to survive as a versatile individual in an unpredictable world. Individuals so educated will keep the society itself flexible, adaptive, and innovative.[17]

Professional preparation in every field of endeavor has just begun when the student leaves school, having earned the right to be a practitioner in his field. Teacher preparation must be a continuous process, beginning during the college experience and extending throughout the teacher's professional life. The health education teacher must follow a constant program of continuing education through extensive reading in professional journals and scientific literature. Current sources of data, such as the periodicals *Today's Health* and *Consumer's Reports* are a must for the specialist and highly desirable for the elementary teacher having health instruction responsibilities. The medical sections of responsible news magazines and newspapers are another good source of new information. To combat folklore and tradition preventing acceptance of new solutions to problems, to eliminate the influence of superstitions and quackery upon health behavior, and to answer the many simple everyday questions related to healthful living requires constant and selective reading of professional materials. To separate truth from fiction and fact from fancy requires the development of ability to discriminate, which can only be achieved as an outcome of broad and persistent reading in the literature of the sciences.

Certainly one mark of the professional is membership in an organization dedicated to furtherance of the goals of his specialty. There are several such associations that serve school health education. The American School Health Association is the only one, however, whose entire concern is in the school health program. The American Association for Health, Physical Education, and Recreation, and the American Public Health Association also have sections with emphasis on school health, and many school health people belong to these organizations as well. Through their journals, publications, annual conventions, and other services, the school health educator can learn much that will help keep him abreast of current trends and programs.

Attendance at relevant lectures, institutes, conferences, workshops, and other such special learning opportunities should be scheduled whenever possible. And it is recommended that teachers return to the college classroom periodically for graduate work and continued exploration of the many subject areas that constitute the multidisciplinary field of school health education. The individual who is committed to his growth as a person and as a professional cannot fail to radiate enthusiasm and confidence. No teaching technique can top a positive, dynamic approach to one's subject area. A climate for learning that reflects the teacher's vitality and fresh, continuing, personal interest is uniquely conducive to learning and translating knowledge into behavior.

NOTES AND REFERENCES

1 Elena M. Sliepcevich, "Implications of the School Health Education Study for Professional Preparation of Teachers," mimeographed paper given at the American Association for Health, Physical Education, and Recreation annual convention, Dallas, Texas, March 21, 1965.

2 ———, *School Health Education Study—A Summary Report,* Washington, D.C.; School Health Education Study, 1964.

3 School Health Education Study, *Directory of Institutions Offering Programs of Specialization in Health Education,* Washington, D.C., School Health Education study, 1970.

4 Richard Grimes *et al.,* "A Systems Approach to the Design of a Model Under-graduate Curriculum for Health Educators"; paper given at the annual meeting of the Research Council of the American School Health Association, Houston, Texas, October 1970.

5 Jessie Helen Haag, "Health Knowledge of Prospective Teachers," *Journal of School Health,* October 1963, pp. 350–353.

6 Joseph Dzenowagis and Leslie Irwin, "Prevalence of Certain Harmful Health and Safety Misconceptions Among Fifth and Sixth Grade Children," *Research Quarterly of the AAHPER,* May 1954, p. 150.

7 Haag, *op. cit.,* p. 350.

8 J. Philip Keeve and Gerald J. Specter, "Responses to a Teacher Health-Knowledge Inventory," *Journal of School Health,* October 1967, pp. 384–386.

9 National Conference Steering Committee, "Recommended Standards and Guidelines, Teacher Preparation in Health Education," *Journal of Health, Physical Education, and Recreation,* February 1969 (reprint).

10 *Ibid.*

11 Dorothy C. Tipple, "Education for Nurses for School Health Service," *Journal of School Health,* December 1963, p. 448.

12 *Ibid.*

13 Loretta C. Ford, "The School Nurse—A Changing Concept in Prepara-Elimination," *Journal of School Health,* March 1970, pp. 121–122.

14 Jane Coleman, "The Changing Role of the Nurse: An Alternative to Elimination," *Journal of School Health,* March 1970, pp. 121–22.

15 Cyrus Mayshark, "A Descriptive and Comparative Study of the Administrative Patterns Operative in Six School Health Programs," U.S. Office of Education project no. 6-8288, Knoxville, Tenn., May 1967.

16 The Joint Committee of the National School Boards Association and the American Association of School Administrators, *Health Education and Sex/Family Life Education* (pamphlet).

17 John Gardner, *Self-Renewal,* New York; Harper & Row, 1965, p. 26.

CHAPTER 8 CATEGORICAL AND CONTROVERSIAL ISSUES

As in every other discipline, curriculum decisions in health education must be based upon careful synthesis of data gathered from analyses of its body of knowledge as well as the needs of the students and the community. The problem is complicated in health education, however, by the very fact that health instruction *is* based upon student needs. Human needs are personal, often intimate, and therefore emotion charged. Probably no other area of the school curriculum finds itself the center of greater community dissension or is pressured more insistently by special interest groups. In the field of health education, special consideration of as many as thirty categorical health problems such as smoking, alcoholism, venereal disease, dental health, drug abuse, cancer, tuberculosis, heart disease, and sex education are being urged upon the schools by as many pressure groups. Other pressure groups are working just as hard to get some aspects of health education *out* of the schools.

There is more than one area of potential controversy in health teaching. One can get into an argument over almost anything, from the trivial question of how much water to drink each day to whether certain aspects of or any sex education should be taught. Principally, however, objections are most likely to be encountered in the broad areas of (1) sex education; (2) treatment of the sick; (3) administration of medical care;

(4) drug-abuse education; and (5) current and local problems such as the fluoridation of public water supplies.

Which point of view or which group should the school administrator heed? And if new subjects are added, what should be taken out, if anything, to make room for them? Choices must be made among alternatives, and choices reflect somebody's values and beliefs. The difficulty lies in designing a curriculum plan for health teaching that fulfills student and community needs and at the same time represents the values and valued knowledge of all those concerned.

Because certain aspects of human behavior are so sensitive in nature, there are some who believe that instruction about these behaviors does not belong in the classroom, whereas others are just as insistent that it does. This kind of conflict is exemplified by sex education programs. Surveys show that the great preponderance of parents favor sex education in schools. So do most physicians, psychologists, educators, and their related professional organizations. Still we find sex education courses being vigorously attacked in some areas by minorities who see it as a threat. One legislator opposing sex education in 1969 added an amendment to a proposed bill banning such instruction in the state of Louisiana which would exclude such instruction in all schools except in adult education courses, and then *only with the permission of parents and grandparents!* Proponents, on the other hand, point to increased rates of illegitimacy, abortion, venereal disease, unhappy marriage, and broken homes as justification for *separate* courses in sex education.

Increased incidence of premarital sex activity among students appears to be linked in many ways to increased use of mind-altering drugs, both behaviors being symptomatic of the emotional disturbances and rebelliousness that so alarm parents and other adults today. Not so many years ago, drug-abuse education was regarded uneasily as possibly motivating rather than preventing drug abuse. Sex education is perceived by some critics in the same way and involves a "What they don't know can't hurt them" assumption.

Today drug-abuse education is the "in" thing and thousands of hastily put together "new" drug education courses have been instituted in schools throughout the nation in an attempt to meet demands being made for such education by a concerned public. No one really knows how many students are using illegal drugs, but there appears to be an increased use of these substances either experimentally or compulsively by some young people. As a result, an avalanche of materials has been developed for use in the schools. Most of these materials describe the drugs of concern and are largely fact oriented. The irony is that study of the harmful effects of alcohol and narcotics is one of the few aspects of health instruction that has been required in most states since the 1890s, thanks to the efforts of the Women's Christian Temperance Union.

That sexual behavior and use of illegal drugs are problems of major proportions in today's society cannot be denied. In 1967 the Curriculum Commission of the Health Education Division of the American Association for Health, Physical Education, and Recreation identified family health (including problems of sexual experimentation, early marriages, early parenthood, illegitimacy, abortions, and the changing role of men and women) as a crucial health problem of the 1960s and 1970s.[1] The commission members did not then perceive the problem of drug abuse (use of marihuana and other hallucinogens, narcotics, barbiturates, amphetamines, and certain volatile substances) as being similarly crucial. However, the School Health Education Study in the same year included both areas explicitly under two of the ten broad concepts comprising the total curriculum. These two concepts were, "The Family serves to perpetuate man and to fulfill certain health needs," and "Use of substances that modify mood and behavior arises from a variety of motivations."[2] The discussion that follows recognizes that teaching about sexuality and family relationships and drug use and abuse is most effectively carried out as part of a comprehensive health education program. The intention is not to suggest that these are such distinct areas that they should be taught separately, but only that there are special problems that tend to be associated with instruction about them.

SEX EDUCATION

– what is sex education? What do we mean when we speak of sex education? Some critics perceive it solely as education in the mechanics of the sex act. "Is the School House the Proper Place to Teach Raw Sex?" trumpets Gordon Drake in a Christian Crusade publication. The implication, intended or not, is that some other place *is.* The John Birch Society urges the formation of local committees to fight "this filthy communist plot." Others have described sex education as a sinister campaign to create an unceasing and dangerous obsession with sex in the minds of children. "I'd rather have my children learn about sex in the gutter, as I did, than from the perverts who teach sex in the schools," said a world-famous satirist in a personal interview recently. Perhaps the attempt to divorce educational programs concerned with human sexuality from the rest of human health behavior invites this sort of attack. To the uninformed, "sex education" sounds as if it is education for sex, and "sex" to many is a dirty word at worst and synonymous with coitus at best. What might help rather than another attempt to sugar-coat such education with a euphemistic title is a clearly stated description of what sex education does encompass and what it seeks to accomplish. Such a description would not only improve public relations but would also clarify the goals of sex education for those who are teaching it.

Is sex education simply the physiology of the reproductive system? Is it a process of telling young people the facts of life and cautioning them about possible unpleasant outcomes of premarital experimentation? Should sex be approached with a "crime and punishment" attitude to prevent premarital intercourse, illegitimacy, or venereal disease? If our purpose is to promote chastity, will giving information about reproduction, describing the diseases transmitted sexually, and warning against the embarrassment of illegitimate pregnancy and the shame of being discovered guarantee the desired behavior choice? For all four of these questions the answer is "no."

The plain fact is that the consequences long used to frighten young people into avoiding sexual contact until after the appropriate ceremony are not as terrifying as they used to be. Rapidly changing abortion laws, the freely dispensed "pill," shifting perceptions of the necessity for chaperoning, quick, available transportation affording instant anonymity in nearby towns, confidentiality rules protecting minors who request treatment for venereal disease from public health agencies, and the effectiveness of modern drugs in quickly curing such infections are but some of the reasons for the change. The statistics on the number of brides who are pregnant before the ceremony attest to growing acceptance of and indulgence in premarital sex activity. Less than twenty years ago, a prominent film star who forthrightly bore a child whose father was admittedly someone other than her husband was so violently criticized that it was many years before she could make another picture in this country, or wanted to, for that matter. Today, this same behavior on the part of film stars is reported in the fan magazines and the press more as a matter of gossip than of scandal and effects no visible change in the popularity of the persons involved.

Not only are the old roadblocks disappearing, but society itself is changing in a way that is a cause and at the same time a result of this increased freedom of choice. Forces fanning natural desires for sexual pleasures are unceasing and unavoidable in an economy that uses sex to sell everything from automobiles to toothpaste. Today, nudity and explicitly depicted sex acts and perversities dominate the subject matter offered by the entertainment industry, and best-selling books and magazines feature what might have been termed simple pornography only a few years ago.

Sex education in its usual and narrow sense has been designed to dispel ignorance of sexual matters and to clarify misconceptions. And this is necessary. But knowledge is not enough. For example, there is considerable evidence to show that illegitimate pregnancy is often neither unexpected nor unwanted. Knowledge of contraceptive techniques or the possible outcomes of premarital intercourse will not deter the young woman determined to punish her parents or capture a husband.

Hoyman suggests that what is more appropriate today is space-age sex education—an ecologic, ethical approach involving the biologic, psychologic, social, and ethical dimensions of sexual attitudes, standards, values, and behavior.[3] Others define a modern view of sex education as education for effective living with an understanding of human sexuality as an integral, inseparable part of it. The creation of satisfying interpersonal relationships rather than simply the exercise of sex would be the goal, and it would involve the whole population and the total life span, going far beyond genital behavior to include roles and intersex expressions of love and affection.[4]

– what are some things we need in sex education today?

Basically, we need to know what we are doing![5] We need to know that delving into this area gives the teacher an opportunity to organize a rich educational experience exploring the most significant and important aspect of life. From childhood to old age man has his problems —both personal and social—as he tries to adjust himself to a society with moral standards proscribing his sexual activity. Good teaching has to be more than the transmission of static information with no relevance to ongoing problems. To affect behavior positively and to help develop an effective family member are in the long run the principal goals of sex education, and to achieve these more than the anatomy of the reproductive system is needed. It is helpful to have information about pregnancy, nocturnal emission, homosexuality, and masturbation. But, more important, it helps to have thought through the implications and responsibilities of sexual activity and determined one's own values and standards as guides *before* one is confronted with the first temptation to engage in sex play. It is useful to know something about such social problems as child neglect, child abuse and abandonment, illegitimacy, and abortion. Discussion in all of these areas is within the broad scope of sex education. How can anyone sensibly discourage the schools from preparing young people to live effectively as adults, to vote knowledgeably, and to counsel their own children in later years? To discuss such prospects as predetermination of sex, the use of artificial insemination, and reproduction without sperm or ovum, to explore the causes and prevention of divorce, or to identify the biological origins (or lack of them) of our religious and moral codes are all a part of sex education. Should we teach about the population explosion, and contraception? By all means, but, of course such discussions should depend upon the age group, existing legal restrictions, and school policy.

We need to understand that teaching in this area is inescapably related to the religious doctrine of every culture found in our pluralistic society. We cannot teach sex education without considering the Christian doctrines relating to chastity, monogamy, and divorce, the

Judaic or Moslem or other religious beliefs about modesty, privacy, or marriage customs. Discussion of boy-girl relationships, parenthood, or names of the sex organs cannot be separated from the influence of twenty centuries of religious and moral teaching. For many people, the church and family are far stronger influences than the school, especially in such a personal area as sex behavior, and to ignore this strength is to invite trouble. An encyclical produced by Pope Pius XI in 1929 still more or less sets the boundaries for Catholic acceptance of sex education, and the reality of this fact is inescapable.

Our society still seeks to preserve chastity in the young unmarried. We still want them, once married, to stay married. Divorce is not yet a totally acceptable solution for marriage problems. And we still do not really condone adultery. Does a sound program of sex education contribute to the preservation of these cultural goals? We must know what we are trying to accomplish and be able to come reasonably close to proving that we do it.

These three cultural objectives—chastity before marriage, monogamy, and the lasting marriage—are the most deeply rooted patterns in our society. They are the rocks upon which our social system is built. They are involved in our whole concept of the family, which is the basic unit of our society. We are what we are with a heritage of puritanical reverence for the word of God, and His word is still a dominant force in the dynamics of our daily—and nightly—lives.

We need to know that we are helping students cope with the so-called new morality. They have problems. There may be nothing new about these problems, but perhaps there are more of them, and they affect more people because there *are* more young people and they have greater freedom today. The new morality brings with it a new set of rules, and nobody seems to be quite sure what they are and which of the old ones are still in force, if any. If the Supreme Court has trouble defining pornography, if censorship of entertainment is disappearing, if local groups do not know what smut is and what is not, then where does that leave the lively adolescent? It leaves him searching for values to assist him in his decision making about sex behavior. "Do I or don't I?" "How far do I go?" The drive-in movie may be the proving ground, or the overnight beach picnic or the love-in. Decisions *will* be made, and it is our job to help these young people make them wisely rather than emotionally, tugged along by urges more powerful than reason. We cannot help young people by giving them unrelated facts about the anatomy of sex, but we can help by relating those facts, if possible, to the whole jigsaw puzzle of values, ideals, appetites, capabilities, hazards, and all the other factors that should be considered by the individual as he chooses among alternatives in behavior.

We need to know that we are teaching everybody, and in this day of high population mobility we are likely to have every kind of person in any given classroom—the rich and the poor, the well and the sick, the genetically favored and the genetically handicapped. We will have children from every religion, race, and educational background. We will have the two hundred thousand youngsters who come before our courts every year. We will have the half million with psychomotor irregularities. What kind of sex education will they receive? For they will learn about sex somehow. Will they be educated or miseducated?

We will have the 10 million hungry youngsters, the 7 million whose life expectancy is shortened by disease and despair. We will have the youngsters who will grow up to become our problem drinkers. Does sex education in the schools have anything to offer these people? Most importantly, perhaps, we will have the 40 percent of all children who drop out before they finish their twelve years of school. Why do they? Because our contemporary programs of education do not motivate them to stay in school. And part of our failure is due to the absence of just such an area of study as we are discussing here, an area that might give a little more meaning to life, help them to learn, who they are, and cultivate a bit more of the self-respect so badly needed by these dropouts.

We teach everybody, yet no one sex education curriculum will fit them all. We need variation in content, approach, and style if we are to do the job right.

And we need to admit that in developing sex education as a part of a broad program of health education, we are not only shattering an old liberal arts tradition but scaring some of our fellow educators. Although our colleges and universities and thus our high schools have made heroic attempts to study man and his society, man and his environment, man and his technology, they have been very chary about studying man himself. Tradition has it that we can talk of man in relationship to his world but not about man himself. We are discouraged from getting personal—and what is more personal than sex behavior? So we need to know that we get less support than we would hope for from some of our deans and principals because they are afraid to break new ground, especially with such a controversial topic as sex education.

Another thing we need is well-prepared personnel in charge of sex education. Ideally we would hope for a reasonable measure of competence on the part of anyone who would presume to accept some responsibility for teaching others about human sexuality. Let us begin with parents. In the first and last analysis they have the key to health education. There is absolutely no need for parents to fear that someone is going to usurp their prerogative in teaching their children about sex. Inevitably parents have the first word, and both by word and by example children are indelibly affected by what happens at home. From infancy on, what is learned about modesty, sex differences, sex roles, family relationships, heredity, love, restraint, dress, chastity, promiscuity, morals, romance, marriage, and the whole gamut of values and attitudes has its origin in the home. The home transmits, from infancy onward, the powerful cultural values and practices that we propose to clarify, supplement, modify or, if necessary, deny with sex education.

All teachers are involved in sex education in one way or another. But we mainly think of elementary teachers, health educators, physical education teachers, science, biology, home economics teachers, and nurses as being specifically responsible for instruction. Are all of them equally well prepared to meet that responsibility? Hoyman says emphatically that we are not preparing enough teachers to meet the need and that those opposed to sex education are attacking at this weak spot.[6]

Bender studied the human reproduction knowledge of 163 prospective elementary teachers assuming that such information was basic to, and therefore indicative of the students' overall sex knowledge. He found that the sampled teachers were poorly prepared in terms of their knowledge of human reproduction. Admitting that this is only a small facet of the teacher's total sex education knowledge he says, "One shudders to think what might be found if we delved into teachers attitudes, misconceptions, methodology, etc., concerning the dissemination of sex education information."[7]

The requirements for teaching credentials set by State Departments of Education are crucial here, but running a close second in importance are the *sources* of teachers and administrators, our college Departments of Education. The prospective teachers now in college need more than one three-hour course to cover the whole field of health education. To handle mathematics adequately they get fifteen or twenty credits in some schools. Is the binomial theory more useful or important than an understanding of adolescent love? Many colleges and universities do not provide teaching candidates with even a basic health course. So it is perfectly true that we have hundreds of elementary and secondary school teachers going into the field every year not knowing a thing about health science and its various components.

Furthermore, the day is long past when we can leave such a vital area of health education to the part-time attention of someone with a combined health and physical education major. As we have pointed out earlier, such majors seldom have much health content at all and most physical education teachers prefer to teach physical, not health education. Health science is a recognized field of its own, and a health educator needs all the preparation he can get in order to qualify as a teacher in what is possibly the most demanding discipline, in terms of its scope, in the curriculum.

We need curriculum directors, principals, and superintendents with enough knowledge and perception of the significance of health education and its noisy member of the family, sex education, to present effectively the case in legislative hearings and before board meetings, community groups, and even their own staff. It is time for graduate schools of administration to incorporate some consideration of the health problems of our people into the course work planned for school administrators. They should be provided practice in organizing educational programs that might help solve some of the problems of health education.

– what don't we need in sex education?

We don't need any more animals to help us in our teaching. Are farm families happier because they know about the mating habits of farm animals? Is the divorce rate lower? Are farm husbands more faithful? Is there less promiscuity among farm-raised children? Fewer illegitimate pregnancies? Are the ingredients of an enduring marriage learned in the barnyard? Does raising animals in the classroom really help a youngster to understand his own problems? Or is this animal approach merely a dodge—a way to avoid the real and delicate issues involved in *human* relations? What does this use of zoological phenomena have to do with friendship, decency, morals, devotion, chastity, and love? Is family life education and homemaking among human beings understood better through watching the male bird bring home the provender to feed the hungry mouths of his young?

We do not need an indiscriminate use of descriptions of the anatomy and physiology of human reproduction. Discriminating use, yes. And the criterion for discrimination is that anatomical and physiological detail is useful only as needed to explain a problem or answer a question or contribute to an understanding of function. The textbook chapter on family life ought not to begin with the anatomy of the reproductive system. Learning facts about anatomy and physiology without relevance to interest, needs, or problems is as starkly empty an activity in learning about life as speed reading a sonnet would be in appreciating poetry. Physiological facts do not provide the beauty of life or the melody of thought. Learning about the Graafian follicle or the prostate gland may or may not have any relation to a life experience. A good teacher is concerned with affecting real life decision-making skills, not with fostering the accumulation of knowledge for the sake of knowledge.

We do not need people who accuse the health educator of everything from immorality to homosexuality if he or she tries to help some student develop decision-making capabilities relevant to sexual behavior. Nor do we need those who punish or ostracize or in other ways make life difficult for young ones with problems. For example, we can certainly get along without those who would refuse to let girls who become pregnant during the school year return after delivering their babies. Youngsters need an open door somewhere, a door that will lead to competent counseling, but on *their* terms and dealing with their problems, which are imposed on them by the world in which they live. We do not need teachers, principals, board members, or citizens who are afraid, or insensitive, or unaware of the problems today's young people must face.

There are a lot of things we don't need! We don't need to have children sent home with questionnaires inquiring into their sex life, or their parents' sex life. We don't need to assign drawing or labeling of the genitals. We don't need graphic descriptions of coitus. We don't need inaccuracy, guesswork, folklore, superstition, or ignorance. If the teacher doesn't know an IUD from the pill, he had better not try to answer any questions about contraception until he catches up on his reading.

Another thing we don't need is continued fragmentation of the curriculum into little subareas relating to health. Sex education and family living is one of these areas. It becomes a convenient target for those who do not understand what we are trying to accomplish in the total field of health education. We don't need a separate treatment for sex education at the elementary or secondary levels any more than we need a semester of environmental health, dental health, or drug-abuse education.

– what do young people say they want to know?

Most of the judgments and decisions about sex education, or any kind of education for that matter, are made by adults: school administrators, school board members, legislators, teachers. Seldom have students been asked what they would *like* to learn. Although there have been careful attempts to ascertain student needs, in the final analysis it has been adults who have interpreted the results and decided in their wisdom which of those needs ought to be met by the schools. But times are changing rapidly and young people are demanding and getting not only a respectful audience for their views but a voice in curriculum decisions in higher education and also at the secondary level.

A city-wide Youth Health Conference in Detroit, Michigan in 1967 explored young people's perceptions about the kind of knowledge needed to cope with social situations, when they thought this information and guidance should be given, by whom they thought it could best be handled, and exactly what kind of help they considered most essential and presently lacking in their environment. Couch reports the following generalizations drawn from the many frank opinions expressed in discussion of eleven categories of relevant topics:

1 Practically no one felt adequately prepared to cope with the sex problems of adolescence.

2 Concern seemed to be focussed mainly on pre-marital sex relations in high school years.

3 Much less thought was given to the total role of sexuality in life situations, or to other related aspects of family education.

4 Ideas about parents were rather ambivalent, i.e., some expressed open hostility or antagonism toward parents for having failed them in an important area of guidance, while others spoke wistfully of help for parents themselves so that when children needed their help, a better job could be done.

5 Although many young persons wanted children to get guidance in sex matters very early (ranging from 4 or 5 years of age when first questions were asked, to the elementary grades) most agreed that the greatest emphasis should be placed on sex education in the junior high school years.

6 Rather than exactly *who* could teach them about sex, discussion focussed on the *kind* of person. Young people felt that they had sought, too often unsuccessfully, for someone they could trust, regardless of age, sex, or functional role.[8]

A survey of over 5000 children from kindergarten through the twelfth grade in Connecticut found that "requests are practical and fervent for an honest sex education beginning in the elementary school and culminating with marriage preparation in grade 12."[9] A 1970 Gallup poll reported that 89 percent of high school juniors and seniors in a sampled population favored sex education courses, 82 percent approved of discussions of birth control, and 57 percent believed that married pregnant high school girls should be permitted to attend classes. Nor were parents asked the same questions far dissimilar in their beliefs, voting approval of sex education in the schools by an overwhelming majority. The vote of parents was 72 percent in favor of such instruction with 60 percent approving inclusion of information about birth control.[10]

A less extensive but interesting survey of students selected from four southern California high schools in the spring of 1970 found them unanimous in wanting sex education. The reasons given revealed their need even more compellingly than their expressed wish.

1 "Because most of them" engage in sexual intercourse at one time or another, and the knowledge of how the reproductive systems work should be helpful

2 So that the students could weigh the facts concerning birth control and sexual intercourse and decide for themselves what they want to do

3 To reduce the number of unwed mothers by placing a lot of emphasis on contraception

Clearly, the opponents of sex education, whatever their motives, are not only effectively and unfairly forcing their personal beliefs and decisions upon the great majority of parents (which is what they claim their opponents are doing), but denying the very real needs of young people. To pretend that if no instruction is offered in the schools, sexual experimentation is not occurring is to emulate the ostrich!

– a problem-centered approach

If we agree that youth want and need help in meeting social situations competently and in learning to cope with the powerful sex urges that are their natural heritage, then the best approach to sex education is through human situations as they arise in life and as they become important and meaningful to the students involved. How a 7-year-old boy would act when going to a girl playmate's birthday party is a human life situation and thus part of sex education. Whether to "go steady" in junior high school or high school, how to conduct oneself at a dance or at a drive-in movie, what legal requirements must be met before marriage, what assets a young man should have before he proposes marriage—these and many similar human problems give the best platform for classroom discussions. These problems should be explored as fully as the students wish and should be identified and chosen by the students themselves.

Here, for example, is one listing of forty-five separate but related questions that came from students, directly or indirectly and that might serve as a basis for discussion in junior and senior high school.

Current Problems

1 What behaviors, manners, courtesies, and customs are desirable among boys and girls in order to exhibit harmonious social relationships within the school (a) Conduct on dates (b) Conduct around the school (c) Language and "horseplay" (d) Dress (e) Drinking on dates

2 What is the basis for attraction and friendship between boys and girls? (a) The nature of sex appeal (b) Similarities in interests (c) The need for attention (d) The relative importance of social status (e) Loyalties

3 How can one go about meeting the boy or girl one would like to date? (a) Introductions (b) "Pickups" (c) Organizations

4 Is it desirable to establish a "steady date" in high school? What about variety in friendships?

5 What responsibilities do a boy and girl have to each other and to the parents of their companions? (a) Arriving home from dates (b) Differences in family standards (c) Safety on dates

6 What knowledge of the reproductive structures and functions is necessary to the establishment of an intellectual understanding of one's own life and life in relation to others?

7 How can a boy or girl control the reproductive urge? (a) The use of intelligence in relation to emotion (b) Interests (c) Moral standards (d) Recognition of consequences

8 What is menstruation and what are its normal characteristics? (a) Purpose (b) Regularity

9 How should girls care for themselves during menstruation? (a) Rest (b) Bathing (c) Exercise (d) Medical care

10 Are complete sexual relationships before marriage justifiable? (a) Moral standards (b) Probable consequences (c) Effect on later marriage (d) The futility of "the conquest"

11 What are the best sources of information on matters of love and marriage which are available to high school students? (a) People (b) Books (c) Movies and television (d) Miscellaneous literature

Premarriage Problems

13 What consideration should be taken into account in the selection of a marriage partner? (a) Maturity (b) Health (c) Background (d) Interests (e) Age (f) Looks (g) Education (h) Job

14 How can one tell when one is ready to assume the responsibilities of marriage? (a) Age (b) Income (c) Maturity (d) Willingness

15 What should each partner know about the health and background of the other before agreeing to marry?

16 How much money should a couple have before they marry (a) Tastes (b) Locality (c) Standard of living (d) Child planning

17 Should opposites marry?

18 Should engaged couples be allowed greater intimacies than others? (a) Local customs (b) Effect on marriage (c) Effects of restraint

19 How long should engagements last?

20 What attitudes should be cultivated regarding the influences of "in-laws" on the forthcoming marriage? (a) Parental decisions and advice (b) Gifts and support (c) Living with parents (d) Visits and vacations

21 What legal requirements must be met before marriage? (a) Health certificate (b) License (c) Banns (d) The minister

Family Planning

22 How can sexual compatibility be established in marriage? (a) Individual differences in response and desires (b) Attitudes (c) Trial and error

23 How soon should couples plan for and have their first child? (a) Financial arrangements (b) Religious beliefs (c) Health reasons (d) Readiness for children

24 How soon should a physician be consulted with reference to pregnancy or family planning?

25 What sort of examination should the prospective mother have before pregnancy?

26 What should be known by the couple about how life begins? (a) Function of reproductive organs (b) Genetic mechanisms

27 Under what conditions would further childbearing be detrimental to a mother's health? (a) Medical judgment (b) Emotional state

28 What changes in diet as well as in rest and other personal habits should be made during pregnancy? (a) Medical judgment (b) Rest (c) Exercise (d) Diet (e) Household work

29 What are the early signs of pregnancy? (a) What are the tests for pregnancy?

30 What sort of care should a mother have following the birth of the child? (a) Medical advice (b) Sympathetic family

31 How long after the birth of a child is a physician's care needed?

32 What sort of adjustment is required of the husband during pregnancy? (a) Patience (b) Sharing of duties (c) Restraint (d) Development of affection

33 What should be known about hospital costs, insurance plans and necessary home equipment in anticipation of a child?

34 What assistance do the federal and state governments give to wives and families of servicemen? (a) The funds for maternal health (b) Sources of information

35 What plan should be made by the family regarding recreational interests, friends, and distribution of time within the home? (a) Planning as a group (b) Selfish interests (c) Income and expenditures

36 How can differences of opinion within the home be reconciled? (a) Frankness (b) Willingness to settle differences (c) Authority (d) Customs and traditions

The Care of Children

37 How much attention should a child have from the parents? (a) The rights of infants (b) Fondling (c) Spoiling the child (d) Decision making

38 To what extent should the presence of a child affect the relationship between the husband and wife? (a) Continuation of joint interests (b) Sharing affection (c) Building the family

39 What medical care (e.g., diet, immunization, control of infections, habit regulations, correction of defects) should be provided for the child?

40 How can one tell if the baby is developing normally? (a) Weight (b) Motor controls (c) Length (d) Vision (e) Hearing

41 How many toys and other playthings should be provided for the child? (a) Overstimulation (b) Purposes (c) Values

42 How should the parents plan in advance for the emotional responses and psychological growth of the child? (a) Response to people (b) Crying (c) Development of character traits (d) Imitation

43 How should the child be prepared for school? (a) Attitudes (b) Skills (c) Clothing (d) Immunizations (e) Sociability (f) Personal habits

44 What attitudes should be developed in the child in preparation for the visits to the physician and dentist?

45 At what age should parents plan for the social development of the child in his relationship with playmates and adults?

From human problems of family and social interactions such as these, a teacher, with the help of his class or a committee, can formulate small units of work as they seem relevant and meaningful to the group.

– guidelines for sex education programs School administrators, health educators, or other concerned persons wishing to improve existing programs or to develop new sex education courses of study can find a sound set of such guidelines in the policy statement developed by the Illinois Sex Education Advisory Board and issued by the State Superintendent of Public Instruction in 1967. Among the principles recommended for a sound and comprehensive program were these:

1 Sex education programs, to be really effective, must be carefully and thoughtfully planned at the local community level, under the general administrative authority, responsibility, and direction of the local board of education and school, with the active, constructive involvement of teachers, parents, and community leaders and groups.

2 Sex education involves the home, school, church, and community, all working cooperatively towards areas of common agreement.

3 Sex education should include the biological, psychological, social, and moral aspects of sex because human sexuality and sexual conduct involve the whole person and his or her life style.

4 Family life and sex education in school should be a continuous process, based upon a sequential, spiral learning progression flexibly planned for grades 1 through 12. The curriculum should be based upon the problems, personal-social needs, and interests of students, and upon the local community situation.

5 Family life and sex education is concerned with both facts and values. It should be broadly conceived and planned as an integral part of education for personality and character development, guided by positive ideals and goals as well as by negative restraints and social sanctions.

6 Youth should be sex-educated, not merely sex-informed or indoctrinated.

7 Sex education must not be an isolated special facet of education but must be integrated into the school program, instead of being departmentalized.

8 Sex education should be planned to take into account individual differences, and to anticipate the developmental needs of children and youth, to avoid the "too little," "too late" approach which has characterized too much sex education in the past.

9 So-called "sex education booby traps" such as teaching students (a) specific methods of birth control, (b) specific methods

of VD prophylaxis, and (c) sexual techniques should *not* be included in sex education. However, it is desirable that appropriate instruction be included on topics such as petting, premarital sexual intercourse, masturbation, VD education, pornography and obscenity, the dangers of world population explosion, and selected legal aspects of sexual behavior.

10 Since instruction is the most important factor in the success or failure of sex education in the school, teachers should be carefully selected and adequately prepared.

11 Family life and sex education may be taught either in mixed classes of boys and girls, supplemented by individual counseling on personal questions and problems, or in separate classes for boys and girls, depending on the school and grade level and upon local school-community conditions. However, it may be desirable to teach such courses in mixed classes in senior high school as one step toward helping boys and girls and men and women to understand, appreciate, and get along better with each other to the end of promoting happy, healthy home and family life.

12 The instructional methods used in family life and sex education should be based upon sound educational principles as related to the established objectives. Educational materials should be carefully selected on the basis of established criteria of acceptability.

13 Sex education films should be viewed only as educational aids, and not as a substitute for a sound program of family life and sex education.

14 Evaluation and improvement of the sex education program on a continuing basis is essential. Because behavioral changes, including attitudes, interests, practices, and sexual conduct are the desired outcomes of sex education rather than knowledge alone, it is recommended that *all* evaluative procedures be approved by the school administrator working cooperatively with a local curriculum committee.

15 Family life and sex education programs should be paralleled by a sound community program of sex education for adults.[11]

– who should teach sex education?

The answer to that question is "everybody" and everybody does. Sex education is going on everywhere and it begins almost at birth. Of course it belongs in the home, and it *is* in the home intended or not. The trouble is, what the child may be learning by example at home is not always a positive concept of his own sex role or of marriage.

When it comes to who is giving young people information about sex, the answer appears to be that neither parents or teachers are providing most of it. Studies show that young people get most of their information from their friends, who in turn got it from other friends. Students say that at home parents are frequently embarassed or uninformed and most do not talk openly and honestly about sex, while at school the information they get tends to be irrelevant, insufficient, or is made available too late. For example, a recent Purdue poll of

1000 adolescents revealed that 53 percent of the boys and 42 percent of the girls got their information from friends. Only 15 percent of the boys and 35 percent of the girls learned the physiological aspects of sex from their parents, and just 6 percent of the group learned these facts in school![12]

The professional teacher, whether man or woman, single or married, who expects to be effective in providing meaningful, objective learning opportunities in this area must be entirely comfortable both with the subject matter and his own sex role. Szasz suggests that the one *must* for such a teacher is that he be an enlightened individual who is able to talk easily with young people. He should perceive the young person as a human being of worth, who is living in a family situation to which he is adjusting with whatever skills and understandings he has been able to acquire. Such a teacher is further described as follows:

> The teacher in this role recognizes the right of his pupil to learn about events of life as they may arise, and he takes steps to offer evidence to show relevance—if any—between events of life and the rules and regulations of society. In this role, then, the teacher provides formal education in a challenging, curiosity-arousing and curiosity-satisfying atmosphere, utilizing moments appropriate for the introduction of certain socially sensitive issues for discussion. The teacher in this role recognizes that wise educational programs must be rooted in an understanding of the nature of man and of the nature of society.[13]

– teacher preparation Teachers qualified to help students seeking answers to questions specific to family and social life situations, as in every other area of health instruction, should have a fairly comprehensive background in psychological, sociological, and anthropological, as well as physiological factors that influence health behavior. Certainly the answers to most student problems will not be found in antomical or physiological facts. Not only adequate background, but continuing study and wide reading are essential. Because the subject is of such paramount and unending interest, related articles and books abound. The health teacher must make searching out and reading about current information, new discoveries, new techniques of teaching, and fresh materials for use in the classroom a way of life, a way of life that must be given even greater emphasis once his professional preparation has been completed and his teaching career begins.

DRUG EDUCATION

We have said earlier that the apparent increase in premarital sex activity among our youth today appears to be linked in many ways to increased use of mind-altering drugs, both being symptoms of the emotional disturbances and rebelliousness that adults find so alarming. Like sex education, drug-abuse education has long been the object of pressures upon the schools, commencing with the Women's Christian Temperance Union in the 1890s and now by concerned parents and adults at every level of government and community involvement. These two health science categories are also those most often taught as separate courses rather than as an integrated part of a total health curriculum, as if it were reasonable to assume that the drug taker has no sexual functions, no family responsibilities, no need for nutrition, or that his drug dependence could be unrelated to his other health problems or, in the case of sex education, as if the social, emotional, and physical sexual problems and needs of an individual were unrelated to his decisions and needs in any other area of health behavior, including drug use.

– what is drug-abuse education?

Educators, like any other group of professionals, tend to develop terminology that might be labeled "jargon." "Drug-abuse education" might be classified as jargon, for although it is intended to describe instruction that, hopefully, will motivate students to avoid illegal or improper use of drugs, looked at logically the term sounds as if it were *education in drug abuse.* Indeed, many specialists in education and medicine argue that such instruction does in fact whet curiosity so that the result is increased interest in experimentation with drugs rather than the reverse. However, there have been so many frightening data reported reflecting drug-abuse practices among students from elementary grades to the university level that schools are racing to purchase special materials, prepare teacher specialists by means of federally funded local and regional workshops, and institute the typical crash programs that are supposed to eliminate whatever problem the focus may be.

– what is drug abuse? what is a drug, for that matter?

There seem to be several interpretations of the word "drug." First, to the lay public, drugs are usually perceived as those chemicals whose use frightens and concerns so many—illegal substances such as heroin, marihuana, and LSD; illegally obtained and abused depressants such as the barbiturates and stimulants such as amphetamines; and certain volatile substances such as airplane glue, gasoline, and paint thinner when used as intoxicants.

On the other hand, pharmacists and pharmaceutical manufacturers, understandably anxious that the word "drug" not take on a totally negative connotation and disturbed by recent FDA rulings identifying certain so-called wonder drugs as not only useless but harmful, urge that students be taught that drugs are basically helpful to man. Viewed in this context, drugs are medicines, harmful only when misused (in amounts or ways other than directed) or abused (taken illicitly for kicks rather than for medical purposes). The recommendation that drugs be disassociated from discussion of tobacco and alcohol in a unit of instruction reflects this strictly medical notion of the word. Accordingly, we can recognize in a paper titled *Drugs in the Health Curriculum: A Needed Area* the pharmacist background of its authors as they report in shocked dismay "We have observed efforts to discourage self medication entirely" with reference to a health education approach to the problem.[14]

Health educators do indeed look at drugs from a third and somewhat different frame of reference. The word "drug" has been defined broadly as any chemical agent that affects living protoplasm. Health education is concerned with the abuse or misuse of *any* substance that modifies mood and behavior. Not just the illegal, medical, and volatile substances, but a wide range of chemicals are included among those classified as affecting human behavior. There are even foodaholics, it must be remembered.

Most of the current crop of so-called drug-abuse education materials concentrate on one or the other of the first two notions of drugs. Few pay much or any attention to the major drug-abuse problem in our society—alcoholism—or to the only somewhat less visibly dangerous drug-abuse problem—tobacco use. Most fail to consider that coffee, tea, and cola beverages, and aspirin, bromides, and a host of other nonprescription medications are drugs and can cause dependence. How often do we hear statements like the following: "I just can't get going in the morning until I've had my coffee." "I'm tired, let's go get a coke." "I can't get to sleep unless I take a bromo to help me unwind." "Where's the aspirin, I've got a headache." It would appear that drug abuse, if we are to judge by the narrow interpretation given it by drug-abuse source books and curriculum guides, is the illicit or improper use of only certain chemicals and that lack of social acceptance or customary usage rather than logic or the degree of harmfulness inherent in a given chemical are the criteria.

Drug-abuse education, as defined by the content of most specifically designed curriculum materials, is a matter of tracing the historical background of the use of the drugs of concern, describing their chemical composition, and detailing their harmful effects upon the body. First and foremost, says pharmacologist George Spratto, the proper approach to drug-abuse education should be straightforward and objective; facts should be given and myths perpetuated for decades destroyed. Paradoxically, however, he also points to the fact that junior or senior high school students are *more apt* to try anything they have heard or read about and that college students "are more sophisticated in this respect and tend to limit their selection of substances to those which they know more about."[15] These two generalizations seem to contradict the assumption that giving students facts about drugs would cause them to avoid their use.

– are facts enough? "Education is not reversing drug use by America's young," says William Raspberry, *Washington Post* columnist. Mike Royko, who writes for the *Chicago Daily News,* says much the same thing. Education that focuses on telling the students the facts can be the solution to drug abuse only to the extent that ignorance is the problem. In most cases, urban teenagers already know more about drugs than their teachers. Royko says,

> After millions of words have been written or broadcast on the subject of drugs, after countless hollow-eyed junkies have told their stories on countless TV documentaries, after the endless stories about those poor little rich girls dying from overdoses, just about everybody would know of the dangers. . . . Everybody seems to agree that they [white, middle-class young people] are the best-schooled, best-informed, smartest, most knowledgeable generation of little creatures that this country has ever produced.[16]

Clearly, facts are not the answer in and of themselves. The crucial dimension of the problem is not the substances and their harmful effects, but the social, emotional, and physical forces motivating their use. It is not as helpful to know that marihuana is technically known as Cannabis sativa or that it contains a drug called tetrahydrocannabinol as it is to know what leads people to use it. The critical time for analysis of the dynamics of drug abuse is not after it has become a problem, or after an individual's value systems are well established, or even in isolation from every other aspect of human behavior. Health education that touches upon behavior in the area of drug abuse should provide students an opportunity to examine real issues, related to the total person, from a rational rather than an emotional or moralistic frame of reference.

Perhaps drug-abuse education, if it emphasizes the benefits and appropriate uses of drug products, might better be titled "drug education." Unquestionably, those drugs that are medicines have many positive uses and need to be taken with as much care as they should be prepared and prescribed. The positive aspects of drugs, and respect for their potential to ameliorate and even cure when used properly, is one aspect of health science. But the facts involved scarcely need to be stretched to the dimensions of an entire curriculum. To cover the subject matter or factual content encompassed in health education would be impossible even given full kindergarten through twelfth grade consideration. Once again, the necessity of selecting teaching strategies that focus on *process* rather than facts is clear-cut. Whether or not we misuse or abuse a substance is a choice that each of us makes not once but many times in a lifetime. Facts are necessary to make a reasoned choice, but an individual with the ability to use those facts logically and to discover new facts as they are needed, independent of a teaching-learning situation, is the goal of health education.

Psychiatrist Seymour Halleck, speaking of what he terms "The Great Drug Education Hoax," says that many people seem to believe that as long as they keep *talking* about the drug problem it will be solved. His own experience, he says, seems to indicate that as long as he presents only objective material about the physical and psychological effects of marihuana, without raising moral questions, the audience seems to become progressively more enthusiastic about the drug. He adds:

> I do not know if raising ethical questions about the general problems of artificial euphoria actually discourages young people from using drugs. Certainly such an approach cannot provide any young person with a clear yes-or-no answer on whether he should experiment with a particular drug. It does, however, provide him with an intellectual framework from which he can make a rational decision unbiased by the exaggerated views of his peers or his parents. And considering the problem of drug usage in basic moral or ethical—and social—terms does seem to minimize the destructive and insane polarization of viewpoints which appears to be an inevitable result of the ordinary drug education program.[17]

– recommendations for teaching

Teaching about wise use of drugs requires no very technical knowledge. The prospective teacher needs a thorough preparation and qualification as a health educator but no special extra studies or techniques. The same teaching strategies described in Chapter 5 apply here. Students in this case need to be allowed to discuss human problems and the role of drugs in attempts to escape those problems along with more constructive solutions that might be employed, rather than told the nature of the chemicals.

Where instruction must be carried out by nonspecialists, Means suggests a progression of general guidelines for elementary and secondary teaching. In his conclusion he recommends that:

1 Drug abuse education be incorporated as only one important phase of a total, comprehensive, and well-planned and organized health education program.

2 More adequate professional preparation be provided in drug abuse for *all* elementary school teachers and those who are likely

to have responsibility for such instruction at the secondary school level.

3 In-service and continuing education, such as workshops and seminars, be planned and organized to help increase the understanding and competencies of present teachers who are likely to have responsibilities for drug abuse instruction.

4 Attention be given to improving the competencies of teachers or prospective teachers and in-service teachers in drug abuse education.

5 Schools and colleges re-evaluate existing curricula to assure that adequate and sequential instruction on drug abuse is assured each student throughout the educational experience.

6 Emphasis in drug abuse education be devoted to the development of wholesome attitudes and sound practices, rather than the traditional devotion to only physiological effects and the acquisition of factual information.

7 Full utilization be made of existing and increasing resources for drug abuse education within the school and in the community.[18]

The curriculum materials developed by the writers of the School Health Education Study examine the problem of drug abuse with this kind of rationale in mind. As stated earlier, concept nine, "Use of substances that modify mood and behavior arises from a variety of motivations," considers every possible substance but in a context of the social and emotional forces that lead to their use. The curriculum begins with the dynamics involved in the use of even simple, commonly used substances and progresses to increasingly more complex or dangerous drugs as the student progresses through school. The teaching strategies correspondingly become more complex as he matures and learns problem-solving skills. He is involved in relevant, meaningful learning situations rather than acting as a passive recipient of factual information. A young person whose values are being modified as a result of a reasoned examination of the real issues and motives of drug abuse is far more apt to make sound decisions relative to the use of drugs.

DEALING WITH CONTROVERSY

The sources of controversy vary. Sometimes there will be individual parents or concerned adults in the community who object to discussion of certain topics such as contraception, premarital sex, or even something as relatively impersonal as fluoridation of water supplies; frown on the use of certain resource speakers in the classroom such as drug "addicts"; or find some teaching technique such as group encounter, or certain audiovisual materials objectionable. Actually, it is nearly impossible to avoid controversial issues, particularly when sensitive areas are singled out for a categorical approach as in the case of the subjects just discussed. Suggestions helpful in meeting any possible objections include the following:

1 Teachers should keep full notes of what they and their students do and say relative to controversial issues. It is undeniably helpful when someone demands to know "What are you teaching these young people?" to be able to show them in detail.

2 Teachers should keep as full a record as possible of the student problems or questions asked about the controversial topics. It could be subsequently important to show that the teacher did not introduce these topics arbitrarily, but that these issues were student concerns and were discussed in class in order to get at the truth rather than allowing attitudes to be shaped and behavior promoted by street-corner or locker-room conversations.

3 Teachers should remember that while they are public servants, they are *professionals* and can stand upon their proven qualifications as does any other professional. However, an attitude of aggressive defense must be solidly based on a scientifically sound position. For example, if a teacher has been discussing religious healing in terms other than accepted knowledge about psychosomatic relationships, he has a much weaker defense. If, in dealing with boy-girl relationships, the teacher has allowed vulgarisms to be used or has made the discussion too personal, then he is vulnerable to criticism. A teacher can meet controversy successfully only if he is sure of his position. Nothing contributes more to such confidence than a thorough and constant preparation in the science of health *and* in the science of education.

4 Much potential objection to teaching about the subjects of sex education, venereal disease, insanity, and other special areas can be prevented if one avoids the spectacular or shocking, uses simple terms, shuns the abnormal or the morbid, is objective, and keeps a sense of humor throughout.

A recommendation of the staff of the Center for the Study of Instruction of the National Education Association summarizes this point very well in its statement about teaching about controversial issues.

> Rational discussion of controversial issues should be an important part of the school program. The teacher should help students identify relevant information, learn techniques of critical analysis, make independent judgments, and be prepared to present and support them. The teacher should also help students become sensitive to the continuing need for objective re-examination of issues in the light of new information and changing conditions in society.

These three questions are posed to sharpen the focus of the issue for administrators and faculty:

1 Does the school board have a clear policy statement on teaching about controversial issues? Are the staff members and the public aware of it? Is it acceptable to them? Does the statement adequately reflect the views of teachers?

2 Do teachers feel free to teach about controversial issues in a perceptive and creative manner? If not, why not? What factors are impinging upon academic freedom? What can be done about them?

3 What criteria do teachers use for deciding whether a particular topic warrants consideration in the classroom? The maturity and backgrounds of the students? The adequacy of human and material resources? The significance of the issue?[19]

Szasz suggests that three guides can assist teachers when problems arise. First, the teacher should not be caught up in the emotions of a person or a group. Second, he should keep an open mind toward the problem rather than make premature judgments based on biases or opinion. Third, the teacher should recognize his own limitations and acknowledge them and utilize the resources of others in meeting problems.[20]

SUMMARY

Much controversy can be avoided if categorical, crash programs are discarded in favor of a comprehensive program of health education. As Henry Bruyn asserts, the current controversy about sex education in schools would certainly have been minimized or even lacking if a broadly based program in health science were already established in all schools and content relevant to man's sexual role and functions in society were just another chapter in the larger health textbook or curriculum.[21]

It is not that controversial or categorical health issues should not be dealt with in the schools. It is that they are not health education of themselves but only *parts* of health education. It is the total human being who uses drugs, lives in a family relationship, and has sexual and a host of other needs. His behavior is influenced by a wide range of interacting forces emanating from the community and his home as well as from himself in the shape of his needs and basic demands. Pieces of health information, however logically presented relative to a specific health problem, cannot effectively modify health behavior unless the impact of those many other forces is also explored.

The Joint Committee of the National School Boards Association and the American Association of School Administrators, speaking of the piecemeal approach to health problems such as separate courses in sex and family life education, says:

> The Committee is unanimous in its firm belief that the only effective way in which the school can fulfill its responsibility for meeting the health needs of youth is through a comprehensive program of health education in grades K through 12. Such a program estab-

lishes the organizational frame work for meeting the health needs, interests, and problems of the school-age group as well as preparing them for their role as future parents and citizens.

Including sex and family life education with the other categorical health topics in one sound, interrelated, and sequential program not only saves time in an already crowded curriculum, but assures that all topics will be part of a long-range program and will receive more complete and detailed consideration at the appropriate level of the student's development.[22]

NOTES AND REFERENCES

1 Curriculum Commission of the Health Education Division of the American Association for Health, Physical Education, and Recreation, *Health Concepts,* Washington, D.C.; Curriculum Commission of the Health Education Division of the American Association for Health, Physical Education, and Recreation, 1967.

2 School Health Education Study, *Health Education: A Conceptual Approach to Curriculum Design,* St. Paul, 3 M Education Press, 1967, p. 20.

3 Howard S. Hoyman, "Should We Teach About Birth Control in High School Sex Education," *Journal of School Health* (November 1968), pp. 545–556.

4 Lester A. Kirkendall and Deryck Calderwood, "The Family, the School, and Peer Groups; Sources of Information about Sex," *Journal of School Health* (September 1965), p. 296.

5 Delbert Oberteuffer, "Some Things We Need and Some Things We Don't Need in Sex Education, 1970," *Journal of School Health* (February 1970), pp. 54–65.

6 Howard S. Hoyman, "Where Are We Now in Sex Education: An Appraisal" (mimeographed), Urbana, University of Illinois.

7 Stephen Bender, "The Human Reproduction Knowledge of Prospective Elementary Teachers," paper presented at Research Council of the American School Health Association, annual meeting, Houston, Texas, October 1970.

8 Gertrude B. Couch, "Youth Looks at Sex," *Journal of School Health* (September 1967), pp. 332–229.

9 Ruth Byler, Gertrude Lewis, and Ruth Totman, *Teach Us What We Want To Know,* Connecticut State Board of Education, 1969.

10 Gallup, George, "The Public's Attitude Toward the Public Schools," *Phi Delta Kappan,* reprint, October 1970.

11 Adapted from the Illinois Policy Statement on Family Life and Sex Education.

12 National School Public Relations Association, *Sex Education in Schools,* Washington, D.C.; National School Public Relations Association, 1969, p. 3.

13 George Szasz, "Sex Education and the Teacher," *Journal of School Health* (March 1970), p. 152.

14 Mickey C. Smith, Robert L. Mikeal, and James N. M. Taylor, *Drugs in the Health Curriculum: A Needed Area,* (mimeographed), paper presented to the annual meeting of the American School Health Association, Detroit, Michigan, November 10, 1968, p. 8.

15 George R. Spratto, "Toward a Rational View of Drug Abuse," *Journal of School Health* (April 1970), p. 195.

16 Mike Royko, "Drug Hazard: A Plethora of Warnings," *Los Angeles Times,* August 2, 1970.

17 Seymour Halleck, "The Great Drug Education Hoax," *The Progressive,* July 1970, p. 33.

18 Richard K. Means, "Drug Abuse: Implications for Instruction," *Journal for Health, Physical Education, and Recreation,* May 1970, p. 55.

19 NEA, *From Bookshelves to Action, A Guide To Using the Recommendations of the NEA Project on Instruction,* Washington, D.C.; NEA, 1964, pp. 12–12.

20 Szasz, *op. cit.,* p. 154.

21 Henry Bruyn, "Drugs on the College Campus," *Journal of School Health* (February 1970), p. 96.

22 The Joint Committee of the National School Boards Association and the American Association of School Administrators, *Health Education and Sex/Family Life Education* (pamphlet) n.d.

SELECTED READINGS

Adams, John B., and Michael E. Sestak, "Sex Education—A Sensible Approach," *Journal of School Health* (May 1967), pp. 222–225.

Advisory Panel (headed by Donald K. Fletcher), *Drug Abuse: Escape to Nowhere,* Philadelphia; Smith, Kline, and French Laboratories, 1967.

AMA, *Drug Dependence—A Guide for Physicians,* Chicago, 1969.

Ausubel, David P., *Drug Addiction: Physiological, Psychological, and Sociological Aspects,* New York; Random House, 1967.

Avery, Curtis E., "Sex Education Through Rose Colored Glasses," *The Family Life Coordinator,* October 1964, pp. 83–90.

Bennell, Florence B., "Eliminating Barriers to Sex Education in the Schools," *Journal of School Health* (February 1968), pp. 68–71.

Boe, Sue, "Drugs: The Tools of Medical Progress," *Journal of School Health* (February 1970), pp. 65–70.

Breasted, Mary, *Oh! Sex Education,* New York; Praeger, 1970.

Commission on Professional Rights and Responsibilities, National Education Association, *Suggestions for Defense Against Extremist Attack: Sex Education in the Public Schools,* Washington, D.C.; NEA, March 1970.

Committee on Drugs of the American School Health Association and the Pharmaceutical Manufactuers Association, *Teaching About Drugs: A Curriculum Guide, K–12,* Kent, Ohio, Committee on Drugs of the American School Health Association and the Pharmaceutical Manufacturers Association, 1970.

Demos, George D., John W. Shainline, and Wayne Thomas, *Drug Abuse and You,* New York; Chronicle Guidance Publications, 1968.

Dezelsky, Thomas, and J. V. Toohey, "Are You Listening to the Lyrics?" *Journal of School Health* (January 1970), pp. 40–42.

Fowler, Evelyn, "Factors Involved in Voting on Fluoridation and Their Implications for Health Education," *Journal of School Health* (September 1967), pp. 345–349.

Gadpaille, Warren J., "Is There a Too Soon?" *Today's Health,* February 1970, pp. 34–35, 71.

Goodheart, Barbara, "Sex in the Schools: Education or Titillation?" *Today's Health,* February 1970, pp. 28–30, 76, 79, 80, 83.

Harms, Ernest (ed.), *Drug Addiction in Youth,* New York; Pergamon Press, 1965.

Hoyman, Howard S, "Sex and American College Girls Today," *Journal of School Health* (February 1967), pp. 54–62.

Johnson, Warren R., *Human Sex and Sex Education,* Philadelphia; Lea & Febiger, 1963.

Juhasz, Anne M., "Characteristics Essential to Teachers in Sex Education," *Journal of School Health* (January 1970), pp. 17–19.

Kilander, H. Frederick, *Sex Education in the Schools,* New York; Macmillan, 1970.

Kitzinger, Angela, and Patricia Hill, *Drug Abuse,* Sacramento, State Department of Publication, 1967 (source book and guide).

Levine, Milton I., "Sex Education in the Public Elementary and High School Curriculum," *Journal of School Health* (January 1967), pp. 30–38.

Lingeman, Richard R., *Drugs from A–Z. A Dictionary,* New York; McGraw-Hill, 1969.

Linner, Birgitta, *Sex and Society in Sweden,* New York; Pantheon, 1967.

Manley, Helen, *A Curriculum Guide in Sex Education,* St. Louis, Mo.; State Publishing Company, 1964.

Michaelson, Mike, "In Search of Sanity: The Man in the Middle," *Today's Health,* February 1970, pp. 31–37, 71.

National Institute of Mental Health, *A Federal Source Book: Answers to the Most Frequently Asked Questions About Drugs,* Washington, D.C.; National Institute of Mental Health, 1970.

Nowlis, Helen H., *Drugs on the College Campus,* Garden City, N.Y., Anchor, 1969.

O'Donnell, John, and John C. Ball, (eds.), *Narcotic Addiction,* New York, Harper & Row, 1966.

Schoel, Doris R., "Sex Education, Family Living, and Human Relations—An Integrative Program That Grows with Youth," *Journal of School Health* (March 1968), pp. 129–139.

Taylor, Norman, *Narcotics: Nature's Dangerous Gifts,* New York; Delta, 1963.

PART TWO FOUNDATIONS OF ADMINISTRATION AND PROGRAM

CHAPTER 9 THE PROMOTION OF CHILD HEALTH

Going to school is a total experience, not just an intellectual one. When a child enters the first grade he will never be the same thereafter. He will be affected intellectually, socially, physically, and emotionally. There are some adults concerned about the expanding scope of education who, preferring to ignore this fact, say that the only function of the school is to develop children intellectually. They say that physical and recreational development belongs to the parents or to the community. This sort of assignment of principal responsibility may be convenient to those who do not know the facts of growth and development, but it must never be forgotten that a child is indivisible and that while intellectual pursuits are undertaken in the classroom, the total individual is being affected. A child is conveniently divisible only in the imagination of those uninformed or malicious people who want to divide him for their own purposes.

Schooling can be helpful or harmful, favor human development or retard it, be an integrating experience or a frustrating and disintegrating one. The school health program is committed to the promotion of the health of children and to their growth, development and individuation.

A TOTAL EXPERIENCE It is a singular mistake to believe that school health education is concerned only with the physical aspects of child health. To be sure, most people think of health mainly in physical terms. Goals of physical well-being or physical fitness are still more clearly understood by the public than those of mental and spiritual health, even though concise and discrete definitions of the former are impossible to formulate. The holistic nature of man makes it impossible to fragmentize him; to be concerned with physical health to the exclusion of the rest of his nature. The sophisticated educator knows that mental health and physical health are merely two aspects of the same being and that there can be no dealing with one without the other.

Mistaken, also, is the idea that the school health program is primarily or solely interested in providing health services to children. The modern school health program is aware that there are many factors which affect the health of the individual child. There are many variables to be considered. Health of children is a vastly complex matter involving the whole child and his environment. Health is a dynamic, ecological resultant involving the interaction of the hereditary endowment, a healthful, safe environment, an adequate standard of living, adequate medical and dental care and public health services and education, resistance to communicable and noncommunicable diseases, optimum nutrition, growth and development, organic soundness, and functional vigor.[1] It involves optimum dynamic motor fitness and suitable exercise throughout life; refreshing rest, relaxation, and sleep; resistance to stress, fatigue, frustration, and boredom; homeostasis and optimum metabolism, repair, and recovery from illness and injury. It involves a resistance to premature aging and death, a healthy, mature personality and healthful living, a will to live, healthful attitudes, beliefs, and practices, useful, satisfying work, and creative achievement. Certainly love and affectionate sharing and belonging, heterosexual adjustment, enjoyable, constructive recreation and use of leisure, enjoyable aesthetic experiences, including those with nature, opportunities for risks, challenges, adventures, and new experiences, spiritual faith, ideals, values, and a search for meaning and freedom for personal social fulfillment through significant commitments to ultimate concerns are all involved. Health is as complex as human life itself and depends upon many interacting variables.

The modern school health program is concerned with all these elements of health, just as it is concerned with the many causes of disease. School health educators should believe in the active promotion of health through all of the processes that go on in the name of education or schooling. Historically, school health programs, along with the programs of other health agencies, have been primarily interested in the prolongation of life and the minimization of incapacity, pain, and discomfort. But the focus on curing of disease has been changed and replaced by efforts to minimize departures from normal physiological functioning. This is the preventive medicine approach. Attention has turned to the precursors of illness, such as genetic deficiencies, latent or incipient illness, poor immunity status, and sex- or age-related physical conditions, and to finding out if there are problems in a person's health status before he is in a state of concern.

The thrust of modern school health programs is therefore toward the promotion of health as we have described it in previous chapters. In this approach, health is not an entity that is lost or gained, nor is it a quantity but, rather, a developmental process involving many levels of response to a total environment. The total environment includes physical, biologic, social, and conceptual components. Healthy responses will be life enhancing. School health education seeks to promote healthy, positive, adaptive responses. Halbert L. Dunn describes high-level wellness as an integrated method of functioning that is oriented toward maximizing the potential of which the individual is capable.[2] Wellness requires that the individual maintain a continuum of balance and purposeful direction within the environment where he is functioning. Implicit in the expression "promotion of health" is the idea that there are gradations of health, that everyone not affected by specific disease or disability is not equally healthy. At present, gradations of health in this positive sense are not measurable, but the concept has definite understandable meaning. Health is not a condition, it is an adjustment; it is not a state but a process. That process adapts the individual not only to our physical but to our social environment.[3] This concept of health as an ever-changing adaptive process leads into that of wellness or quality of life.

THE ROUTE TO WELL-BEING

If "environment" can be defined as the sum of external forces that act on the individual and if one recognizes the simple truth that no organism can exist without an environment, then it becomes clear that the child and his environment are aspects of one interacting system, the child's ecosystem. The school becomes part of each child's environment and abdicates its responsibility if it does not play a strong role in the promotion of his well-being. The school plays an enabling role in helping each child to accomplish his unique developmental sequence, a development that allows each child to fulfill his individual goals, which expand, change and are perfected with increasing maturity and individuation. Fortunately, the routes to the performance of developmental sequences that lead to well-being can be described.[4]

– kindergarten through grade three

The late preschool and early elementary years constitute the time period in which most children are attempting to establish a favorable ratio between initiative and guilt.[5] This is the period of time when the child begins to grow together in body and mind and comes to realize that he has a personality all his own. There is great interest in adult heroes and uniforms and in tools, toys, and weapons. Activity of all kinds is pursued for the sake of the activity itself and not for the sake of production. Children engage in large-muscle activities involving running, hopping, skipping, jumping, and hammering and learn to do many personal activities for themselves such as washing, dressing, and tying shoes. Small-muscle activities such as pasting and coloring and some drawing begin. Height and weight are gained, although relatively slowly. Deciduous teeth are lost and primary teeth develop. There is a high level of activity and, in most children, constant talking. The child who does not accomplish the skills and attitudes of initiative will come out with an unfavorable ratio in favor of guilt. These children are recognized by their anxiety, jealousy, and aggressive behavior, which are categorized as immaturity. The school has the opportunity to enable children to develop favorable ratios of initiative versus guilt and, in Erik Erikson's words, develop method and competence.

– late childhood

The latency period, or the childhood period of late elementary school years, is characterized by attempts to develop a favorable ratio between the sense of industry and the sense of inferiority.[6] During this time the child will attempt to win recognition by producing. Tasks are attempted for the purpose of producing something. It is the time of the tool world, the time of developing concern over right and wrong. Hand-eye skills are developed, and there is interest in speed and ability to perform tasks accurately. Reading is improved, as are the communication skills of handwriting, speech, and listening. The child who is unable to accomplish the tasks presented to him during this period will develop feelings of inferiority and inadequacy and will feel that his future is determined by factors outside of himself, such as race, background, clothing, and economics.

–early adolescence

The period of early adolescence and late childhood is particularly notable for the "endocrine revolution" that begins to take place. It is a time of rapid gain in height and weight and of changes in the distribution of body fat and the development of an adult figure—a time of breast development, menstruation, peach fuzz, and voice change. The task of developing a sense of industry is superseded by the quest for identity. The child's primary question is Who am I? and he may be concerned with idols, young love, and ideals, clans, and fads. Adolescence is a period of extremes of behavior and a time of questioning. Schools have the opportunity to help young people find out who they are or, conversely, to add to their role confusion and cause them to freeze into delinquent behavior and fail to develop an occupational identity. Pupils who have the opportunity to develop a favorable ratio between identity and role confusion will develop devotion and fidelity.

– late adolescence Well-being in the late adolescent period involves a continuing struggle to develop identity but is superseded by the development of a favorable ratio between intimacy and isolation. The beginnings of genital love occur. A sense of commitment and ethical strength develop. It is a time of developing affiliations and of physical combat; or on the other hand, when the environment is unfavorable, it is a time of isolation, self-absorption, and the beginning of character problems. This, then, is a time of vocational planning and counseling, pair dating, and concern over appearance. Rebellion and negation of parental control may also develop. It is a period in which adult bodily proportions develop, as well as high-level coordination and athletic ability, beard growth, and regularity of menstruation. Youth brings together the beginnings of the adult personality.

When the school years are over and the young person must meet life, he will have accomplished certain developmental tasks if his ecosystem, that environment within which he lives and interacts, has allowed.[7] If he has so matured he will probably have acquired the following through his growth period:

1 adequate strength and vigor

2 well-formed habits of eating, sleeping, exercise and health protection

3 sufficient command of bodily skills to
   a insure exercise enough to keep well
   b make for efficient work and restful play
   c encourage general self control through bodily control

4 a satisfactory appearance and manner

5 a well developed intellect and good background of facts and ideas and good habits of clear thinking, adequate diction, vocabulary and the ability to express himself well

6 a progressive weaning from childish behavior and from excessive dependence upon others

7 a widening range of interest and creative outlets

8 increasingly adequate social skills, ever widening insights, tolerance and understanding; general consideration for others

9 a well balanced moral and ethical code of behavior and the ability to live up to it[8]

He will have developed the so-called strength and basic virtues of direction and purpose, method and competence, devotion and fidelity, affiliation and love and will be prepared to enter the adult world of economic independence and social adjustment to the people with whom he works and lives.[9] He will be able to function as a citizen of his community and adjust to marriage or to the lack of it. He will be able to live successfully with himself and with his place in life and will be able to use these skills to pursue the fulfillment of his unique goals.

Because of the compulsory attendance laws of our culture, the school is an important part of the environment of each child. The school has a responsibility to help the child through his stages of development along the paths of well-being, and the activities of the school must be directed to that end.

THE SCHOOL'S RESPONSIBILITY TO PROMOTE WELL-BEING

One of the strange omissions from twentieth-century educational practice has been the idea that an understanding of the nature of the learner is basic to teaching. It is folly to suggest that teachers can be prepared by four years of subject matter with a fifth year added for a few courses in methods, if there is nowhere a mention of the study of the nature of the pupils. The unsuspecting and innocent 6-year-old has the right to enter an institution that is concerned about him as an individual and about him in relation to the environment into which he, by law, has been pressed. School personnel have a responsibility to understand, as well as possible, the nature of the child's ecosystem. In the psychosocial sphere, it is necessary to know the nature of the home and the people in it, the nature of the peer group with which the child associates, and the type of community that surrounds the home environment. It is necessary to know the relationships between the people in the home and the people with whom they associate. A teacher should know who the important others are in the child's living process.

The child's physical environment is equally important to know. What is the nature of the atmosphere that the child breathes? Is it filled with particulate matter, with allergens, or is it adequate for the development of good health? Is the water supply similarly pure and desirable? Does the child have enough space and adequate shelter? Are there harmful animals in his environment? The school must know all of these if it is to help in the promotion of well-being.

Further, a great deal of information must be gathered on the nature of the learner himself. What is the nature of the child's heredity? Is he biologically adequate for the performance of duties in school? Are his life style, habits, personality, and living skills such that he will be able to grow and develop in a way that will give him a chance at successful living? Does his world of ideas and personal knowledge and facts give him the type of stimulation that will be necessary for him to take part in the learning process and to take part in life? How does each child function in the area of feelings? Intellectually? Socially? How does he function in the home, in the school, and with peers? The school personnel have the responsibility for understanding all of these things in order to promote the child's well-being.

The teacher must also understand the developmental status of the child. Many teachers consider that the child comes to school as a blank slate on which the teacher will write the wisdom of the ages. Others assume that the child is an empty cup to be filled with knowledge. Nothing could be further from the truth. Every child who comes to school has a wealth of experiences behind him. The child in his new clothes and shiny shoes and cleanly scrubbed face who comes to school on the first day has gone through the trauma of the birth process and the entry into the cruel, cold world. He has had the learning experiences of walking and talking and toilet training, and he has grown from the helpless infant to the child who is ready, hopefully, for separation from his home and entry into the world of school. How well the child has fared in the birth process and in passing the developmental landmarks in his growth process must be taken into account by the teacher as the child enters school. There is a probability that in each classroom a wide range of developmental patterns will be seen—a range that will go from children who have been unable to learn to speak, walk, or control their bladders successfully, to those whose development would correspond to that of late childhood. Children cannot afford to have teachers who do not take into account their environment and their unique developmental status.

– the schools in promotion of well-being When the child comes to school, he meets a sensory overload that is sometimes overwhelming. He is propelled into a world of noise, of strange sights and sounds, of new faces and new companions, of rules he never heard of and finds constraining, of books and homework, of track systems and recitations, of graded and ungraded classrooms, of marks and report cards. He is separated from home for the first time and feels anxious about this. Unless the people in the school, the physical environment of the education system, and the teaching-learning process are consciously planned for the promotion of his well-being, schooling can be a harmful, disintegrating experience for the child. If, however, the school has organized in order to enable the child to travel along the pathway to well-being, schooling can be a helpful experience that favors human development and integration.

What is the environment that the child meets when he goes to school? What can be designed to promote his well-being? Who and what does the child meet when he goes to school?

He Meets Teachers / First, and principally, he meets teachers who will become his alter parents for a time and who will have an influence second only to his parents. Teachers and principals, nurses and doctors, custodians and cooks, bus drivers and lunchroom managers—the whole wonderful, and sometimes terrifying, personnel of the school will help to shape his life. Later on it will be guidance counselors and coaches, deans and professors, and campus functionaries of all kinds who will mold and shape and affect in a real way the adolescent becoming a man or woman.

What kind of people are these? For the most part they are good, substantial, well-prepared and well-intending persons. They are victims of no particular occupational hazards, nor are there any particular selective factors operating for their entrance into their professions. They become ill—and die—of the same maladies others do, at about the same rates. They suffer from nervous and emotional disturbances at the same rate as the general population.

The fact of the matter is, however, that society seems to expect the teacher to be perfect—to be a perfect model of emotional and psychological stability, never to be absent and always able to keep his head in time of stress. The teacher is expected to be some kind of intellectual and emotional paragon.

For these reasons a good school health program will do everything possible to secure the emotional stability of teachers. The teacher is in a position, through sheer presence and influence of personality, to affect the development of a variety of emotional and intellectual responses on the part of his pupils. Teachers who are in good mental health have more stable pupils than teachers who are not. The behavior of the teacher has an effect on the pupil's sense of security, his freedom from tension, his resourcefulness, and his search for social recognition. Furthermore, a teacher relatively free from problems of his own can be more alert to the problems of others and can devote more time to creating a classroom atmosphere in which children can develop socially and creatively.

The teacher whose economic life is secure, who likes his job, who is physically well, and who participates with satisfaction in the social and recreative life of the community is a better teacher because of these satisfactions. A teacher who is able to handle criticism and gossip and not be depressed by it, who faces the onset of sedentary life with resources able to meet it, and whose own emotional life is in order is a far better teacher because of these attributes. The harassed teacher, worried over finances, insecure in his position, nettled by students, disturbed about personal matters, resentful of his sex, fretful in the classroom, lacking in resources for self-entertainment, and bored with life is the one most likely to be a deterrent to the best psychological program for students and to be an impediment to their emotional growth. The well-being of the teacher, therefore, is a fundamental concern to the process of promoting the well-being of pupils.

The Child Also Meets the Teaching-Learning Process / Most of the effect of the school experience is made through the teaching-learning process, that interaction between pupils and teachers, organized knowledge and activities which confront the child year after year. He can get used to teachers and perhaps learn to take the physical environment for granted, but the inexorable, constant, and sometime baffling demands of the curriculum remain with him as a source of growth and development or, unfortunately perhaps, of frustration and sometimes failure.

The Curriculum / In this remarkable society where universal literacy is demanded, universal education is offered, and a high premium is placed on a college education, the pressures on the young to do well in school are only now beginning to be studied and understood.

There is a considerable lack of understanding on the part of many as to the potential relationship between the curriculum and the promotion of the health of children. It can be safely stated that to ask millions of children to conform to a relatively fixed curriculum in order to gain diplomas is to produce dropouts by the millions whose health problems of a psychological and physical nature are appalling. Whenever education is reexamined, some politicians, military officers, businessmen, and even educators fall back on a disproven, unsound concept of the nature of the educable human being. They seem to believe the child is like a sack, to be held by the throat while the goods of education are poured into him, "to the limits of his intellectual capacity." Actually, no such impersonal treatment of individuals is profitable. The teaching-learning process, the curriculum, must be individually constructed not only with the idea of increasing the intellectual capacity but also in order to improve the health of the individual. When one realizes that 40 percent of the children who enter school at the first grade leave before they finish the twelfth *for one reason or another,* one wonders why. It is entirely possible that we have constructed an educational program with a curriculum that is clearly unsuited to our young people.

Our country is devoted to the development of the individual as its central ideal. In our democracy, dedicated to the supremacy of the individual, to his right to development, to his search for self-determination, we must make sure that school curriculums are developed that will make such attainments possible and that do not shatter the psychological stability of those who are forced into its molds.

What educators and laymen alike must comprehend is that the community can provide the best schools, the best teachers, the best curriculum conceivable, but unless all of these resources are designed to meet the needs of the child, the benefits will not be received. This is another way of saying that schools and teachers and curriculums had better be developed for children, adolescents, and college-age people to further their growth as individuals.

Curriculums cannot be developed just to satisfy national pride or to keep us ahead in the space race or to appease someone who found a misspelled word in an application form from a college graduate. There is no surer way to perpetuate the dropout, the current high rate of student unrest, violence, and other less spectacular forms of maladjustment.

Of all the influences bearing upon the students in the school environment, the teaching-learning process is the most significant in influencing the development of a self-image, the stimulation of ambition, and the preservation or destruction of self-confidence. Theoretically, at any rate, the curriculum should be designed to teach and motivate children to work at the upper limits of their powers. Personnel in health education should, above all others, be aware of the program's influence and should be sensitive to the growth and development needs of young people. G. Wagner states there are four significant observations that should be noted, especially by teachers and committees planning curriculum guides.

1 Teachers, before they plan their school programs, should understand the characteristics and needs of the children they are to teach and their patterns of development.

2 The curriculum guides should be so well organized that the characteristics of children clearly have their implications in the curriculum content and design. It is desirable in such guides to list the characteristics of children for each grade level and follow these by an outline of goals, content and implementing activities for the several curriculum areas.

3 All children have an innate compulsion to develop to their fullest capabilities. For this reason curriculum guides should be designed to foster the potentialities of each child, thus minimizing the too common practice of regimented, "lock step" progression.

4 It appears as though committees and certain curriculum areas such as art, homemaking and physical education (and to a degree at the elementary school level) have been more concerned about relating their knowledge of child development to the curriculums they prepare than are other curriculum committees. Perhaps committees in all curriculum areas should give more thoughtful at-

tention to the building of programs based upon a clear and empathetic understanding of the pupils they are to teach.[10]

Any teacher should ask himself the following questions when a new group of children enter his classroom at the beginning of a school year:

1 What academic achievements do the individual children bring to my classroom?

2 How fit for the tasks ahead is each of my pupils?

3 What experiences will I need to give those who are emotionally unstable or socially inept?

4 What are the common, and also the individual, needs and interests of my pupils?

5 How do the characteristics of these children differ from their characteristics when they entered the preceding grade?

The principal motivator to learning is success. Just as recognition must be given to fast moving, superior children so that they will not suffer boredom and frustration, destructive not only of their best talent but conceivably of their life, so also must we provide a wide range of experiences so that all can achieve success in learning. Special pathways to diplomas and degrees should be developed for the exceptional student. As a general guide, a curriculum that is adapted more to individual needs than to mass administration will contribute more to the health of children than other types of curriculums.

Relevance, too, has become a key word in the development of curriculum. In the past, too often the concepts taught through the learning activities were pertinent more for the past or for the needs of the teacher than for the learner. Modern educators are making forecasts of the future of our country in order to determine the kinds of competencies and skills present-day students will need in order to be successful adults. Such curricula then become relevant not only for the present well-being of the pupil, but also are designed to improve his success in the future.

THE DAILY ROUTINE The task of the school would be facilitated if children could be prepared at home for the school experience. Principally, parents should depict the school not as a combination correctional institution and labor camp but as an opportunity and as a time for growth and development and joy. Teachers are, by and large, rather nice people. The attitudes that children bring to school and the feelings toward school that they have developed from their parents frequently determine the quality of their adjustment to school and to the life for which school prepares. Parents who can give their children a good start in life, who can prepare them for being away from home, who provide a preschool range of experience and some participation in sharing the discipline needed for group life, and who can teach them to follow rules and agreements will give their children an advantage in coping with the demands of the school today.

What goes on in the classroom will have a major bearing on the well-being of students of all ages. It is not enough that the classroom merely creates no additional problem. The classroom experience can be a positive influence—it can not only solve some of the student's problems, but develop those substantial qualities that make for successful adaptation to his environment. The atmosphere of the school and of the classrooms should be such that the child will learn to tell the truth instead of lie, be courageous instead of cowardly, be polite instead of rude, be honest and not deceitful, be companionable rather than antagonistic. A teacher who seeks these positive, desirable qualities rather than merely trying to correct the undesirable ones, will make a great contribution to the integration of the student's personality. Ralph Ojemann states that "In general teachers control the behavior of the children in class by disciplinary measures based on the overt behavior of the children and without taking into account the causes of behavior. The individual teacher's attitude toward the children and the intensity of his own needs to control them determines his response—that is, the type and severity of the discipline."[11] Professor Ojemann thought it probable that if a teacher learned to understand the causes of behavior, his attitude toward the children would change and he would not simply inhibit the children's behavior but would deal with it in a way that would be more mutually satisfying. This hypothesis was tested, and it was demonstrated that when the conflict between teacher and pupil was lessened, the children did better work. The teacher had become more effective because he had approached the pupils' behavior through an understanding and appreciation of their backgrounds, ambitions, and worries. The teacher thus dealt with his pupils in a dynamic, rather than a static, manner.

The relationship of the teacher and his students, the purpose that he inculcates within the class, and the kind of discipline and the way it is carried out in the classroom form the basis for the positive influence on the health of the children. Once the teacher can accept the point of view that his influence can and should go beyond the dispensing of knowledge and enter the realm of total development, he then recognizes infinite possibilities in teaching. He can teach children to face reality, to seek value from things inherent in the act, to respond to motivations, to seek and get a clear estimation of self without delusions, to enjoy fair appraisal, and to cultivate those study values that will be productive.

ACTIVITY

Closely related to the way classroom business is carried on and the discipline that is preserved is the balance of the kinds of activities which go on in the classroom. The classroom is at best a highly artificial and unnatural environment. The human being must learn to be as inactive as classroom and study hall require him to be. Teachers who know the nature of the learners in their charge will provide for a variety of activities and for a change of pace in the physical expenditure of the energy that goes on in the classroom. Children in the late preschool and early childhood age-range will need large amounts of big-muscle activity balanced by periods of rest and relaxation, when the amount of stimulation is at a low level. Children in later childhood will profit by proper ratios of activity using small- and large-muscle skills. Even the adolescent who seems quite mature and settled performs better in the classroom and develops more positively when given the opportunity to stretch his muscles in vigorous physical activity.

Our puritan tradition gave little credence to the belief that play and fun were quite all right. Schooling had to be a grim, serious, no-nonsense business. This tradition lingers. That is why the "hard" subjects are generally considered better for the young person than the easier ones—and this attitude also partially explains why many people have a short-sighted view of the kind and quality of learning and personal development that can come out of a well-organized physical education program.

The area of play has long been underrated as an influence in meeting experiences of success and failure, joy and disappointment. A well-conceived program of physical education will give its participants an opportunity to feel the satisfactions of achievement, and such satisfactions are of prime importance to many. There is opportunity within physical education, when its activities are carefully selected, for cultivating the objective and extroverted outlook as contrasted to the subjective and often the introverted. There is ample opportunity to establish status among one's fellows, to understand self, and to find those satisfactions that come from a feeling of identification with a group. Above all, there is an opportunity to have fun, to enjoy life, to know pleasure. The physical education program should not be a grim business, sober, formal and serious, nor angry and irritating as it sometimes becomes when competition incites bad behavior. Children need and deserve the free, joyous interest of dancing, singing, games, and sports. Many will find in physical education, including the athletic program, their only opportunity for the cultivation of leadership. Children's games are replete with experiences of being leader and its converse of being just one of the team. Such experiences should be developed for all they are worth. To view physical education as only a strength building or physical fitness program is to overlook its richest potential, that of contributing to the psychological and social development of its participants. Motor activities—games, sports, and athletics of all kinds—can be rich educational and developmental experiences when they are conducted not for the glorification of the coach but for the enrichment of the lives of the students.

TIME SCHEDULE

Not only must the classroom atmosphere be evaluated carefully in terms of the pupils' health, and not only must the activity carried on within the classroom be varied and offer a change of pace, but also the time schedule of the classroom is important. The length of the school day must be compatible with the children who are in the classroom. A study by the NEA indicates few schools have made major changes in the length of the school day.[12] Further, it was shown that there is a gradual increase in the amount of time spent in school by children as they go from grade to grade. Double sessions born from the necessity of caring for variance of school enrollment when adequate facilities are not available, as well as busing in districts that are spread out geographically may increase the length of the school day to proportions where children will become overfatigued and their health and learning jeopardized.

Pupil time in school is often increased by voluntary participation in interests and activities during the after-school hours. These activities may be intramural or interscholastic athletics, music or dancing lessons, or various kinds of club meetings. Some pupils fail to participate in any of these available programs; others tend to be involved in too many school-sponsored activities. Counseling on an individual basis by teachers, parents, and guidance personnel can help pupils work out a balanced program.

Consideration must be given to differing individual and group needs in determining the length of the school day. The healthful and stimulating effect of variety in the daily program and the differences in fatigue levels among various age groups should receive attention. A decision concerning the length of the school day should take into account the importance of avoiding fatigue and boredom as well as the fact that these conditions are influenced by pupil interest, the alternation of sedentary and active forms of learning, and the emotional climate of the classroom.

THE WORLD AROUND THEM

It was clear to those attending one of the national conferences for physicians in schools that "the physical aspects of the school environment should have priority in developing a health program. . . . Provisions should be made for a safe water supply and sanitary disposal of waste . . . adequate heating, ventilation and lighting . . . safety of the building and grounds and transportation . . . ."

These are elemental considerations taken for granted in many urban communities but so fundamental everywhere as to make their mention imperative. Perhaps no disaster is more disturbing than a school fire, sickness arising in a school lunchroom, or a school bus accident.

– architectural considerations

In the last century and early in this, school buildings were constructed merely to house students. Little thought was given to function or to the promotion of the child's health. The child was and is expected to adjust to the environment. Flexible though a child may be and liberal though nature has been in giving him an abundance of energy and strength, he cannot conform to some of the architectural monstrosities and community monuments that are used for schools.

Even though there are many thousands of very fine schools, the ideal school has probably never been built. To apply all that is now known about lighting, ventilation and sanitation, paint and acoustics, and fire protection will require architectural advances far beyond the traditional ones. Architects are required who are willing to study children, not just prepare a blueprint, who are willing to think through the problems of function and not merely prepare plans to fill a specified physical area or to satisfy the requirements of the adult staff.

Some forward-looking communities desiring to construct buildings commensurate in value with the children who will inhabit them are designing structures that reflect architecturally the uses to which they are to be put. They are built for children, not to fit a building already established. They are built by architects who are as sensitive to the health of children as they are to the structural requirements of the building. The blueprints are not taken from the top drawer and used over and over again. They are created fresh for each community, for each site, for each conception of the purposes of the school and of the children who are enrolled in it. Such an architectural approach is organic; it is functional. It is useful and not monumental. It is different from what we are used to. Some typical differences in approach are shown in the comparison on page 250.

Modification from the traditional can be made indefinitely. The school of the future will contain even more adaptations developed for function, for health, and for location. The building will be built by architects of imagination and ingenuity. The product will be a place in which children will find pleasure and stimulation and where they will be able to read and see, grow and develop.

As investigation and experience mount up relative to the influence of the physical plan and the welfare of the student, standards begin to

Traditional	*Functional*
1. Poorly ventilated and damp gymnasiums and locker rooms in the cellar	1. Above grade in air and light
2. Shops in cellar or inside	2. Shops, like gymnasiums, above grade
3. Two or three main exits	3. Exits from each room
4. Two or more floors	4. Rambling one-floor plans
5. Limited play space	5. Large areas for outdoor work
6. Fixed room areas resulting from permanent wall construction	6. Expandable room areas through the use of movable partitions
7. Horizontal ceilings	7. Tilted ceilings for better air and light
8. Sameness in room and laboratory colors	8. Liberal use of color, contrasting danger colors, reflecting colors, pleasing colors
9. Harsh-resounding walls and ceilings	9. Acoustically treated walls and ceilings
10. Rooms straightaway	10. Diagonally placed rooms for better light
11. Sharp-angled stairways	11. Safer ramps and curves more expedient for passage
12. No facilities for exceptional children	12. Facilities, handrails, wheelchairs, special rooms, and so forth, for the handicapped
13. No health suite for nurse or physician	13. Space for the nurse and physician
14. Blackboards	14. Light-reflecting chalkboards
15. Miscellaneous heating	15. Radiant heating

appear. Professional groups of school people and architects have in some instances collaborated on studies which are helpful in school-building construction. Many of these standards are published, but they fill more pages than could be used here to reproduce them. Teachers and administrators need but to turn to them, however, to secure valuable assistance in planning for lighting, ventilation, room and laboratory location, fire protection, sanitation, construction materials, paint and color, acoustics, and other physical elements so important in school construction.

– all for the sake of the individual

Children can reap the best harvest from their educational opportunities only when every phase and facet of their educational experience contributes and none detracts from their best interests. Personnel, curriculum, administration, buildings, atmosphere, color, field experiences, activities, everything in the school environment must fit together to the end that the student emerges as well integrated an individual as the influence of the school can make possible within the child's total environment and within the constraints of his heredity.

There is an earnest purpose for this concern about the impact of the school experience. This purpose is best expressed perhaps in a cogent quotation from the National Society for the Study of Education:

> In our society the individual is the unit around which we build and naturally then we lean toward a concept of integration which involves the organization and the meaning which an individual is able to perceive and the experiences he has. We are desirous that he develop a concern for organizing and inter-relating his entire experience to the point where he will consciously work to make things "fit" while still maintaining sufficient flexibility that new patterns for organization and interpretation are welcomed and actively sought. We desire also that the individual develop certain skills which, at the present incomplete state of knowledge of the process of integration, seem to be valuable. We desire that he become acquainted with the attempts made and the bases used by others in organization of their knowledge and experience, not so much for the sake of knowing these as for providing an experience and critical analysis and judgment preliminary to making his own integration. We desire that he relate his developing knowledge and skills to the world about him and get satisfaction in doing it.[13]

The school health program takes a holistic view of the child and his environment and attempts to mobilize the resources of the educational system, his family, and the community to the promotion of his well-being.

REFERENCE BIBLIOGRAPHY

1 Howard S. Hoyman, "An Ecologic View of Health and Health Education," *Journal of School Health,* XXXV, 3 (March 1965).

2 Halbert L. Dunn, *High Level Wellness,* Arlington, Va., R. W. Beatty, 1961.

3 *President's Commission on the Health Needs of the Nation,* Washington, D.C., 1953.

4 Erik Erikson, *Childhood and Society,* 2nd. ed., New York, Norton, 1963.

5 *Ibid.*

6 *Ibid.*

7 Robert Havighurst, *Developmental Tasks and Education,* 2nd ed., New York, McKay, 1961.

8 Breckenridge and Vincent, *Child Development,* Philadelphia, Saunders, 1965.

9 Erikson, *op. cit.*

10 G. Wagner, "What Are Schools Doing; Pupil Growth Characteristics and the Curriculum," *Education,* 86 505–29 (April 1966).

11 Ralph Ojemann, *Committee on Preventive Psychiatry of the Group for the Advancement of Psychiatry, Promotion of Mental Health in the Primary and*

Secondary Schools: An Evaluation of Four Projects, Report no. 18, January 1951, p. 8.

12 NEA, Research Division, "Length of School Year and School Day," *Research Bulletin 43;* December 1965, pp. 103–105.

13 Nelson B. Henry, *The Integration of Educational Experiences,* 57th Yearbook, National Society for the Study of Education, Part 3, Chicago, University of Chicago Press, 1958, p. 22.

SELECTED READINGS

Breckenridge and Vincent, *Child Development,* Saunders, Philadelphia, 1965.

Dunn, Halbert L., *High Level Wellness,* R. W. Beatty Ltd., Arlington, Va., 1961.

Erikson, Erik, *Childhood and Society,* 2nd ed., Norton, New York, 1963.

Fit to Teach, American Association for Health, Physical Education and Recreation, The Association, Washington, D.C., 1957.

Havighurst, Robert, *Developmental Tasks and Education,* 2nd. ed., McKay, New York, 1961.

Healthful School Environment, Joint Committee on Health Problems in Education of the NEA and AMA, The Associations, Washington, D.C. and Chicago, 1969.

Hoyman, Howard S., "An Ecologic View of Health and Health Education," *Journal of School Health,* 25:3, March 1965.

CHAPTER 10 HEALTH AND DEVELOPMENTAL PROBLEMS OF CHILDREN

Knowledge of the desirable patterns of child growth and development and the goal of providing appropriate activities and supplies to enhance this process provide the basis for planning and implementing the school health program. When the school environment, programs, and personnel are planned to meet the needs of the largest proportion of children, we may expect well-being to be promoted. We cannot assume, however, that such programs and personnel will be appropriate for all children.

We can no longer be satisfied merely with planning to serve the "average" or "normal" child. Averages force us to ignore differences and emphasize likenesses. It is wiser to plan for the various children always present in school populations who fail to reach, or who exceed the standard developmental levels. Programs should be planned to reflect those children who are ill, handicapped, normal, retarded, or gifted.

Consideration of differences characteristic of various age groups affords a functional approach to planning the health programs that deal with variations. Knowledge of the foreseeable variance in growth and development and information about illnesses that have increased incidence and prevalence relating to age groups can help in planning appropriate health services for children. There are differences in health needs among children and differences in their capacities to respond to a health program at the varying ages. Just as knowledge of optimum growth patterns and needed contributions to health can serve as a stimulus for a program to promote well-being, so, too, can knowledge of illness and maldevelopment characteristic of age groups help us in planning programs for variant children.

This chapter will provide a brief overview of the health and developmental problems of children by age level and will conclude with a description of several problems of particular concern in the school age population. No attempt is made to be exhaustive. Further information may be obtained by rereading Chapter 1.

HEALTH PROBLEMS BY AGE LEVEL

Whenever we attempt to serve a child, we should begin by asking ourselves the question, "What's going on here? In what way at this moment is the child growing and developing physically, mentally, emotionally, and spiritually? What is he trying to do? Which of his present patterns of behavior are signs of strength (and will readily be perceived as such) and which are signs of strength that can be misinterpreted by the uninitiated?" A negativistic 2-year-old who is developing into a very independent person may appear to be "uncontrollable," or the child in kindergarten who is merely exercising his healthy large muscles may mistakenly be called "pathologically hyperactive."[1]

What then are the developmental and what are the common health problems in the school age conformation?

– early childhood

The most frequently found health concerns in the elementary school years are overweight, underweight, short acute illnesses, dental problems, visual and hearing defects, and limitations in strength and stability. Many children come to school carrying the burden of the problems which they acquired during birth or early infancy. These include congenital defects, undescended testicles, mental retardation, cerebral palsy, epilepsy, asthma, allergies, and, on occasion, the rare metabolic diseases such as phenylketonuria. The acute health problems of childhood relate to poisoning, injuries such as burns, falls, bruises, cuts, and fractures, and all of the childhood infectious diseases including ear infections, colds, flu, and pneumonia. Some early schoolchildren are more like preschool children than like schoolchildren. There are many developmental levels at every age. Among the developmental problems that are still of concern from kindergarten to grade three are thumb sucking, wetting and soiling, immature speech, including lisping and stuttering, fatigue, picky eating, masturbation, and changing sleep and rest patterns. School health activities should reflect the diseases that are of most severity or that occur most frequently in this population.

– late childhood Children in the upper elementary years are, by and large, in a very healthy period of their lives. Some may continue to have chronic problems such as speech problems and dyslexia. Some may have identified hearing problems or vision loss, and a very small proportion of children may have chronic rheumatic heart disease or kidney infection. The acute problems are at a very low ebb during this period, but accidents continue to be a major source of morbidity and mortality. Parents, and children, too, will ask many questions about growth and development. Such things as nail biting, urinary frequency, grimaces, and anxiety over growth will be among the subjects that will be discussed most often. In many cases beginning menstruation, vaginal discharge, and easily aroused sexual feelings will present a problem to a child and should be taken into account in planning school health programs.

– early adolescence Children in grades six to nine have, as a general rule, very good health. They do, however, have the adolescent overconcern with somatic complaints. Generally they are quite concerned with overweight, underweight, tallness, physical fitness, acne, and poor eating and sleeping habits. There is experimentation with alcohol, coffee, tobacco, glue and other drugs, and often there is fear of disease and death. This is, of course, the time of great physiological change and the beginning of the search for identity that sometimes leads to extremes of behavior in the quest for an answer to the question, Who am I?

It should be remembered that adolescents' difficulties are often a reflection of the conflicts and patterns of their early experiences. The prevention of adolescent problems begins at the time of birth and not at the time the child enters junior high school. The problems which an adolescent is having can be profitably viewed as reactivations of the experiences of infancy or childhood. By viewing adolescent behavior as such, it is sometimes possible to help or prevent the problems that sometimes seem overpowering to the teenager.

The search for identity often leads the adolescent into extremes of behavior ranging from friction between them and their parents to rebellion and even violence. Sometimes an identity crisis leads to severe anxiety states or to delinquency, and there is much concern over masturbation, early heterosexual behavior and, on occasion, experimentation with homosexual activities. Daydreaming is at its peak and often is so real to the adolescent that he begins to believe his fantasies. While developing activities to help in the control of teenage problems, the health services and health education program must also take care not to participate in activities that freeze teenagers in bizarre behavior patterns, when what their behavior amounted to was merely experimentation with a different life style.

– late adolescence Perhaps the division into early and late adolescence is an undesirable one, for all of the problems of early adolescence continue on into late adolescence. At this age there is a particularly wide span of developmental patterns. The late adolescent, of course, is more mature and more responsible and has had the opportunity to answer more adequately the question, Who am I? Those planning programs for youth in the high school age group will have the opportunity to consider such late adolescent problems as venereal disease, car accidents, athletic injuries, toothaches, malocclusion, hepatitis, and mononucleosis. Rising problems of sexual experimentation, teen-age pregnancy, depression and suicide, use and abuse of drugs, and anxiety over social acceptance constitute challenges for those seeking to deal with variant behavior as well as promote the well-being of children.

The National Health Survey and other sources show that children have a large accumulation of illness and disabilities at the time of school entry and that these conditions tend to become more numerous with passing years.[2] The following table indicates an increase, between 1960 and 1970, in the number of children with common health problems.

	1960	*1970*
Epilepsy (under 21)	360,000	450,000
Cerebral palsy (under 21)	370,000	465,000
Mentally retarded (under 21)	2,180,000	2,720,000
Eye conditions needing specialist care including refractive errors (5–17)	10,200,000	12,500,000
Hearing loss (under 21)	360.000–725,000	450,000–900,000
Speech (5–20)	2,580,000	3,270,000
Cleft palate-cleft lip	95,000	120,000
Orthopedic (under 21)	1,925,000	2,425,000
Congenital heart disease	About 25,000 born each year, of whom 7,000 die in the first year	
Emotionally disturbed (5–17)	4,000,000	5,400,000

Source: *Health of Children of School Age,* Washington, D.C., U. S. Department of Health, Education and Welfare, Children's Bureau, 1964.

POVERTY'S CHILDREN The Commission on Civil Disorder has the following to say about the health of ghetto residents:

> The residents of the racial ghetto are significantly less healthy than most Americans. They suffer from higher mortality rates,

> higher incidence of diseases and lower availability and utilization of medical services. They also experience higher admission rates to mental hospitals. These conditions result from a number of factors. From the standpoint of health, poverty means deficient diets, lack of medical care, inadequate shelter and clothing and often a lack of awareness of potential health needs. As a result, about thirty percent of all families with less than $2,000 per year suffer from chronic health conditions that adversely affect them as compared with less than eight percent of the families with incomes of $7,000 or more.[3]

Statistics from Headstart programs across the nation indicate large numbers of children with rampant dental cavities, recurrent ear infections, iron deficiency anemia, and less than average height and weight for their age. The child who is apathetic because of malnutrition and whose experiences may have been modified by acute or chronic illness or whose learning abilities may have been affected by damage to the brain by trauma or poisoning cannot be expected to respond to opportunities for learning in the same way as the child who has not been exposed to such conditions.

The child who is a product of either urban or rural poverty, the child who is a member of an ethnic minority that has suffered discrimination chronically, and the child who is disadvantaged in his total environment is at great risk in the area of health problems. Such children must be identified and not merely additional but special educational opportunities effective for them must be provided. Groups of children from any of these backgrounds must be differentiated into meaningful subgroups for purposes of remedial, supplemental, and habilitative education. Whenever conditions of risk to the child can be identified, principles of public health and of current biosocial knowledge should be utilized to reduce learning handicaps in future generations. It is not enough just to provide additional teaching-learning opportunities.

Concern for the socially disadvantaged cannot, in good conscience, restrict itself to the provision of either equal or special education or preschool opportunities for learning. It must concern itself with all factors contributing to educational failure among which the health of the child is a variable of primary importance.

Such an argument is not new. The basic relationship between poverty and illness and educational failure has long been known and more recently devastatingly documented.

Few factors in the health history of the child have been as strongly associated with later intellectual and educational deficiencies as prematurity of birth and complications of the pregnancy from which he derives. The premature infant not only has a poorer chance of surviving than the infant born at term, but when he does survive, he has a higher risk of being handicapped. Prematurity is associated with a large number of neurological, mental, sensory, and other handicapping conditions, which results in a large representation of prematures among the retarded and educationally backward children at school age. Prematurity and its complications in regard to learning have a high representation in the poverty segment of our population. This is true not only in classes for the retarded but also among children classed as minimal brain dysfunction.

A higher proportion of children from poverty families than from more affluent parents are likely to have survived complicated births or serious illnesses and threats during the period immediately after birth. These may have lasting effects, which the child will bring to school. Malnutrition is a problem that is more and more being connected to malfunctions in learning and disturbances of behavior. Study after study of the nutritional habits of people of our country indicate that poor nutrition is highly related to the income and educational level of the family. Children of deprived environments are very likely to be suffering from malnutrition.[4]

> Studies on experimental animals appear to demonstrate that either nutritional or sensory deprivation at an early age when the brain is still developing result in learning handicaps. The possibility that many of the world's underprivileged children are being permanently retarded in their ability to learn and to adapt to the demands of a modern society is a matter for serious consideration.[5]

School health programs must take into account the health conditions of the child and also the environment from which he comes in developing the special activities in the school and in the community that can help the learner. The school program must plan with the family and with the community for changes in the environment from which the child's difficulties came, if handicaps resulting from a disadvantaged environment are to be remedied.

PROBLEMS OF SPECIAL CONCERN IN SCHOOL

Certain problems sometimes occur in a large enough percentage of children to cause schools particular concern. These include problems that are directly destructive to the learning process and also those conditions that occur frequently enough to upset the functioning of the educational program and that have an indirect effect on the child's learning ability. Included are learning disabilities, accidents, communicable diseases, mental health, and poor nutrition. The nature of these problems will be described below, and programs of control and remediation carried on by schools will be described in later chapters.

– learning disabilities

The term "learning disabilities" provides us with a broad rubric under which we can group all of those problems that seem to inhibit learning. The very shortness of the term and its seeming simplicity should not lead us to think that this is a very simple subject. Learning disabilities are extremely complex and controversial and are now in the process of being studied intensively. Learning disabilities include all manner of learning deficits, such as dyslexia, difficulty in reading, and dyscalcula, difficulty in arithmetic. These are the most common, followed by problems in spelling, writing, and music, all of which have their own technical descriptions. These problems are caused by a multitude of factors. Ray Barsch ascribes learning problems to intellectual deficits, which may themselves be caused by many things: parental rejection or affective neglect; sensory impairment of sight or hearing; excessive anxiety (parent generated); social disadvantage, which has impoverished the intelligence; physiologic dysfunction; and poor teaching.[6] Looking behind each of these categories and determining the many causes for them gives some idea of the overlap and complexity and difficulty of this particular area.

Most people, however, when they speak of learning disabilities, are using the term to mean reading problems. Because of the varying definitions that are used in deciding whether or not a child has a reading disability it is difficult to know what a given person means by dyslexia. For this reason statistical statements on the incidence and prevalence of problems will vary as much as 15 to 20 percent. Estimates of children in the school population with reading problems will vary anywhere from 5 to 15 percent. It is most often stated that boys outnumber girls in a ratio of 4 to 1. Reading is the most frequent area of learning disability among the children listed by teachers as having learning problems. At least half of the children with reading problems are described as hyperactive and nervous or significantly immature. A large percentage of them appear to have significant difficulty in motor coordination. Subjective appraisals include "poorly motivated," "poor worker," "lazy or slow." "Immature" is probably the favorite adjective that teachers use to describe such children.

There are many classifications of reading disabilities. The following is one of the most functional.[7]

1 Dyslexia (sometimes referred to as congenital dyslexia). It is a condition characterized by an individual's inability readily to acquire, and subsequently to use, one or more language skills with a facility commensurate with his intelligence. Dyslexia is associated with an individual's tendency to reproduce language in an unusual fashion. It is often found to be familial in occurrence. In general, this diagnosis is applied to those young people who have found it very difficult to learn to read and spell but who are intelligent and learn arithmetic more readily.[8]

2 Slowness in learning to read (sometimes referred to as secondary dyslexia or bradylexia). The child in this category is slow in his reading or slow to learn to read because of any one of, or a combination of, many factors such as low intelligence, faulty vision

or hearing, emotional disturbances, poor cultural background, or poor instruction.

3 This category is a mixture of the first two and is the largest group. Not only can emotional disturbances cause reading problems, but it is very rare indeed for a child with congenital dyslexia not to develop rapidly a secondary emotional problem.[9]

Gerald Jampolsky sums up the problem well when he states:

1 Inadequate diagnosis leads to inadequate treatment.

2 The majority of children who are over two years retarded in their reading have psychological problems that inhibit their total adjustment to life. These psychological problems may be primary in that they may cause a reading problem or they may be secondary in that they are brought about because the child has trouble learning to read.

3 The either/or battle of organic versus psychologic etiology of reading disabilities has little merit. It is more rational to view disorders as a symptom on a continuum with many complexities entering into the problem. Emotional factors are only some of the many factors at a varying degree.

4 Anxiety as a result of intra and interpersonal conflicts may play a varying but important role in inhibiting children from learning to read.

5 With regard to the socio cultural factors that contribute to the reading problem the three C's can inhibit the learning of the three R's. By this it is meant that misinterpretation or over or under emphasis of Competition, Conformity, and Competency can actually inhibit the learning process.[10]

There may be no field in medicine or education that is so challenging or difficult to deal with than dyslexia because of the multitude of interacting causative factors, each bearing independently, though sometimes cross-related and varying in degree. In spite of all these difficulties we must do the best we can. It seems obvious that the investigation of a child with reading difficulties can best be done through the team approach, that is through interaction and correlation of several disciplines. It seems best to view dyslexia as multifactorially "caused." Treatment, therefore, must almost always be a multipronged approach that attempts to develop a special environment in which a given child can function and flourish.

– mental illness and behavioral disorders

What is mental illness, maladjustment, or unsocial behavior? What is mental health? These questions are not easy to answer, but the problems are there (teachers and others see them) and Sherwin S. Radin has roughly placed them in categories as follows:

A Academic problems—underachievement, erratic, uneven performance.

B Social problems with siblings, peers—such as the aggressive child.

C Relations with parental or other authority figures, such as defiant behavior, submissive behavior, or ingratiation.

D Overt behavioral manifestations, such as tics, nail biting, toilet problems, sleep and feeding disturbances, exhibitionism, aggressive and sadistic behavior, phobias, fire setting, interest more befitting to the opposite sex, such as the tomboy girl or sissy boy, bizarre or unusual behavior expressions, speech peculiarities, such as delayed immature speech development, neologism, echolalia, and psychosomatic disorders.[11]

Placed in the larger perspective of the population as a whole, mental disorders have been classified by the American Psychiatric Association as follows:

1 Mental retardation—subnormal general intellectual functioning which originates during the developmental period and is associated with impairment of either learning or social adjustment, or maturation, or both.

2 Organic brain syndromes—disorders caused by, or associated with impairment of brain tissue function.

3 The psychoses—patients are described as psychotic when their mental function is sufficiently impaired to interfere grossly with their capacity to meet the ordinary demands of life. The impairment may result from a serious distortion in their capacity to recognize reality.

4 Neuroses—anxiety is the chief characteristic of the neuroses. The neurotic person, as contrasted to the psychotic, manifests neither gross distortion nor misinterpretation of external reality.

5 Personality disorders—characterized by deeply ingrained maladapted patterns of behavior that are different in quality from psychotic and neurotic symptoms.

6 Psycho-physiologic disorders—this is a group of disorders which are determined by physical symptoms caused by emotional factors and involve a single organ system. For example, a psychophysiologic skin disorder applies to a skin reaction caused by nervousness.[12]

Other classifications are perhaps of less interest to those in school health. They include special symptoms, transient situational disturbances, and terms used for administration.

It is of considerable interest, however, that the American Psychiatric Association, in its latest edition of the *Diagnostic and Statistical Manual of Mental Disorders,* has added a classification called behavior disorders of childhood and adolescence. This major category represents disorders occurring in childhood and adolescence that seem to be less fixed than the psychoses, neuroses, and personality disorders. Perhaps this is due to the great changes in all behavior that appear at this age and the relative malleability of children and adolescents. The most common of the behavior disorders are hyperkinesis, withdrawal, and overanxiousness.

Rather than attempt to delineate each of these categories specifically, it seems desirable because of current interest in the problem to give a picture of the hyperkinetic child.

Hyperkinesis is characterized by overactivity, restlessness, distractibility, and short attention span, especially in young children. The behavior usually diminishes in adolescence.

Perhaps the best way to describe the condition is through the use of a case history. The story of Billy gives some idea of the dilemma and frustration that parents, teachers, and the community face in dealing with a hyperactive or hyperkinetic child. Billy seemed basically to be a well-meaning boy who was generous and thoughtful of others, but when he was with a group of children he tended to become over excited, throw tantrums, and get into fights. He was bright and curious but strangely enough, was not able to concentrate on a project for very long. Developmentally, he could run and jump and climb and throw easily enough, but he had difficulty with his finer motor coordination in such activities as cutting, pasting, printing, and painting. He was able to attend kindergarten, but even in that relatively unstructured situation, his restlessness and short attention span became a problem for the teacher. He did not finish his work and spent most of his time wandering around the room distracting other children and the teacher as well.

The teacher's first reaction was that Billy needed more discipline at home. The parents felt Billy needed more structure and a more understanding teacher at school. However, no amount of reasoning, sending him to his room, sending him to the school office, spankings, or other forms of discipline had any noticeable effect. About the only time Billy was calm was when he was alone with his parents or when he was carrying on some childhood activity in his own room with little distraction or stimulation. He always became excitable and nervous and angry when he was in school or with other groups of children.

Because of these difficulties the child was examined by the family physician, whose initial impression was that with decreased stimulation and increased tender, loving care, Billy would tend to grow out of his undesirable behavior. The parents were instructed to ignore temper tantrums or at least try to be objective about them and to provide firm structure and support. Hopefully, the doctor felt, the unusual behavior would disappear by the time Billy entered school.

When this turned out not to be the case, the family physician referred Billy to a specialist who was able to confirm the physician's diagnosis—hyperkinesis. In this particular case it was possible to try one of the stimulant medications which have been found to have a paradoxical effect in that they seem to calm a large percentage of the children who are diagnosed as being hyperkinetic. With the use of the medication and with continued cooperation and support on the part of the teacher and the family, Billy has begun to do considerably better in school and has been able to develop a moderate amount of self-control. He is at least approachable at this point and the prognosis is that he will continue to improve. If it is possible for him to complete the early school years without feelings of failure and with a good self-concept, it is likely that few long-range deficits will occur.

Unfortunately, it is not always the case that a child such as this receives care in time to prevent the psychological problems that develop from being a failure in almost all areas of childhood endeavor.

Concurrent with interest in the hyperkinetic child, there is concern for children who have been labeled "brain damaged" or "minimally brain damaged." There is a large amount of literature concerning children with disturbed perceptual-motor function. It is beyond the scope of this book to discuss each of these problem areas in depth, but it should be noted that all of them are seemingly related to each other, at least in their external manifestations, and that they all relate to learning disabilities, either directly or through unusual classroom behavior that retards the child's progress. Some of these children show frank neurological signs on physical examination, others show unusual activity on the electroencephalogram.

Estimates of the number of children with significant emotional problems varies anywhere from 20 per thousand[13] to 20 to 40 percent of all children. Obviously the statistics quoted depend entirely on the definitions of the author. However, we can be assured as we plan school health programs that the emotional and behavioral problems of children present a large area of concern to the personnel of the school district. The teacher is usually the first one to see evidences of maladjustment or overt behavioral differences. The daily demands of the classroom are likely to reveal the child's inability to cope with them as expected. Every pupil may exhibit types of behavior indicative of emotional problems at one time or another. Some types of behavior, even in exaggerated form, are on occasion entirely normal reactions to physical and social situations. For example, a pupil may be irritable because he is hungry, sleepy because he was up all night, or foul-mouthed because that is the way everyone in his family talks, or fearful for realistic reasons.

Any observation needs to be interpreted and evaluated. No teacher should base her judgment on a single observation without considering all factors that influence a pupil's emotional health. Observations that provide clues to the emotional health of pupils may relate to educational progress, physical appearance or behavior, social behavior, personal behavior, or violations of rules. The teacher should be alert to each of these categories.

Perhaps in the long run it is more profitable for the physician, teacher, and nurse to understand normal childhood and adolescence and to understand the variations in such traits as tolerance, restlessness, friendliness, confidence, stability, and tenseness that are compatible with their effective living, than it is to be able to move gracefully in those circles where "schizoid," "paranoid," and "cyclothymic" are equally common terms.[14] The function of school health personnel is to attempt to distinguish the patently abnormal from those variations from the usual that only temporarily interfere with the child's ability to do his schoolwork and get along with people. The school health personnel will do best if they think of most children in the terms one associates with normality. It will then be less likely for personnel to mistake eccentricity for abnormal behavior and transient disturbances of emotional growth for serious disorders or to join forces with those who would have all students exhibit similar behavior.

– accidents

If we measure the importance of a child health problem by its mortality rate, accidental injuries qualify as high priority. They are by far the greatest threat to life in the school ages. As a matter of fact, the leading cause of death for all ages up to age 34 is accidents. When accidents are compared with all causes of death combined, we find that nearly half the deaths among boys at ages 5 to 14 and about one-third of the total among girls in this age group result from accidental injuries. During the later teen years, 15 to 19, the percentage rises to more than three-fifths of the total mortality among boys and to about two-fifths among girls.[15]

The Public Health Service estimates that more than 17 million children under 15, or at least one-third of the entire child population in the United States, are injured each year seriously enough to require medical attention. Statistics on the number of nonfatally injured school age children are somewhat difficult to find. Most accidental-injury studies either include or concentrate on preschool ages, during which accidents take a still greater toll of life than during the school years.

Data from the National Health Survey, at present our main source of information on school age nonfatal accidents on a national scale, indicate that each year about 12 million children between the ages of 6 and 16 years suffer injuries requiring at least one day of restricted activity or medical attention. Based on this survey, the time lost from school annually is 39.2 days per 100 boys, and 23.3 days per 100 girls.[16]

According to *Accident Facts,* published by the National Safety Council, at the high school level there are about 18.6 accidents for every 100,000 school days. At the junior high school level the rate falls to about 15.9 per 100,000 school days, whereas at the elementary level the rate is 6.4 accidents per 100,000 days of attendance.[17]

The leading types of accidents for school age children in the United States continue to be motor vehicle accidents, drowning, fires and explosions, firearms, and falls. The child is at risk from accidental death and injury in all portions of his environment and in all of the activities that he undertakes.

The greatest hope in the field of accident prevention lies in education. Effective safety is far more than a matter of limitations and restrictions. It is a matter of learning how to live and act in a safe way. Schools have the opportunity to provide both direct and indirect education to students to help them appreciate and utilize protective devices. Education can also help them anticipate and overcome hazards in new and unfamiliar situations.[18] The school health program has a clear responsibility not only for the educational approach, but also for making sure that the school environment is as safe as it can be made for children. A comprehensive and well-planned school health program will include education, a safe environment, and proper enforcement and supervision.

– nutrition

Studies of children's growth and development have long been used as an indication of the interaction between nutrition, income level, and various other environmental factors. Recent studies on the effect of early nutrition on subsequent mental development have renewed interest in this subject. That malnutrition in early life adversely affects mental development is regarded as truth, although the duration of the effect, the separation of this effect from other environmental factors such as social stimulation, and the best methods of correcting the situation remain speculative. It is now thought that during certain critical periods, malnutrition sufficient to produce retarded growth, as shown by such measurements as height and head circumstance, is correlated with retarded mental development.

The national nutrition survey currently being conducted under the auspices of the Public Health Service is the first large-scale survey to be made in this country that includes clinical and laboratory data as well as information on diets. When completed, the initial phase will focus on low-income areas including some 70,000 persons in 10 states. In the preliminary report Schaeffer stated that the findings in children, especially in the preschool group, indicate an alarming prevalence of signs of malnutrition including gross retardation, anemia, unsatisfactory blood levels of albumin, vitamin A, and ascorbic acid and unsatisfactory levels of urinary riboflavin. Some outright cases of deficiency disease such as rickets and protein deficiency (kwashiorkor) were found.[19]

Recommendations for children's diets must now take into consideration the 1968 revision of the recommended dietary allowances of the National Academy of Sciences, National Research Council.[20] The recommendations include many additional age categories for children and changes in the recommended daily allowances for many nutrients as compared to the recommendations of 1964. Notable are the increases in requirements for iron and calcium among adolescents.

Many factors in the home and community life complicate the problem of nutrition enormously. Nutritionists agree that were it not for the competing attractions that lure many persons, particularly children, away from a rational diet, we would have healthier children in our schools. Apparently resources are available to feed the population well; it becomes a matter of educating parents and children and providing economic resources that make the purchase of good food possible and its use desirable.

Generally speaking, it may be said that our population is well fed. Compared to people in many other countries the family in the United States is in a favorable position nutritionally. Nevertheless, there are hundreds of thousands of parents and children who have poor dietary practices, who have a low intake of vegetables and fruit, who rely too heavily upon sweets, and who do not know how to choose food for their own good. Far too many persons omit breakfast, choose a poor lunch, overeat, follow some nutritional fad, or in some other way handicap themselves because of nutritional stupidity.

The school has a responsibility to accept in this area. Not only must it discharge its traditional educational function in regard to the problem, but also because millions of children eat about one-fourth of their meals on school premises, the school must provide good food and demonstrate proper food preparation. The school is in a position to influence nutritional behavior even though it has stiff competition from commercial advertising, family customs, ignorance, and perhaps above all, individual taste, which, when selection is limited, does not always lead a person to eat what is good for him.

– communicable disease In spite of the development of safe and effective vaccines that have wide-spread use in the United States, infectious disease continues to be the most common cause of absence from school among children. Respiratory infections account for a major portion of the infectious diseases. The common cold is the most common cause of illness among children and accounts for almost 50 percent of all illness. Presumably because of the wide-spread use of vaccines to prevent diphtheria, whooping cough, polio, and measles, influenza now occurs more frequently than the total of all of the common childhood diseases. If the population continues to have its children immunized and to keep their boosters up to date, and with the introduction of rubeola and rubella vaccines, the common childhood diseases should become almost nonexistent. There have been clusters of families who have neglected to keep their immunizations up to date or have neglected them altogether. In these situations there have been outbreaks of diphtheria, whooping cough, and polio. These diseases can be kept under control, but only if strong vigilance is maintained in keeping the population immunized.

Venereal disease is a continuing problem, especially in the teen-age years. At the writing of this book, gonorrhea was increasing in almost epidemic proportions in all parts of the United States and drastic measures were being taken to establish some sort of control. For this disease no immunization is available. There is the additional problem that girls who have gonorrhea often do not have symptoms that let them know they are in need of care. Several states have passed legislation that allows children age 14 and over to come to health departments for treatment without parental permission. This is an effort to make it easier for children to accept treatment.

Tuberculosis presents a continuing threat to all age and class levels but more particularly to the lower socioeconomic groups. A more detailed account of tuberculosis and control measures in the schools is included in Chapter 14.

Another disease which in the past has been relatively low in incidence appears to be on the increase. This disease is infectious hepatitis, which is increasing among children and young adults as well. Attempts to develop a vaccine for this disease have to this date been unsuccessful.

Infectious disease has continued to be of very great concern to school health programs but over the years has decreased in its relative importance because of the many measures of control and the general increase in the standard of living. Some illnesses have been decreasing over the last thirty years. These are rheumatic fever and rheumatic heart disease, osteomyelitis, mastoid infections, streptococcal illness, and meningitis of all kinds. Infections of the kidney, too, occur less frequently. Even though communicable disease is relatively less important in the overall school health picture, it is still a field in which school health personnel must be very active. Expert programs of control of these conditions are outlined in Chapter 14.

SUMMARY

This brief review of the health and developmental problems of children has presented an idea of the proportions of children who may be expected to have specific kinds of problems. The relation of illness and developmental problems to age group, and their relation to learning and to socioeconomic groups, provide the basis for planning realistic school health programs. The review of certain conditions that are of critical importance to the child and to his functioning in school presents further information on the multifactorial causation of the problems of children. Particular concern must be paid to the nature of the school environment and the special situations that must be provided for that proportion of children who do not fall within the central group of "well" children. These adaptations are outlined in Chapter 13. School health programs must plan for the promotion of well-being and for the control of variance.

NOTES AND REFERENCES

1 Pauline Stitt and Karl Shultz, "Fivefold Focus on Child Health," *Nursing Outlook,* 15, 8 (August 1967).

2 Clara Schiffer and Eleanor Hunt, "Illness Among Children; Data from the U. S. National Health Survey," *United States Children's Bureau Publication,* no. 405, Washington, D.C.; Government Printing Office, 1963, p. 13–16.

3 *Report of the National Advisory Commission on Civil Disorders,* Washington, D.C., Government Printing Office, 1968, p. 136.

4 "Malnutrition, Learning and Behavior," *Archives of Environmental Health,* 19 (July 1969), 3.

5 Herbert G. Birch, "Health and The Education of Socially Disadvantaged Children," *Developmental Medicine and Child Neurology,* 1968, pp. 10, 580–599.

6 Ray Barsch, "Perspectives on Learning Disabilities: The Vectors of a New Convergence," *Journal of Learning Disabilities,* 1, 1 (January 1968).

7 John V. V. Nichols, "Reading Disabilities in the Young," *Journal of School Health,* XXXIX, 6 (June 1969).

8 J. Roswell Gallagher, *Medical Care of the Adolescent,* 2nd ed., Des Moines, Iowa, Meredith, 1966.

9 Nichols, *op. cit.*

10 Gerald G. Jampolsky, "Psychiatric Considerations in Reading Disorders," *Reading Disorders,* Richard M. Flower, Helen F. Gofman, and Lucie I. Lawson (eds.), Philadelphia, Davis, 1965.

11 Sherwin S. Radin, "Mental Health Problems of School Children," *Journal of School Health,* XXXIII, 6 (June 1963), 252.

12 *Diagnostic and Statistical Manual of Mental Disorders,* 2nd ed., Washington, D.C., American Psychiatric Association, 1968.

13 *Report of the Committee on School Health,* Evanston, Ill., American Academy of Pediatrics, 1966, p. 36.

14 Gallagher, *op. cit.*

15 Schiffer and Hunt, *op. cit.*

16 *Ibid.*

17 *Accident Facts,* Chicago, National Safety Council, 1965.

18 George Wheatley, "Accidents and School Children in School Health Problems," Pediatric Clinics of North America, 12, 4 (November 1965), p. 941–956, Saunders, Philadelphia, 1965.

19 "Current Developments in Childhood Nutrition," *Dairy Council Digest,* 40 2 (March-April 1969).

20 *Recommended Dietary Allowances,* 7th rev. ed., Washington, D.C., Food and Nutrition Board, National Academy of Science, National Research Council, publication no. 1694, 1968.

SELECTED READINGS

Accident Facts, National Safety Council, Chicago, yearly.

Diagnostic and Statistical Manual of Mental Disorders, 2nd ed., American Psychological Association, Washington, D.C., 1968.

Gallagher, J. Roswell, *Medical Care of the Adolescent,* 2nd ed., Meredith, New York, 1966.

Kosa, John, Aron Antonovsky, and Irving Zola, *Poverty and Health, A Sociological Analysis,* Harvard University Press, Cambridge, Mass., 1969.

Optimal Health Care for Mothers and Children: A National Priority, U.S. Department of Health, Education, and Welfare, National Institute of Child and Human Development, Washington, D.C., 1967.

Report of the Committee on School Health, American Academy of Pediatrics, Evanston, Ill., 1966.

Report of the National Advisory Commission on Civil Disorders, Washington, D.C., 1968.

Schiffer, Clara, and Eleanor Hunt, *Illness Among Children: Data from the U.S. National Health Survey,* Children's Bureau Publication #405, Washington, D.C., 1963.

Scrimshaw, Nevin, and John E. Gordon, *Malnutrition, Learning and Behavior,* M.I.T. Press, Cambridge, Mass., 1968.

CHAPTER 11 THE PERSONNEL OF THE SCHOOL HEALTH PROGRAM

The school meets its opportunity to help children by developing a program of health services and environmental care to match its program of instruction. School people know that much of their educational effort will be enhanced when it does. School people know how difficult it is to teach a partially seeing, tired, or sick child, and the school attempts to identify those children and help them receive care.

Out of this rather simple and logical point of view have grown extensive and valuable programs involving the cooperative effort of many persons, professional and otherwise. These programs range from the rather uncomplicated use of the town doctor to immunize children in school against diphtheria to the full-fledged programs of services found in many of the large cities.

The professional people who attended the National Conference on Coordination of the School Health Program stated the interest and responsibilities of schools in pupil health as follows:

The school's responsibility for health education and health promotion rests upon four principle premises: (1) the obligation of the school to aid and maintain the pupil's optimum fitness to learn; (2) the obligation of the schools to maintain conditions that promote healthful living while pupils are under school jurisdiction; (3) the obligation of the school to help assure optimum health for each individual; (4) the obligation of the school to enable young people to make intelligent decisions about personal, family and community health.[1]

In a fully integrated school health program the child as a whole takes the center of the stage. Objectives of child health development are agreed to and sought. His health and welfare, his psychological and social development, his safety and wellness all become prime considerations along with his intellectual and academic advancement. It becomes imperative that all that goes on within the school experience contributes to and does not detract from the total development of the student. To bring this ideal to its fullest maturity obviously requires the highly coordinated effort of many persons, none working in isolation from the others but all working within a master plan to the ultimate benefit of children.

SOME BASIC CONSIDERATIONS

In a program as complex as school health has come to be, cooperation and coordination mean face-to-face relationships in the solution of problems. These do not in every instance result in productive achievement, particularly if those concerned have given little or no thought to the cooperative requirements of a good school health program. To this end it would be well to consider several factors that are basic to the attainment of the cooperative action needed:

1 *Many talents are needed.* There is a place in the total health program for physicians, nurses, and teachers. Teachers of physical education, sight saving, speech and reading, home economics, psychologists, dental hygienists, dentists, social caseworkers, immunologists, dieticians, sanitary engineers, school administrators, and still others of specialized and non-specialized abilities are useful. Their counterparts from the consumer's side are, of course, the children and their parents. Little can be done without some of the key professionals; likewise little can be done without the full participation and cooperation of the consumers. A school health program is truly a large experiment in group action aimed at the improvement of the life of the individual child.

2 *The talents must be used in an atmosphere of mutual respect and professional confidence.* Success in school health education comes when each profession recognizes the worth of the contribution of the other, refuses to usurp more responsibility or more credit than is due, and shares in the thinking, planning, and execution necessary to get the job done. It is not always easy to get a group of individuals to work cooperatively. Sometimes the teacher assumes far too much prerogative in the guidance of the child or, worse, discounts the efforts of others as they try to effect the life of one of her children. Sometimes the physical education teacher assumes far too much in the sphere of diagnosis or fails to make

use of the best scientific information in giving health instruction. Sometimes the physician or nurse, prepared in highly individualized professional traditions, finds himself unable to appreciate the work of others or, worse, insists that all school health work must be considered a private reservation and that all other participants must be subject to his direction. Any of these manifestations are always unfortunate. They jeopardize the attainment of the objectives of child development.

3 *A program of school health education should not be an object of charity.* Contributions to it should not be sought on that basis. In the early days many physicians and some nurses were asked to donate their time for examinations or screening. Other people were urged to donate books, equipment, or time. Private practitioners were asked to examine children or give the summary of their findings to the school. With rare exceptions this charitable approach to administration has been a failure. Physicians have their professional competence to sell, others have specialized talent that cost them years to develop. Such skills should be bought and paid for by the schools if they expect to make good use of them. No part of the program that involves any measure of professional competence should be performed without adequate compensation.

4 *A school health program is an educational enterprise, not a medical one.* It is not in competition with the practice of medicine, it is complementary to medicine, supports it, educates school children to patronize it, discovers individual needs that are referred to it, but does not compete with it. School health education has no eventual aim to substitute its services for those of a private physician.

There is evidence to show that where complete school health education programs have existed there is not less but more demand for the services of physicians and public health workers. The school has a legitimate purpose in concerning itself with the health of the child. The school realizes that education cannot go on fully and constructively unless the child is in good health, and it tries not to waste public funds in attempting to educate children who are unable to receive an education. Finally, to teach about health, to organize experiences pertaining to it, and to carry on education in a healthful environment are the basic purposes of the school. The school must give its students control over the means of existence, over life. Certainly learning about health and healthful living can be considered in no other way than as a means of furthering our existence and theirs within the scope of education. There is no infringement upon the province of the physician, the hospital, or the clinic. There is thus no grounds for discoordination. School health education programs deserve the cooperation of all professional personnel united to serve within it.

5 *The school is in no position to finance extensive curative or remedial medical or dental programs at public expense.* Principally the school acts as an interested community agency willing to stimulate others to find the means to provide the needed resources for the benefit of handicapped or ailing students. Of

course exceptions are made but in nearly every instance the exceptions are endorsed by the medical and dental groups of the community who appreciate the fact that only through these means will the children involved be properly cared for.

It is well recognized that there are millions of people unable financially or unprepared intellectually to seek and find medical service. The school sees their need, at least insofar as the need is expressed through children, and is in a position to encourage social and public agencies in efforts to bring medical aid to them.

6 *The emphasis on school health education has moved from the mass to the individual.* This is a general trend in all of education. It becomes no longer important to survey thousands and thousands of children in an annual physical exam unless within such a program each child is given thorough attention and his individual status and needs are discovered and adequately dealt with. School health is individual centered, not program centered.

HEALTH PERSONNEL OF THE SCHOOL

School health education depends upon the qualifications of the personnel involved and the way in which they work together. School health education is actually a fascinating and massive experiment in group cooperation. Each person within the program relies to some extent upon someone else or upon many others. When all are well prepared for their tasks and can fulfill their interdependent responsibilities effectively, the total program will reach its goals.

Many people contribute their time and skills to the success of a school health program. Some participate as generalists; for example, the school administrator and the teacher. Others are specialists, such as the nurse, physician, and dental hygienist, who have chosen to work in schools because of a commitment not only to the goals of health, but also to the compatible goals of the education system. The representative members of the school health team will be discussed below.

– the administrator

Basic to the work of any health program is a sympathetic, interested, informed, and willing school administrator. Nothing can go on successfully in a school without his supporting consent and in turn the administrator knows that he must accept final responsibility for all that goes on. Hence, many principals are cautious about the element of school health education until they are sure of the merits of the program.

To develop an outstanding health program the administrator must secure the funds for the program, employ adequately trained personnel or establish inservice training programs, establish an adequate public relations program with the communities so the patrons of the school will understand the processes and details of the health program, establish personnel records and evaluate programs, provide for health and sick-leave programs for school personnel, and guide architectural personnel so that all new facilities will be constructed with thoughtful regard for the health and welfare of the children and teachers.

These are his basic responsibilities. He may allocate some of them to other people, but in the end the success or failure of the enterprise comes back to the principal or superintendent. School health education can develop just as far and no further than is agreed to by the principal administrative officer of the school or district.

– the teacher The teacher at any level from kindergarten into college is essential to the instruction program in health and to the screening and observation program. There is no one quite as influential as the elementary or secondary teacher in shaping the concepts and in imparting the knowledge relating to healthful living. No teacher falls outside this category. The biology teacher in high school, like the teacher of English or social studies, has a large bearing on the formation of life's patterns as they relate to health. The elementary teacher is as influential in the development of these patterns as she is in the development of reading skills.

The teacher is the first line of defense in school health services programs. She is in a position to observe children over a period of time and to observe changes in their health or in their behavior. She also has more frequent talks with parents about children. She has the opportunity to pass on to nurses and to physicians or parents the information that she has acquired through observation, screening, or daily contact with pupils on such matters as vision, behavior, fatigue, hearing, appetite, relations with peers, and anything else bearing upon the health of the child that would indicate a need for assistance. She can also note needed improvements in the environment and suggest alterations in curriculum and in the organization of the school day that would react favorably upon children. The teacher as an educational expert can, if she is aware of the holistic nature of the child, throw considerable light on possible reasons for scholastic difficulty, behavior problems, and even delinquency.

As is the case with any other worker in the school health program, the classroom teacher has the opportunity of receiving assistance from the specialists on the school health team that will help make her work with children more effective. She can expect advisory assistance regarding the health and welfare needs of all pupils as well as specific help in assisting children who present special health, behavioral, or welfare problems that interfere with their school adjustment and progress, or that influence adversely the class group activities. Specialized health personnel often can provide understanding and insight into causative factors within and outside the school that affect the child's adjustment in school and can give suggestions of ways the teacher can work with children who need further help. The classroom teacher may also ask for and receive help in understanding the nature of services that are available to the child through the community and in understanding ways of preventing certain types of problems.

– the nurse The nurse has come to be an integral part of the school faculty. Although it is true that only a few schools have the services of a full-time nurse, slightly over 85 percent of them have at least part-time service and this situation is improving. Where nurses are not employed as faculty members by boards of education, their services are being provided to schools by public health departments.

The services of a nurse are literally vital to a complete school health program. She participates in so many ways and performs so many functions that a description of all of them here would be impossible. A detailed report has been published by the School Nursing Committee of the American School Health Association. This distinctive and helpful report, which recommends policy and practice, summarizes the role of the nurse in the school health program as follows.

> 1 The school nurse works as a member of the school staff under the administrative direction of the school to which she is assigned. The school administrator has the responsibility for the development, interpretation, and maintenance of the school health program as part of the total school program. The nurse has the leadership role in developing the essential elements of the school health program in cooperation with the administrative staff, school personnel and representatives of the medical profession and appropriate community agencies.
>
> 2 The school nurse assists in providing inter-related health and educational services to support and stimulate the learning process. This is accomplished by a variety of broad functions designed to promote, protect, maintain and improve the health of pupils.
>
> 3 The school nurse has a leadership role in integrating all health activities within the school into a coordinated health program, in relating the school health program into the total school program and in coordinating the school health program with the total health program of the community.
>
> 4 The school nurse plans for a continuous evaluation of her professional skills and assists with the evaluation of the total school health program in terms of accepted standards and changing needs.

5 The school nurse recognizes that the health status of the school staff is a significant factor in the promotion, protection and maintenance, and improvement of pupil health.

6 The school nurse has a dual professional role as a member of the teaching profession as well as the nursing profession.[2]

An equally authoritative statement of the functions and qualifications for school nurses has been published by the American Nurses' Association.[3]

In a study of the role and functions of the school nurse as perceived by public school teachers, Orcilia Forbes found that teachers perceive the nurse as performing most frequently in the areas of health appraisal and follow-up, and in health protection and safety.[4] Time studies indicate nurses in New York City schools spent, before reorganization, about a third of their time on nonprofessional activities such as clerical procedures, while health appraisal and case finding were the activities in which they spent most of their professional time.[5]

Elizabeth Stobo summarizes the work of the present-day school nurse very well:

> In school health work the clients are children. This makes it essential for the nurse who works in the school to have a good understanding of normal growth and development. She also needs to be knowledgeable about various clinical deviations, especially those that directly influence learning. Just as it is important to know about clinical deviations from the medical point of view, it is essential to have knowledge about learning deviations from the educational point of view. In the school the nurse has an overarching responsibility between nursing and education. Her knowledge of medical problems does not make her a junior physician; her knowledge about education does not make her a junior teacher; but her ability to take this knowledge, synthesize it and apply it in her work with children, does make her a competent nurse to work with school age children and youth.[6]

The same competence makes her a valuable helper to the teacher in the classroom situation.

– the physician

In an ideally developed program of school health education, a physician serving the school is a requisite. Much of the success of the health activities program revolves around him and his services. Originally brought into the schools to examine for hearing and vision, the physician has had the scope of his work enlarged to insure him a key position in the entire educational program. His duties extend far beyond the routine and hasty examination of children and the compilation of statistics. He has become in every sense a member of the school staff participating uniquely in the development of school health programs. His potential duties have been described by the American Academy of Pediatrics:

> The school physician should function as a medical advisor as well as a specialist employed for a professional job. The physician in the school, however, is primarily a health advisor rather than a source of medical care. To community health agencies and physicians he has the role of liaison with the schools. He advises the school staff on medical matters. An important function is to analyze with the nurse the information she has gathered about pupils and their families and to prepare her for leadership in securing follow-up. He also advises parents and children as to the facilities which exist for solving their medical problems. However, he should not replace or substitute for the child's own physician or other community health services. In the medical examination his primary aim is toward effective counsel rather than in specifically stated diagnosis or in treatment. The school physician should not give treatment except of first aid and emergency type. He should discover the child who needs medical attention and attempt to make a correct evaluation. Using the knowledge gained by his evaluation, he can without discussing specific diagnosis, guide the parents to their private physician or other community health services.[7]

The school physician can aid and supplement the private physician in his care of the child. More intimate knowledge of the school environment and his greater opportunity to suggest and recommend needed educational and recreational modification are of help to both private physicians and parents. He should have a good knowledge of available community resources and thus be able to tell the family and the private physician what these resources are when they need them. The school physician also has an opportunity as part of the organization staff to act as a counselor on health curriculum content, health instruction, and environmental sanitation.[8]

There are other opportunities, of course. The physician can contribute his professional skills to the evaluation of all materials used in the health instruction program, serve as a resource person in health classes, participate actively in the program of the school-community health council, aid in the development of inservice training programs for teachers in relation to their function in school health programs, and supervise the conditions under which competitive athletics are played and the conditions under which food is served at school. The school physician must be able to work cooperatively, not only with school administrators, but also with teachers, dentists, nurses, dental hygienists, counselors, health educators, psychologists, lunchroom managers, teachers of special education, physical educators, parents, representatives of professional organizations, and voluntary health and welfare agencies.[9]

Many physicians serving the schools are finding a useful function in their opportunity to contribute medical information to help school people in their understanding of the learning process itself. Coming from medical science in the last few years is important information about physiological states that contribute to or hamper the child's ability to learn. Learning involves obviously more than intellectual capacity and the biochemistry of endocrine secretions, nutritional states, sexuality, and other physiological factors have a bearing on problems associated with learning.

The unique position of the physician in the educational program has not been easy to establish. The idea of having a physician serve the school was not readily acceptable to medical groups, and the educators were prone to misunderstand the function and use him in a short-sighted way. The cooperation of medicine through physicians, nurses, dentists, and psychiatrists is today welcomed and deemed necessary in the better educational programs. Its success depends largely upon the acceptance of the following practices:

1 Teachers must understand and function within the principle of privileged communication. Information about pupils must be held in confidence and used for professional purposes only.

2 The physician serving the school should, with the school administrator, inform local medical and dental societies of the nature of school problems and programs and utilize the judgment and resources of those groups.

3 Remedial treatment should be carried out by personal physicians. In instances where it is not possible to make such arrangements, school authorities should arrange to have the work done through public agencies and clinics.

4 The medical advisor should obtain all needed data on a child from the personal physician's examination. But in instances where these data are incomplete or the examination is of a type not helpful to the school program, the medical advisor should make the examination a part of the school program.

5 A great deal of the medical advisor's time could be well spent discussing with parents and teachers at school the health needs and development of school children. The advisor should demonstrate what good medical service is and assist parents and teachers in the development of their own conception of the value and nature of adequate medical care.

6 The school physician should be a component of the school system and a direct participant, not "an outsider looking in."

– the dental hygienist Increasingly school districts are hiring dental hygienists to be responsible for conducting a school program of effective dental health education. Such a program aims to help children and youth appreciate the importance of a clean mouth, free of disease and abnormalities, and to help them learn to assume responsibilities for personal care and for securing periodic professional attention.[10] The dental hygienist's role in achieving these objectives involves direct instruction and counseling. Well prepared dental hygiene teachers will be professionally knowledgeable in both the fields of preventive dental hygiene and education and can be of great assistance to teachers either by helping in the preparation of their own study units or by entering the classroom for short periods of teaching. Additionally, school districts often offer services of general inspection and dental prophylaxis as a part of the individual dental counseling program that the hygienist carries on.

– the custodian The school custodian is an important person in the school system. He not only carries a heavy responsibility in operating and protecting valuable school buildings, grounds, and equipment, but he is also a vital factor in promoting school health and safety. The school custodian promotes the health and comfort of pupils by effectively operating the heating and ventilating equipment, cleaning walls, ceilings, and artificial lighting fixtures to secure the best possible illumination, providing temperate water on tap, liquid or powdered soap, and paper towels on hand at all times for handwashing, systematic checking all playground equipment and keeping it in good repair, removing broken glass and other playground hazards, keeping all required exit doors and hardware in good operating condition, keeping all lines of travel through required exits free of obstacles, inspecting safety devices on boilers and pressure vessels to make sure they are always in good operating condition, periodically checking fire alarm systems and fire-fighting equipment, and carrying on a continuous program of fire prevention.

The work of the school custodian is no small task. In a large measure the custodian, as well as the teacher, promotes appreciation for orderliness and cleanliness and promotes good health practices by pupils. Because of his close connection with factors in school health and safety, the school custodian should obviously be a member of a school health committee. His understanding and appreciation of his responsibilities and his competence in doing his work have a direct bearing on pupil health and safety.

– the nutritionist The school lunch manager is responsible for a feeding program that is an integral part of the school's curriculum and health services. Such a program should operate efficiently to provide an adequate and nutritious lunch under sanitary, attractive, friendly conditions and at the lowest possible cost. The manager must also be able to train and supervise the other school lunch personnel that he has helped to select. With these responsibilities the manager must have an understanding of nutrition, food buying, and food preparation. He should also have the ability to work with all other personnel in the school.

The size of the program determines the kind of school lunch manager to be employed. For a large school lunch program in a school system the director should have completed a period of training qualifying him as a dietitian or nutritionist.

The current rebirth of interest in nutrition and the proliferation of research on the relationship between malnutrition and learning have stimulated experimental programs in public school nutrition which would be analogous to that of the dental hygiene program. Public health nutritionists are being hired to serve an educational role as well as to provide individual guidance to teachers, children, and families to better meet their nutritional needs.

– the school health aide or health center clerk

The practice of hiring school nurse assistants has grown out of the need to supplement meaningful health services for the hard-to-reach and the lower socioeconomic segments of our society. This, plus the stimulus of the federal government in providing more training and jobs for poverty groups, has led to the emergence of a force of competent paraprofessional personnel.[11] Paraprofessionals can, with careful creative supervision and training, ease the burdens of the professional and perform many neglected and/or new services. The activities that the assistant has to this point carried out have been maintenance of the nurses office, participation in health appraisal activities, individual child health supervision, record keeping, responsibility for health education materials, and others. The position of the school nurse assistant has been a developing and changing one. It can, therefore, be assumed that her activities will change with experience, new knowledge, and evaluation.

– the consultants

The Psychiatrist / A psychiatric consultant in the schools potentially could play many roles. Among these would be the organizing and implementing of programs for the emotionally disturbed, providing a service program for selected children, or serving as consultant for all personnel of the schools.[12] Perhaps all of these roles could serve a valuable function to the school system. However, the recent emphasis of psychiatric consultation in the schools has been to bring psychiatric insight into education and to broaden the understanding of educational personnel of the psychological dynamics of learning.[13] It would appear that psychiatrists participate most successfully when they apply such insight to the educational problems of specific children and thereby assist teachers and administrators in the handling of the everyday behavior problems in the classroom. Direct psychiatric therapy of teachers and of students is ordinarily considered to be a function of the therapeutic community rather than of the educational system.

The Dentist / The dentist is consultant to the school system in all matters relating to the oral health of boys and girls.[14] In this capacity he advises, assists, and interprets to school authorities and health staff the organization, administration, procedures and policies governing the dental health program in the school. When given administrative responsibilities, he has a responsibility for the professional supervision of the dental hygiene teacher. He might explain how to carry on dental inspections or suggest improvements in the more or less expensive use of dental prophylactic instruction. He might advise in the use of visual aids, resource material, dental equipment, and supplies. In general, he acts as an advisor and consultant to whom the dental hygiene teacher can turn for guidance or assistance.

The school dentist also has the responsibility of working with the dental society locally or with county or state dental groups. In this regard he is in a key position to promote cooperation between the school dental health program and community programs. He must work closely with public health officials and voluntary clinics, particularly to insure adequate dental care for indigent families.

The dentist should also serve as a resource person and see that visual aids, dental literature, and other suitable materials are made available in the classroom. Teachers of health, science, and guidance classes can be particularly instrumental in promoting the dental health programs. The dentist often can help them directly in their teaching by appearing before classroom groups.

As an advisor to the superintendent and board of education in all matters relating to the school health dental program, the dentist may be consulted on such matters as facilities, dental equipment, and selection of dental health personnel. He would be consulted in the preparation of a budget for and financing of the school's dental health program. His role, too, must be seen in relation to the total health service and other pupil services of the school.

ADMINISTRATIVE PATTERNS OF SCHOOL HEALTH

There are three major administrative patterns used in the United States for providing school health services from nursing service to complete health appraisals on school children. In a "specialized" school health service the local board of education operates its own health service and the school nurse is an employee of the school district. In a generalized program the local board of health operates the health service within the school system. Public health nurses working in the schools are employed by, and are responsible to, the health department. A third administrative pattern involves some form of joint authority for financing and administrating the school health programs by the board of education and the board of health.[15] Approximately two-thirds of all school health services programs are administered by boards of education while less than 10 percent have dual administration. The remaining are supervised by a board of health. Superintendents of schools prefer to have school health service programs administered by boards of education because of more: (1) efficiency and simplicity in a single agency administration, (2) success in obtaining funds for school health services, (3) understanding of the total school situation by the health service personnel, (4) complete integration of the health services and health education, (5) emphasis placed on school health, and (6) improved service to school age children.

Regardless of the administrative pattern followed in carrying out a school health program, educators, private physicians, and public health officials must not lose sight of the importance of close and continuous cooperation among all involved.

PUPIL PERSONNEL SERVICES

As the schools have increased their efforts to provide every child with the maximum opportunity for a successful learning experience, an increasing number of persons have been hired from the clinical professions. Often they were organized administratively into groups such as guidance and counseling, health services, and school social work. Unfortunately, many of these functioned autonomously and relatively independently of each other. During the last few years these services rendered by physicians, psychologists, counselors, nurses, dental technicians, social workers, attendance coordinators, and speech and hearing clinicians have been organized into the administrative category and concept called Pupil Personnel Services. This has been an effort to see that Pupil Personnel Services are an integral part of education—a program to facilitate the full development of each pupil. The purpose is to see to it that the clinical professional personnel, teachers, and staff work jointly to achieve the objectives of the school.

Teachers confronted with the public's demand that all children be adequately educated are faced with large numbers of children with reading disabilities, speech disorders, health problems, adjustment difficulties, and the need to promote the well-being of the child. Except for the guidance counselor almost all the personnel coming into schools have had their preservice training in clinical settings. Pupil personnel activities strengthen the school's efforts to identify and understand the educationally significant characteristics of each pupil, to provide information and insights to help the pupil's teachers and parents and the pupil, himself, in his educational progress.[16]

– what does the program cover?

The scope of Pupil Personnel programs varies from one school system to another. There is general agreement, however, that the program includes services in the area of attendance, guidance, health, psychology, and social work. Basic objectives for each of these services can be stated as follows:[17]

Attendance Services / Attendance Services are intended to insure the regular attendance of all children who should be enrolled in school. Efforts are made to promote regular school attendance, to account accurately for pupil attendance, absence, or tardiness, and to carry out proper exemptions and employment certification procedure. Another very important aspect is the effort to discover and remedy the causes of nonattendance. Modern attendance services involve primarily guidance personnel rather than persons and methods represented by the caricature of the "hookey bull" or truant officer.

Guidance and Counseling Services / Guidance and Counseling Services assist all pupils in assessing and understanding their abilities, aptitudes, achievements, and educational needs; help pupils and parents to know about educational and career opportunities and requirements; help pupils make optimum use of these opportunities through planning and progress toward well formulated long-range goals; foster satisfactory personal and social development of the pupil; and provide information useful in planning and evaluating the educational program.

School Health Services / School Health Services aim at helping each pupil attain and maintain the highest possible level of health; providing educational experiences aimed at the development of sound attitudes toward health; fostering understanding and practices that will help these people become more self-reliant in maintaining and improving their own health and the health of others; and promoting healthy and safe school environments.

School Psychological Services / School Psychological Services attempt to identify the learning and school adjustment characteristics of pupils. Psychological evaluations are made of pupils with acute problems of development in school and remedies are suggested on the basis of this diagnostic information. These services also function to assist the school staff in understanding the psychological needs of pupils and in responding in ways which support pupil learning and development.

School Social Work / School Social Work focuses on pupils with problems of a social, emotional origin or nature which interfere with normal progress in school. The casework method is used extensively as are the resources of social institutions and agencies. Social work services include the identification and interpretation of environmental influences on pupil behavior, collaboration with teachers and others in adjustment processes, and strengthening the home influence on the pupil's school progress.

Many Pupil Personnel programs also include Speech and Hearing Services in order to remedy or relieve communication disorders of pupils. These and other remedial services as well as the many phases of school programs for exceptional children are considered by some as parts of the instructional program rather than as additional phases of Pupil Personnel programs. In any case, Pupil Personnel Services should have very close and supportive relationships with all phases of education.

– professional roles in teamwork The specialists who work in the programs listed above serve as resources to administrators and others to provide education adapted to the needs of pupils and give direct assistance to pupils and parents in promotion of the pupil's growth and development. As they go about their tasks the specialists perform many activities in common. All of them will gather and use information about pupils or consult with others in the school or contact parents in school and at home and will work with many resource people in the community. Most of the members of the Pupil Personnel Services team will talk with individual pupils and with groups of pupils and will participate with follow-up and evaluation activities. In the same way principals and teachers perform many of the activities that have been related to the specialists in Pupil Personnel.

In addition to the shared methods of functioning each of the professions brings a unique background and way of working to the school setting. The Pupil Personnel Services administrative structure has been designed to allow a maximum of coordination and cooperation among the generalists and the specialists as they work together to support a pupil's growth or adjustment in the school.

ROLES OF PROFESSIONAL WORKERS

– the school social worker The school social worker performs a specialized form of social work focusing on pupils with problems of a social-emotional nature or origin that interfere with normal progress in school. One of the school social worker's most unique contributions is his skill in the use of social casework methods. Another is his extensive knowledge in the use of various social institutions and agencies. He contributes to the study and adjustment of pupil problems through facility in the use of school and community resources, through an understanding of human growth and behavior, and through an ability to share his professional competencies with others in the school.[18, 19]

– the school psychologist At the moment there appears to be no unanimity of opinion as to the role of the school psychologist. The problem is compounded when one divides, on the basis of the training, the personnel into school psychometrist and school psychologist. Most statements on school psychology emphasize that the psychologist studies and assists the individual pupil, using extensive and intensive psychological techniques and on the basis of this study recommends appropriate education and psychological remediation for exceptional children. The psychologist also plays a role in determining eligibility for pupil placement in special programs or classes and he also participates in planning, executing, and assessing programs of education and reeducation of pupils.[20, 21, 22]

In most school districts he provides appropriate inservice training and consultive services. Where such programs are supported the psychologist may play a strong role in educational research projects, particularly those that relate to the improvement of the educational program. As with most Pupil Personnel specialists he serves in a liaison relationship between the schools, the community, community agencies, and the clinical profession from which he came in order to interpret the educational and psychological program of the schools in relation to children's learning and behavior problems.

J. N. Schiebe describes the psychologist as a clinician who is concerned with direct services to the child in the identification, diagnosis, prognosis, and recommendations for treatment of a child's school connected problem, as a coordinator who coordinates school, home, and community facilities for helping children, and as a consultant to teachers and to administrators in regard to the mental health aspect of the school situation.[23]

– the school counselor Although the role of the guidance counselor in the schools has not crystallized, perhaps the statement by the Joint ACES-ASCA Committee on the Elementary School Counselor will provide a good idea of the current role. They state:

We envision the counselor as a member of the staff of each school. The counselor will have three major responsibilities: counseling, consultation and coordination. He will counsel and consult with individual pupils and groups of pupils, with individual teachers and groups of teachers, and with individual parents and groups of parents. He will coordinate the resources of the school and community in meeting the needs of the individual pupil. The counselor will work as a member of the local school staff and as a member of the team providing Pupil Personnel Services.

We believe that guidance for all children is an essential component of the total educational experience in the elementary school.

By guidance, we mean a continuing process concerned with determining and providing for the developmental needs of all pupils. This process is carried out through a systematically planned program of guidance functions. These guidance functions are a vital part of the school's organized effort to provide meaningful educational experiences appropriate to each child's needs and level of development.

By counselor, we mean a professional person educationally oriented, highly knowledgeable in the area of child growth and development, with a broadly based, multiply disciplined background in the behavioral sciences and a high degree of competence in human relations.

By educationally oriented we mean having a knowledge of the elements of the school program including curriculum, the learning process and school organization. We recognize the value of teaching experience in the schools but feel that knowledge of the school program and processes can also be gained through a planned program of experiences in the schools as a part of the counselor's preparation.[24]

Much of the work of the school guidance counselor is concerned with helping the pupil and parent develop a better understanding of the pupil's personal characteristics and potentialities and working in a developmental way with individual pupils and groups of pupils.

– the speech therapist In most instances the speech therapist is involved in group therapy. He is concerned with auditory training, speech-muscle coordination, visualization, voice training, phonics and phonetics, phonetic or kinesthetic placement for accurate sound production, spontaneous and directed speech, and mental hygiene. He is also involved in the identification of those children who need help and with carrying out a systematic pattern of follow-up consisting of referral, scheduling, and direct therapy.

In many school districts, the speech therapist will also be involved in the identification of hearing loss among children. Hearing programs essentially follow the pattern of mass screening of large numbers followed by tests of hearing sensitivity for those with suspected hearing problems. This more detailed test by specially trained personnel leads to the identification of those who should be referred to an otologist or other physician for a complete diagnostic workup. Although still an area of controversy among speech therapists themselves, speech improvement and its application to the classroom situation has become an increasing part of speech therapy in the schools. Through this means the speech therapist is able to influence the communication problems of children who have borderline difficulties and who would not otherwise be able to benefit from the direct services of a speech therapist.[25]

– role delineation among pupil personnel services specialists

As has been stated in previous paragraphs, the overlap in function among the Pupil Personnel Services specialists is sizable. Questions are being raised as to whether or not satisfactory and professionally meaningful distinctions can really be made among these professions. Each professional feels that he brings a unique point of view and way of functioning to the child and the teaching-learning situation. There is a substantial corps of functions among the professions which are essentially the same. These include knowledge of human growth and development and responsibilities for coordination and consultation. Whatever professional rivalry exists among the specialists in Pupil Personnel is inappropriate in the light of this fact.

The functions of each of these professions can be determined only by the objectives that are established for the school district within which they are working. The goals of the program should be established before the professional roles are delineated. This can only occur through coordination and communication among the members of the Pupil Personnel Services team and other school personnel.[26]

Pupil Personnel specialists, in order to be the most effective, must have a good understanding of the philosophy and purposes of the school as an institution in cooperative efforts with other educational personnel. All are receivers as well as givers. In the teaming of services, competencies and contributions are different and complementary, not hierarchical.[27]

RESEARCH ON PUPIL PERSONNEL SERVICES

In a survey of more than one hundred systems with a coordinated program of pupil personnel services,[28] it was found that more money nationwide was being spent for guidance than for any other service, an average of $12.77 per pupil per year. Health service expenditures ranked second at $4.13, then psychology at $2.47, speech at $2.41, social work at $2.13, and attendance at $1.08. In the systems surveyed, an average of 4.2 percent of the schools' operating budgets was being spent for pupil services. Although the wealth of the school district was positively related to expenditures for pupil services, many other factors were also involved.

Nurses account for one-sixth of all pupil personnel services employees and represent 92 percent of available staff time in the health services personnel directly employed by school systems. In a stratified random sampling of schools and systems across the nation, it was found that 89 percent of the elementary schools and 83 percent of secondary schools were served by school nurses employed either by the schools or another agency. About 40 percent of the schools reported they had a school physician.

THE PUPIL PERSONNEL SERVICES SUITE

The concept of teamwork and the interrelatedness of the professional disciplines in pupil personnel services should be reflected in the building facilities housing these personnel. Areas assigned to social workers, guidance counselors and psychologists should be designed to permit maximum availability to students and staff while having the flexibility to provide privacy when it is needed in personal interviewing or psychological testing. The pupil personnel services suite should be separated from the administrative function of the school, although in small schools it may be necessary to have these offices closely related in order to provide adequate supervision of those who are waiting.

The health center portion of the suite should reflect the functions of the school nurse. There should be an area for children to rest as they are waiting for transportation home, having suffered an acute illness or accident at school, or while they are resting from a temporary upset or disturbance. Lavatory facilities and sinks should be available to the rest area. There should be an area for first aid activities and for the storage of first aid supplies. The nurse will need a quiet office for interviewing children as well as for screening activities. A waiting room area should be available for the use of medium-size groups. This area should be large enough to permit vision screening either through direct use of 21 feet or for the use of the Snellen chart with a mirror.

SUMMARY

Knowledge and experience with the growth and developmental needs of children and of the problems of variant children have led school districts to hire a large number of personnel trained in clinical activities. Among the most frequently employed are nurses, physicians, dental hygienists, social workers, counselors, psychologists, and speech therapists. In the past such organizational departments as health services and guidance and special services have functioned apart and autonomously. The modern trend is for grouping all of the clinical specialities into a category called Pupil Personnel Services, emphasizing coordination, teamwork, and interdisciplinary effort on behalf of the learner as well as in support of the educational specialists of the school district. Although the roles of the social workers, psychologists, counselors and speech therapists have been described, it is not within the scope of this book to pursue their activities further in detail. The following chapters will describe the activities and programs that are ordinarily included as part of the school health education program. It is recognized that these are now generally a part of Pupil Personnel Services and must be designed to mesh with all of the activities of a school district.

NOTES AND REFERENCES

1 American Association for Health, Physical Education, and Recreation Report on the National Conference on Coordination of the School Health Program, Washington, D.C., NEA, 1962.

2 Committee on School Nursing, "The Nurse in the School Health Program," *Journal of School Health,* XXXVII, 2a (February 1967).

3 The American Nurses Association, "Functions and Qualifications for School Nurses," New York, 1966.

4 Orcilia Forbes, "The Role and Functions of the School Nurse as Perceived by One Hundred Fifteen Public School Teachers from Three Selected Counties," *Journal of School Health,* XXXVII, 2 (February 1967).

5 Lester Rosner, Grace McFadden *et al.,* "Better Use of Health Professionals in New York City Schools," *Public Health Reports,* 82, 10 (October 1967).

6 Elizabeth Stobo, "Trends in the Preparation and Qualifications of the School Nurse," *American Journal of Public Health* (April 1969).

7 American Academy of Pediatrics, "A Report of the Committee on School Health," *School Health Policies,* XXXIII, 1 (January 1954), 76–77.

8 American Academy of Pediatrics, "A Report of the Committee on School Health," *School Health Policies,* 1966.

9 Milton Senn, "Role of the School Physician," in "School Health Problems," *Pediatric Clinics of North America,* 12, 4, (1965).

10 Rosemary Ann Frost, "The Role of the Dental Hygiene Teacher in Pupil Personnel Services," *Journal of School Health,* XXXVI, 9 (November 1966).

11 Doris Bryan, "The School Nurse Assistant," *New Dimensions in School Leadership,* Washington, D.C., National Council for School Nurses, American Association for Health, Physical Education, and Recreation, 1968.

12 Knabel Lylton and R. W. MacNeven, "The Function of the Psychiatric Diagnostic Unit in the School System," *American Journal of Orthopsychiatry,* Digest of Papers presented at 36th Annual Meeting, New York, American Orthopsychiatric Association, 1959.

13 L. C. Hirning, "Some Experiences in School Psychiatry," *Teachers College Record,* 66 (October 1964), 64–70.

14 Gerold Natiella, "Role of the Supervising Dentist in Pupil Personnel Services," *Journal of School Health,* XXXV (September 1965).

15 James Wolf and Howard Pritham, "Administrative Patterns of School Health Services," *Journal of the American Medical Association,* 193, 3 (July 1965).

16 Gordon P. Liddle, "The Pupil Personnel Concept of School Health," *Journal of School Health,* XXXV, 4 (April 1965), 153.

17 Bruce Shear, "Team Action in Pupil Personnel Services," *Bulletin of the National Association for Secondary School Principals,* 324 (January 1968).

18 Council of Chief State School Officers, "Responsibilities of State Departments of Education for Pupil Personnel Services," Washington, D.C., Council of Chief State School Officers, 1960.

19 California State Department of Education, "Guidelines for Pupil Personnel Services in the Elementary Schools," Sacramento, California State Department of Education, 1967.

20 H. L. Silverman, "School Psychology: Divergent Role Conceptions," *Psychology in the Schools,* VI, 3 (1969).

21 Merville Shaw, "Role Delineation Among the Guidance Professions," *Psychology in the Schools,* IV, 1 (1967).

22 Council of Chief State School Officers, *op. cit.*

23 J. N. Schiebe, "School Psychologist: Clinician, Coordinator, Consultant," *National Elementary Principal,* 45 (September 1965), 43–44.

24 California State Department of Education, *op. cit.*

25 T. Mandell, and E. L. Walle, "Hearing and Speech Conservation in Schools," *Bulletin of the National Association of Secondary School Principals,* 326 (March 1968).

26 Shaw, *op. cit.*

27 Shear, *op. cit.*

28 Gordon P. Liddle, "Findings from the Health Related Research of the Inter-Professional Research Commission on Pupil Personnel Services," *Journal of School Health,* XXXIX (May 1969).

SELECTED READINGS

Functions and Qualifications for School Nurses, The American Nurses Association, New York, 1966.

"The Nurse in the School Health Program," Report of the Committee on School Nursing, *Journal of School Health,* 37:2a, February 1967.

"Progress in Pupil Services," *Bulletin of the National Association for Secondary School Principals* #324, January 1968.

"School Health Problems," *Pediatric Clinics of North America,* 12:4, 1965.

Teamwork in School Health, Report of the National Conference on Coordination of the School Health Program, American Association for Health, Physical Education and Recreation, Washington, D.C., 1962.

CHAPTER 12 HEALTH APPRAISALS

The whole program of school health education is planned and administered in relation to a realistic appraisal of the well-being of children, their needs, and the nature and extent of their problems. A basic aim, therefore, is to identify early the health problems of the individual children and then work constructively to ready the child for school or to restore the child to such a state that he will be able to profit from the school experience. Additional aims are to provide appropriate learning environments and to work cooperatively with parents and family members. The modern, scientifically constructed program seeks to learn through careful individual appraisal the status of its students and to construct whatever kind of program is necessary on the basis of the findings.

PURPOSES OF APPRAISALS

Why does the school want to appraise the health of its children? Is this not a private affair between the home and family doctor? Is not the school stepping out of its field in seeking data about health? The answers to these questions can be learned by studying carefully the nature of the appraisals the school sponsors, or recommends, and their purposes in relation to the educational program.

Schools now sponsor or recommend a program of screening tests, periodic medical examinations, special examinations for special cases, examinations for athletes, and continuous observation of the health of children by teachers and nurses. Why? There are five reasons:

1 Appraisals provide information that will lead to constructive alterations in the life of the child. It is good sense (and a wise expenditure of public funds) to assure the child's fitness to receive an education. Industry and business recognize the value of fit workers over the sick. The school also finds it more profitable to teach well children and thus seeks out those who suffer from impairments in the hope that constructive action can be taken to remove the cause of the condition.

An appraisal often indicates that the child should be examined further for more careful diagnosis by the use of tests not ordinarily found in school examinations or be referred to the personal physician for attention to the conditions found. This is one of the earliest purposes of appraisal to appear historically and the one most commonly thought of today. It is, perhaps, the most important and the one that takes the appraisal efforts of the school into the home and community in order to get the action necessary to make the discovery worthwhile.

Appraisal establishes a chain of action that will find the children who are in need of medical, dental, psychological, or social services and get them promptly to adequate care. For several million children such activity by the schools may be the only chance they will have for the discovery and care of impairing handicaps.

2 Appraisals provide the basis for adjustments of the school program to meet individual needs. Teachers who want to assist in the total development of the child must know of those factors that are retarding learning or that are likely to interfere with growth. To teach most effectively, teachers must know their children—their possibilities and limitations, their physical as well as psychological status.

Only with such information can teachers and others modify the school study program and adapt it to individual needs. Children with partial vision can be moved forward in the classroom or be given special sight training; hard-of-hearing children can be seated where they can hear; cardiacs can be scheduled only on lower floors; rest periods can be arranged to relieve tensions. There are a great many ways in which the school program can and should be modified to the advantage of individual boys and girls if the data can be found and made available.

3 Appraisals provide the basis for individual compensation for irremediable handicaps or deviations. There are many children who have defective hearing or sight, are abnormally short or tall or fat, have burns or scars or malformations, or are handicapped by other

conditions serious enough to interfere with living life to the fullest. These deviations create social, psychological, or physical problems in their lives. School personnel are in a strategic position to help them compensate for these conditions. The short can be made to feel more comfortable and secure, the tall less conspicuous; the obese can be helped to find success, the crippled to achieve desired ends. These compensations need not be wholly medical. Many of them are social and psychological and teachers have an obligation to help in achieving them. The child must be taught to live well in spite of an irremediable condition.

4 Appraisals provide the basis for classification in a modern program of physical education. Neither election nor assignment to physical activity or active recreational pursuits can be made well without some health appraisal. Physical education has long since passed the day of mass exercise given without benefit of health information about each participant or competitor. The student who has a hernia or a heart defect, who is psychotic, fatigued, or rheumatic, or who has dysmenorrhea must be located, and a physical education program suited to his limitations must then be developed. No elementary school child or high school or college student should ever be excused permanently from physical education. Given adequate information about the student and medical advice as to his possibilities and limitations, a physical educator should and does proceed to construct a program in light of the needs and capacities of the student. Health data are the first screen used in modern physical education. A good program cannot be built without them.

5 Appraisals serve as educational experiences. School health examinations, tests, and other appraisal procedures may serve to teach the student many things about himself. He may learn the nature of his own health condition, his weakness, or his deviations. He can learn to compensate for his handicaps only if he knows about them. The chances are very good that the first contact many children will have with health professionals, that is physicians, dentists, and nurses, will be in school. It is important that the first impression be a good one.

The very procedure of appraisal often brings students into a clearer and more intimate understanding of the nature of competent professional health service. Students learn from any and all of their daily experiences. Certainly they learn much from their out-of-classroom experiences. Every time the nurse or physician comes to the school, every time the doctor calls at home or the child is taken to his office, the child learns something about health services—about nurses and doctors. He may develop confidence, respect, and a sense of the great good that medical services perform. He may gain the impression, on the other hand, that doctors are slipshod, impersonal, vague, and noncommunicative. He may learn what good medical practice is or he may learn the reverse.

These, then, are the five reasons why health appraisals in their various forms should be made part of an educational program. A careful study of these five purposes will indicate that health appraisals of the kind described in the following pages do not mean that the school is in the practice of medicine. Information gleaned from appraisals is needed so as to facilitate the educational process. The school's business is to practice education, not medicine, but medical advice is needed in order to develop the best educational program.

WHEN DO THESE APPRAISALS START? The appraisals should start as early as possible. The preschool appraisal has proven its usefulness in early case-finding so that remedial treatment or special educational procedures may be begun before the child enters school. Whenever Well Child Clinics or periodic health supervision by a physician can be established for preschool children, valuable results will occur.

The screening and appraisal program should continue throughout the school and college years. The frequency of testing and the kinds of intervals at which they are conducted are determined by the kind of appraisal.

KINDS OF APPRAISALS Several kinds of appraisals are used by many modern schools. These range from nondiagnostic appraisals by teachers and parents to thorough medical and laboratory tests by physicians. The various kinds are described below.

– continuous observation The teacher as a member of the school health team has a unique opportunity to observe children and to assess their health status. She sees the child on good days and poor days, witnesses his successes and failures, observes his reactions to other children, and is aware of any changes in appearance and behavior. The Joint Committee states the following:

> Health observation reflects the teacher's sensitivity to the developmental needs of children. The teacher skilled in observation detects deviations without interference to the usual classroom responsibility. Singling out those children who seem to have something wrong with their health is an essential teacher responsibility.

Depending upon the problem, the teacher will make a mental reminder of those children who need further observation or he will make immediate referral to the nurse or person delegated to receive such referral.[1]

The range of teacher observations is extensive. The following list though incomplete, includes conditions that may be noted:

General appearance—Very thin or obese, noticeable change in weight, unusually pale or flushed, poor posture, unkempt look, change in gait, lethargic and unresponsive or hyperactive

Eyes—Crossed eyes; inflamed or watery eyes; squinting, frowning, scowling; holding the book too close to or too far away from eyes; frequent sties and persistent unnecessary wearing of colored glasses

Ears—Discharge from ears, turning head to hear, failure to hear well as indicated by unusual replies or failures to respond

Nose and Throat—Persistent mouth breathing, enlarged glands in neck, frequent colds, persistent nasal discharge or sniffing, odor from nose or mouth

Skin and Scalp—Rash on face or body, sores on face or body, numerous pimples, excessively dry or oily skin, nits on hair, bald spots, frequent scratching

Teeth and Mouth—Irregular teeth, stained teeth, cracking of lips at corners of mouth, pale or blue lips, inflamed or bleeding gums

Behavior When Playing—Tires easily, becomes breathless following moderate activity, lack of interest or loss of interest in sports and games, unusual clumsiness or poor coordination, unusual excitability

General Behavior—Docile and seclusive, drowsy, aggressive, depressed and unhappy, excessive daydreaming, remote, difficulty in working and playing with others, excessive thirst, frequent use of the toilet, unusual tenseness

In addition to observing pupils, the teacher should give careful attention to pupil complaints. These may include pain, headache, feeling hot, dizziness, buzzing in the ears, sore throat, toothache, blurring of vision, or itching of the skin or scalp. Such complaints should never be discounted. These may be due to acute disease or to a physical impairment. Pupils with health complaints should be brought to the attention of the parents in the same manner as those whose appearance or behavior deviates from normal. Usually parents are notified by the nurse or other personnel.

Such a sequence of observation cannot and should not be used to diagnose or identify disease but should merely set in motion a chain of action for the benefit of the child. One of the following may occur:

1 The teacher makes an immediate adjustment in the room or in the instructional program.

2 The child with symptoms of a respiratory disease or one of the common childhood illnesses is excluded from school so that he may receive care and so as not to expose the other children and the teacher.

3 The teacher communicates her findings to the home with the recommendation (but not a diagnosis) that the matter be looked into further by a physician. Teacher/parent conferences are extremely useful at any level of education. Both sides may exchange information about the health and behavior of the students. Sometimes teachers discover danger signals which parents thought were normal. Parents should explain prolonged or frequent absences.

4 The teacher refers the child to a member of the Pupil Personnel Services team who may be serving the school. This person may make further and more extensive observations before reporting to the parents or recommending further study and/or treatment to the family.

5 When the suspected condition warrants, the matter should come to the attention of the parents, who are helped to seek further diagnosis or treatment. Having reported and urged action, the teacher has discharged her initial responsibility but still should be aware of the recommendations that are made so that the classroom learning situation can be modified when necessary to fit the needs of the child's unique situation. Schools and parents do well in including the family medical advisor in getting at the origin of the problem and bringing about an effective solution.

Occasionally schools concentrate observations on one day of the month or semester. The implication here is not good—teachers should be constantly vigilant and constantly aware of the development of their students and ready to help by reporting the first signs of difficulty rather than waiting for any specific day of the month or year to carry out their observations. The teacher in the classroom is a full-time member of the school health team.

– screening Screening tests as a part of health appraisal are preliminary evaluations of the state of development and function of various body organs, performed by teachers, nurses, technicians, nurses aides, or trained volunteers. These procedures select children needing diagnostic examination by professional health services personnel. The popularity of community-wide screening tests, the concept of multiphasic screening, and the computerized performance of various blood tests and related procedures has raised the question, among health administrators, of whether or not it is desirable to introduce into the school an appropriate battery of tests similar to those used for the discovery of chronic disease in older populations. The answer to this question hinges on certain factors, each of which must be weighed in relation to the specific procedure being evaluated.[2]

1 Is the test applicable to the health problems of children of school age? The incidence of some conditions detectable by screening procedures is extremely low in boys and girls of school age. To give all pupils a test that reveals so few who have the condition is an inefficient method of case finding and may be unsound health education. Screening for gout or cholesterol might be desirable in adults but a waste of time in children.

2 Is the test medically sound? Does the procedure provide information that is significant in determining health status? If findings are positive will they lead to diagnosis and suitable treatment when referred to the family physician? If findings are negative, will parents interpret this to mean that their child is "all right" in every way and neglect consultation for conditions not involved in the test? The possibility of overreferral, the proportion of missed cases, and the faulty interpretation of tests when school age children are screened are important considerations. Only those tests should be performed for which a follow-up has been planned. Posture screening, the way it is usually performed, would not pass this test.

3 Is the test educationally sound? Is the test within the province of an educational institution? Can the test procedures be incorporated into the teaching program of the school and can teachers prepare pupils properly for it? Will giving the test in the school lead to useful health practices and improve the child's educability? Testing of blood, urine, or feces are usually not practical in the school setting.

4 Is the test economically feasible? The costs of screening tests will vary in terms of the equipment needed, the technical personnel required to perform them, and the number of tests given. What will be the cost of the test in the terms of the incidence of the conditions being screened among school children? Are there less costly case-finding procedures? Since the school health program has a limited budget, health service functions must be justified financially.

5 Will giving the test in the school promote good relations among the school, health department, the practicing physician, the child himself, and the family? Because a significant number of children have no family physician and receive little or no medical care, it is argued that exposing these children to screening procedures will be educationally worthwhile even though the case-finding value of the tests may be disputed. Others think that screening tests enhance the opportunity for the school to exercise its responsibility for education concerning intelligent selection of a personal physician or other source of treatment by the child and family and to encourage the family to seek needed preventive treatment services for the child.[3] Pregnancy tests or serological tests for syphilis might fail the criterion of acceptable public relations.

Screening for Vision / About one child out of every four of school age has an eye problem making referral for compensatory or therapeutic care desirable.[4] In the population at large an estimated 70 million have eye defects of which 9 million are children in need of eye care. Errors of refraction (nearsightedness, farsightedness, astigmatism) are the most common disorders. Perhaps one-half of the cases discoverable in any given school situation will represent refractive problems. The others will involve developmental abnormalities (cataracts, albinism), 18 percent will have defects of muscle function (strabismus) and another 11 percent will have diseases of the eye. Not all of these situations are remediable by prescriptions of glasses. This is an important fact to remember when undertaking an educational program with parents and children.

The aim of the school's interest in vision is two-fold: to find those pupils whose vision is impairing their schoolwork and to instruct everyone in vision and its care so that the pupils can be prepared to deal with the problems of vision as time goes on. As a matter of routine, there is apparently no need for an annual visual screening test for every pupil. Perhaps biannual screening is sufficient throughout the school years. Screening every two years seems to be adequate but should be available and used for any pupil at any time. Children should be referred on the basis of such symptoms as squinting, impaired reading, red lids, rubbing of the eyes, or tilting of the head. A vision test and observation are useful only to the extent that problems are found and children with problems receive proper care.

Teacher observation, and the types of vision screening normally used in school, are designed to sort out those students who *probably* have abnormalities from those who do not. These tests by nonmedical personnel are tests of visual effectiveness or acuity but *are not* diagnostic tests that indicate the kind of treatment (glasses, surgery, medication) needed to correct the handicap found. The Snellen eye chart test, the Massachusetts Vision Test, and the Modified Clinical Technique (or modifications) are screenings only; they will be effective in finding the pupils or preschoolers who need a thorough eye examination by a competent specialist. Only from such an examination can intelligent therapy be derived. The indiscriminant recommendation or purchase of glasses following the use of one of the screening tests is certainly not recommended.

It is important that teachers develop a high competency in observation of children for visual symptoms. In those schools where no specialist is available to do the screening, teachers should develop competency in using one or more tests currently used for this purpose.

Teachers are also an important part of the referral process and should be aware of the limitations and advantages of each of the screening techniques. As teachers report to parents, they should be able to give the results of the screening test and some indication of the difficulties the child is having in school and to make intelligent recommendations as to the type of professional attention that might be sought by the parents.

The Snellen Chart / The Snellen chart is the most commonly used screening technique for vision. With experience and parental cooperation its use will select well over 80 percent of the children needing vision care. It is a chart made up of letters, symbols, or numbers graduated scientifically in size, and is to be read at specified distances. Children with normal visual acuity should be able to read the majority of the letters or symbols at the standard indicated distance. A 20/20 vision, for example, means the child can read at 20 feet the majority of letters or symbols which he should read at 20 feet; whereas a 20/30 vision means the child has to be 20 feet away to read what he should read at 30 feet. If the child has 20/15 vision it means he sees at 20 feet what one ordinarily would see at 15 feet.

The Snellen chart is inexpensive and can be purchased from any optical supply house. It should be hung on a wall, eye height when seated, and should be well illuminated (20 to 30 foot candles, no glare). Before the test is started young children should be taught how to indicate the direction the lines point (if the usual *E* chart is used) and cards should be available to cover those parts of the chart not being used. The testing at 20 feet usually, or 10 feet using a mirror, proceeds one eye at a time (right eye first) and without glasses. Usually testers begin at the 40-foot line on the chart and work down to the 20-foot line. If the child strains to see, becomes nervous, tilts his head, or squints badly, all such additional facts should be recorded along with the numerical record.

The Snellen test has several distinct advantages for use in school; it is inexpensive, requires no special electrical apparatus, is easy to administer, and takes an average of only about a minute per child. If the Snellen screening test is combined with careful parent and teacher observation, the majority of children who need to be referred for eye examinations will be identified.

Although there is some difference of opinion among experts in vision testing as to who should be referred, the Joint Committee on Health Problems in Education recommends (1) those who consistently exhibit symptoms of visual disturbance regardless of the results of the Snellen test, (2) children eight years of age or older who have a visual acuity of 20/30 or less in either eye with or without symptoms, and (3) children seven years of age or less who have a visual acuity of 20/40 or less in either eye with or without symptoms of eye trouble.[5]

Standards for referral are not absolute. The economic status of the community and the availability of professional personnel to perform eye examinations may suggest alteration of standards. Referral criteria should be set on the basis of advice received from professional personnel in the local area.

The limitations of the Snellen screening technique should be well known to all teachers. It is in no sense an eye examination, but it is reported to be a reliable screening procedure when carried out carefully and with proper illumination. It does not test the coordination of both eyes working together, nor does it test for astigmatism. It may not screen all children with serious defects and, of course, it does not screen color sensitivity. Nevertheless, when combined with teacher observation and within these limitations, it is a useful screen for teachers and will indicate with sufficient accuracy the children who deviate from the norm in their vision.

Some of the other frequently used tests are the Massachusetts Vision Test, the Atlantic City Vision Test, the Modified Clinical Technique, the test of color identification, the convex lens test, and tests for muscle balance. Because of the popularity of the Snellen test it is the only one described here. Information on other tests may be readily procured from the Joint Committee on Health Problems in Education of the National Education Association and the American Medical Association, or The National Society for the Prevention of Blindness (Vision Screening in School).

Screening for Hearing / When a child is deprived of hearing, his social growth and education may be seriously impeded. The hard-of-hearing or deaf lose so much under normal conditions that to help them compensate for their handicap is an important health and educational enterprise. Loss of hearing may retard normal speech and language development and emotional immaturity is not uncommon among these children. When deafness is present, the child lacks a basic source of contact with his environment. His capacity for memory and conceptualization is affected adversely. In addition there are psychological problems associated with deafness or partial hearing that are very serious. Whatever the effect, the child with impaired hearing needs to be found and given every assistance. Early screening for hearing is very important. The most advantageous time would be before the child begins his language development. However, the earlier the loss of hearing can be found, the better it is for the child, and thus preschool hearing screening is an advisable procedure.

As with vision problems, case finding is the first step in the development of a program to aid those with impaired hearing. Case finding begins with the observations of parents and teachers and aims at the location not only of children with impaired hearing but also of those who have potential ear trouble or those for whom hearing difficulty may be prevented.

A child with impaired hearing will show many signs: being inattentive in class, being more aware of movement than sounds, asking for a repetition of questions, frowning or straining to hear, losing much of a class discussion, articulating poorly or inaccurately, having frequent ear discharge and headaches, and developing an unusual voice quality.

Not only children showing such signs and symptoms but also all other children in school should be screened using a puretone audiometer. Watch and whisper tests have been discarded. The goal is to locate children who have even minimal hearing problems so that they may be referred for medical treatment at the earliest possible date. Programs should be designed to identify children with a chronic disability and also children who have difficulty during only certain times of the year.

In newly established programs an effort should be made to test all of the children during the first school year. Thereafter an adequate program includes aggressive attention to the possibility of hearing problems in the early school years. This can be implemented by annual testing in kindergarten and grades one, two, and three. Less frequent testing can be planned in subsequent school years, with particular emphasis on testing children who are new to the district, those who are referred by parents, teachers, and the medical profession, as well as those who have frequent absences with respiratory infections or allergies.

Experience has shown that the puretone audiometer applied individually as a sweepcheck is the most efficient technique for finding impaired hearing. This method is superior to the group phonograph test or the group puretone test.

Two types of tests are generally used when individual testing is done: a sweep test and a threshold test. The sweep test is administered at an intensity of 25 decibels ISO and frequencies of 250, 500, 1,000, 2,000, 4,000, and 8,000 cycles per second. The child who fails to hear two or more tones in either ear is asked to take a second sweep test. If he fails again a threshold test is given. The threshold test is used to determine the amount of hearing loss for each of the frequencies used in the sweep test. In recent years certain school districts have been using abbreviated sweep tests at 1,000, 2,000, and 4,000 cycles per second.[6]

Hearing screening is generally not the duty of the classroom teacher. It is usually carried out by specially trained personnel under the supervision of an audiologist who is certified by the American Speech and Hearing Association.

Referral to a physician should be based on the following factors: results of the threshold test, significant observations of the teacher, or history of previous illness and ear disorders.

Many patterns of screening are used as a part of a conservation of hearing program. Once such a program is faithfully and efficiently conducted by persons competent in hearing case finding, between 5 and 8 percent of all children in a school district will be found to have impaired hearing.

– growth and weight Measuring height and weight are two of the oldest techniques for observing children over a period of time. Since the very beginning of health work in schools, the relationship between height and weight and normal development has been the subject of much speculation. For many years, for example, there was assumed to be a "normal" weight for every height and age, and by consulting the tables one could tell whether a child was above or below the "normal" for his age. More recently, however, new techniques based upon a recognition of the individuality of growth have sought to plot height and weight in terms of its quality and detect as early as possible the deviations from the growth pattern which is normal for each particular child. Several of these techniques are currently being used by schools. They are sufficiently complicated in nature to prohibit description here but materials on them should be read.[7, 8]

By periodically plotting the height and weight of a child on already prepared charts or grids one can roughly compare his actual current status with his expectancy. The relation between a child's height and weight curves as he grows up to the appropriate norm throws light on his growth progress. As deviations begin to appear they may be interpreted as growth abnormalities or failures, and the reasons can be sought through appropriate medical or psychiatric examinations. Such records, although useful in long-term observation, do not appear at this time to meet the criteria for appropriateness of screening devices. The yield of referrals does not appear to justify the expenditure involved.[9]

– dental case finding It may be assumed that all students in school need dental care. The problem, then, becomes one of getting students into the hands of a dentist at annual intervals. The person who screens for dental purposes among younger students will examine the teeth for obvious evidence of decay, unclean teeth, and gum inflamation or ulceration. When such cases are found arrangements should be made to secure appropriate dental treatment for them.

– histories and inventories Histories and inventories round out, in fact are indispensable to, a good screening program. An inventory filled out by parents has been shown to be very useful and reliable in supplying teachers and pupil personnel service personnel with data they need and otherwise would not get. From the replies of parents, school personnel receive useful information on needs and capacity, previous illness, behavior problems, immunization and other personal matters. Older secondary school students and college students are themselves capable of supplying historical data. A reading of such histories has become important to teachers of physical education and other active areas in adjusting the program to fit the student.

– other screening procedures Additional procedures for evaluation of pupil health and determination of need for referral are frequently used, especially in larger schools with well-established programs adequately staffed. Some of these procedures are more extensive than is implied by the word "test," and some may be placed administratively in school departments other than school health services. Nevertheless, as a contribution to the appraisal of a whole person, these procedures should be considered by health service personnel.

Physical performance tests are procedures that measure motor skill, muscle strength, endurance, and other related factors as a part of evaluation and classification for physical education activities, including athletics. Batteries of tests bear the name of the person or organization designing the specific test. They vary considerably in content and intent, so should be selected for a specific purpose. Such tests are recognized as having value for these purposes as well as having a place in overall pupil appraisal.

There is little agreement as to how well such tests measure physical fitness. Those who interpret physical performance tests must be aware of their limitations and avoid attaching undue significance to any particular procedure. It is unfortunate to label an otherwise apparently normal child as physically unfit merely because he fails in an arbitrary performance test that may have little relationship to a total concept of fitness. Physical performance is only one part of total fitness, which in its broad sense includes mental, emotional, and social, as well as physical facets. Fitness is an individual matter and should be evaluated in terms of individual potential as well as group norms.

Psychological, personality and intelligence evaluation by a variety of procedures is usually administered by such school personnel as psychologists, social workers, counselors, and occasionally teachers. Because these people are infrequently found in the health service office, every effort should be made to obtain the records involved so that they may be correlated with the findings from screening procedures during the physician's evaluation.

Serious emotional problems present symptoms that cannot be ignored by the school and should be identified early. Symptoms such as truancy, lethargy, failure to attempt assignments, aggressive or provocative behavior toward teacher or school authorities, behavior dangerous to other children or to the child in question, theft, cruelty, promiscuity, legal delinquency, or persistent failure to learn in spite of evidence of adequate ability may be difficult to understand but certainly are easy to recognize.

Only a few schools have adopted formal screening programs for the early identification of emotional problems. Available instruments for screening children who are potentially vulnerable to maladjustment are newer than those used for other kinds of health problems and have been less well validated. Useful rating scales that teachers can check are now available for specific age groups. Inservice training and preservice training in recognizing symptoms justifying referral of a pupil to members of the health team in the school, to community agencies, or to the medical profession are available to teachers. The fear of false identification may be dissipated if results of screening for emotional difficulties are treated as strictly confidential material for professional use only.

Certain indications of emotional problems are readily observable by teachers. When any important observations are noted on pupils' cumulative records, the descriptions should be precise in terms of data directly observable by the teacher. Specific objective behaviors rather than subjective descriptions based on opinion are noted. The teacher does not make a diagnosis.

SPECIAL PROBLEMS

Unusual or special health problems in a community may warrant a screening procedure that, under ordinary circumstances, might not be justified. When such tests are needed to protect child health, a decision to add a specific screening device to the school program as either a temporary or established practice should follow discussion of its need and value by school, medical, and public health personnel. The discussion should consider the incidence in the local community of the problem which the test will screen, the cost of the test in terms of case-finding potential, the hazard of the condition involved to the child population, and the suitability of the procedures for use in the schools. For example, mass examination of specimens of blood, urine, and feces is rarely warranted in a school health program. However, under certain circumstances, examination of a school population by laboratory procedures may be a necessary facet in the epidemiology and control of endemic or epidemic disease.

It is unwise to introduce new procedures into the school health program without general acceptance by the parents involved and approval by the local medical, public health, and educational authorities.[10]

THE PHYSICAL OR MEDICAL EXAMINATION

The physical examination or medical appraisal seeks to determine the status or quality of health of a student through the use of the examining and diagnostic skill of a physician. Though a teacher or nurse may frequently assist, a physician is required. The procedure requires time, money, and effort and is helpful when findings are used to satisfy the five clear purposes of such appraisals mentioned earlier. If the examinations are to be given, the findings should be used for the benefit of the education and the health of the child.

These examinations go by various names depending on local custom; "physical examination," "medical examination," and "health examination" are the terms most frequently used. What they are called makes little difference as long as they are well done and the findings are used. There are several features of such examinations and their administration that must be secured for greatest effectiveness:

1 A health history is a vital part of any examining procedure. The physician and other personnel concerned with the child should secure the history of any previous experience with communicable or other disease, accidents, emotional maladjustment, nutritional difficulties, immunizations, operations, routine practices of sleep, elimination and eating, moods, fatigue, menstruation, birth abnormalities, and dental history. Dates, places, and duration are important in the history of our parental observation, questions, and comments. Data of this kind are vital to the examining physician and other counselors in determining a course of action to be recommended for a given child.

2 The history should be obtained on a standard form, usually one recommended by the examining physician, prior to the examination, by mail or in person from the student and his parents. School districts will do well to work with local medical societies in preparing a form that is acceptable not only to the schools, but also to the medical community.

3 The physical examination should include evaluation of the whole child, from the hair to the tips of the toes, and should include, as well, the behavior of the patient during the examination.
Examinations conducted at school by physicians who are in the employ of the school are not intended to be explicit in their diagnosis. They represent the tentative evaluation of a condition and the information should be sent to parents or a family physician as a matter of referral.

4 Arrangements for the medical evaluation should match the standards of a private office. These include adequate space, good lighting, ventilation, and privacy. Examinations should not be con-

ducted in one end of a noisy gymnasium where the whole procedure may be open to public view. Preferably an examining or nurse's suite should be set aside where children can move through a waiting room, dressing room, and examining room. Adequate personnel should be assigned to assist the physician so that he may perform his medical functions and be able to delegate routine or nonmedical functions to assistant personnel. Physicians should be paid. If there are no regularly employed school. personnel to perform these examinations, then community personnel can be used but at a fee mutually agreeable. State laws and local ordinances should be consulted to determine whether the employment of physicians and nurses is permissable.

5 Parents of elementary children should be present at examinations whenever possible. If this is not feasible, then conferences should be arranged later between parents, teachers, and physicians and other counselors so that all will understand any problems that arise and a constructive program for the benefit of the pupil can be worked out.

6 The pupil should be informed of the meaning, findings, purpose, and general importance of the examination. Occasionally physicians will deem it wise to withhold some information from the examinee. That is the physician's business and prerogative. Generally speaking, however, physicians experienced in school examinations are finding it educationally useful to be communicative, helpful, and informative with the children. Strong as well as weak points should be noted. If a personal program for an existing disability is to be worked out, the child will need to know a great deal about his condition. To face his problem realistically and intelligently he will need to have a clear knowledge of the nature and prognosis of his handicap.

7 Cogent information must be made available in understandable form to school personnel. It is no longer reasonable to expect the teacher to struggle to educate slow-moving children when their slowness is due to disease, defective hearing, or malnutrition, since, had such information been given to her, she might have handled the children in a wholly different manner. Four of the five purposes cited for appraisal are principally educational in outcome and require action from the educational personnel. Physicians and educators must arrange for a two-way transmission of information. Neither can safely withhold information from the other without the child being the loser. The teacher must have advice from medical personnel as the base from which school programs are to be modified, physical education programs developed, compensations cultivated, and understandings about professional health services communicated. These are educational purposes. The data from physical examinations are important to their attainment.

8 The frequency with which such examinations are given is important. Ideally, of course, every child would have access to medical care consistently and should be examined frequently. Unfortunately, such ideal conditions do not prevail, so lesser provisions have to be arranged. Most medical and educational groups today recommend a minimum of four complete medical examinations

during the twelve years of school, at transition points between school levels and at times of great physiological change. It should be said in passing, however, that the emphasis in school health programs is less on routine examinations and more on special examinations, for example, for learning disabilities, than it once was.

– examinations for athletic teams or physical education classes

Examinations for athletic teams or for physical education classes should vary little from routine health supervision examinations. There is strong opinion that school boy and girl athletes should have an examination prior to and at the end of every school year. Certainly the safest and most informed supervision can be given to athletes only when such frequent examinations are made. The eligibility of athletes as the result of these examinations is generally determined by the local medical community and by the body that controls school athletics on a state or local level.

FOLLOW-UP

No appraisal is particularly significant unless action is taken in light of the findings. Children with cardiac disorders should avail themselves of public or private consultative and rehabilitative services. Children with diabetic, asthmatic, or orthopedic conditions need medical care. Children with speech or voice disorders or cleft palate need the aid of a speech-corrective clinic or service. Follow-up is necessary in almost every case and yet actual experience shows considerable neglect of this important process.

Health appraisals have limited value unless an organized follow-up program is established that insures the best possible use of available health facilities to meet the health needs of children. Effective school follow-up programs encourage, rather than replace, parental responsibility. As a matter of fact, there now appears to be "wide general agreement" that (a) the parent has primary responsibility for the health of the child; (b) an organized school-community group should plan policies and study methods and procedures to be used in the school health program; and (c) school and community representatives must work as a team to provide a good follow-up program."[11]

A successful follow-up program creates a favorable attitude on the part of the child toward his own health and helps parents, teachers, and others concerned with the health of children to appreciate and fulfill their individual responsibilities and develops understanding of the value of continued health care throughout life. In most programs school personnel assume the major responsibility for initiating programs to follow-up on health appraisal because of the schools' continued and immediate contact with the children.

In successful programs the school administrator provides staff, time, and funds for the follow-up program and delineates the responsibilities of school personnel at all levels of the school district. It is vital for the school to establish policies and procedures for the promotion of working relationships between school and the home as well as between the school and community agencies. Many procedures have been used to stimulate successful follow-up to health appraisals in schools but among the most frequently recommended are the following procedures:

1 Teacher-Nurse Consultation—Immediately after appraisals have been conducted and significant findings reported, all records should be carefully examined and discussed by the nurse and teacher. Cases that require special attention should be tabbed on the teacher's records to facilitate follow-through work. Cases that require a modification of the school program but not particular medical care should likewise be noted so that the teacher can make sure recommendations of physicians are carried out as intended.

2 The Teacher-Nurse-Parent Conference—In cases that indicate the need of specialized medical care, it is desirable to have the school nurse, teacher, and parents discuss the educational implications of the health appraisal and any recommendations. In some communities it may be necessary for the teacher to assume the responsibility for follow-up. Whenever possible it would be well to have parents visit the school to review findings of the health appraisal with the teacher and the nurse. Adequate time should be taken for these conferences. They should not be conducted informally while parents and teachers are standing around after a meeting of the Parent-Teacher Association.

3 Home Visits—In cases where the parent does not respond to the invitation to visit the school for the purpose of discussing the health appraisal with the teacher and nurse, either the nurse or teacher should assume the responsibility of visiting the home to explain the findings and urge continued parental action.

4 Teacher Follow-Through—When the recommendations do not involve specific medical care but rather an adjustment of the school program to fit the needs of the individual child, the follow-through can best be done by the teacher.

5 Special Cases—When the needs of the child are adequately interpreted to the parent there is usually the desired cooperation, but when parental neglect or poor economic circumstances or on the occasions when other family problems assume a priority ahead of that expressed by the school, it may be necessary for school personnel to be of special assistance to the family. Sometimes it will be necessary for the school to help arrange for financial assistance for a family. Other times the school may be in a position to know where assistance can be obtained without publicity that might embarrass the child. On other occasions the nurse or

> teacher may have to help the family solve the overriding problem that has prohibited action on the child's health complaint. It is not enough to make a referral and consider that the action will be carried out.

In each school it will be necessary to have personnel assigned to recheck on all referrals resulting from health appraisals and to take educational action that will help the family in the accomplishment of care of the suspected health problem or in carrying out the family's responsibility.

Direct personal contact is desirable in the carrying out of follow-through procedures but is not always necessary. On many occasions a well written, professional letter to the parents will be sufficient to secure the desired action. School personnel also successfully use phone calls. The extent of school efforts in the area of follow-up will be determined by the nature of the community in which the school exists, by recommendations of the community, and by the amount of resources that can be assigned to the correction of health problems.

RECORD KEEPING Data from any of the health appraisal procedures should be recorded clearly, intelligibly, and in a standard form. They should be cumulative and made part of the school record of the child, to be available only to professional personnel and parents. The health records should contain: (1) data from the preschool examination; (2) findings and recommendations from school evaluations; (3) findings and recommendations from any other pupil personnel services personnel; (4) communications and summaries of conferences with parents, child, and school personnel; and (5) a chronological record of adjustments, corrections, and developments pertaining to the child's health.

Much of the success or failure of health appraisal procedures and follow-up in the schools will depend on the accuracy of record keeping and the kind of information flow that exists between the schools, parents, and the therapeutic community. Because school health records should be treated in a confidential manner, there is a great need for carefully setting up the mechanics for handling the records and information flow. Health information should be imparted to other agencies or individuals only on the request of parents and at the discretion of the school administrator. The best interests of the child should always be the foremost consideration.

> There should be agreement on methods of interchanging information among school, physician, dentist, parents and others who may be concerned. The policy seems clear cut when the family physician who sent in the child's examination record asks for information, but in other situations teachers should refer requests for

> information from the health records through appropriate administration channels.
>
> Health records should be readily available to those who need to use them, but not accessible to unauthorized people. This limits their accessibility to professional staff and selected, supervised clerical help. The administration should be encouraged to employ clerical staff sufficient to take care of the records. A minimum of professional time should be devoted to clerical duty. Coordination of the services provided by various agencies involved in the school health program is desirable and whenever feasible, duplication of services should be avoided. While it is felt that children's health records could not be assembled in the files of a single agency, coordination might be furthered through informal clearance between agencies, through an inter-agency committee, or in larger areas, through a central clearing agency. For example, a social service exchange which would have information as to the other agencies serving the individual or family, might fill this role.[12]

Information about a child must remain the confidential property of the professional personnel concerned and the child and his guardian. This is known as the principle of privileged communication. In the early days of school health work physicians looked with dismay upon the request of the educator for the results of the physical examinations of children. The physician had not been in the habit of giving any information about a patient to anyone, save parents and other interested medical personnel. The relationship of the patient and his physician was a restricted or privileged relationship and still is.

The principle itself is as old as the confessional. It is observed by ministers, lawyers, and physicians and must be observed by teachers if they wish to share in the confidential information possessed by physicians as a result of their evaluations. When we go to a lawyer with a legal problem, we know that the secret will not be divulged without consent. The secrets of the confessional are not made common property. A physician does not violate the confidence of his patient. This is the operation of the principle of privileged communication.

Its place in the school health program is clear enough. No one should ever make public, or make the subject of common talk, anything about the health status of a given child. If a teacher is told that one of her junior high school girls has dysmenorrhea, which is affecting her work, her happiness, and her social life, the fact is no one's business except that of the professional personnel in a position to help the girl. The whole school staff need not know this fact. Other children need not know it. If a boy has 20/100 vision it is no one's business except that of his family, his teacher, his oculist, and himself. Teachers are expected to maintain high standards of professional conduct in regard to knowledge about a student's health and family.

SUMMARY

A successful health appraisal program in schools consists of a chain of activities. Among the activities are observation, screening, testing, and examination procedures that assess the needs of children, that are professionally sound, and that are appropriate to the school and community. They are carried on by personnel who are qualified. The results are recorded accurately and maintained in a confidential manner. The chain of activities includes follow-up to involve parents in cases of individual needs and includes teamwork among school, community, and family in the provision of resources and in provisions for information flow sufficient to allow each party to do his job well. Follow-up includes remediation and treatment with information flow back to the parents and school sufficient to provide adaptations and compensations for those problems that cannot be quickly resolved.

Appraisal leads to constructive alterations in the life of the child and adjustment of the school program to meet the individual needs of the pupils and provides the basis for individual compensations for irremediable handicaps or deviations. The kinds of adaptations that occur in school and are based on appraisal procedures and knowledge of the health needs of children are pursued in Chapter 5.

NOTES AND REFERENCES

1 Joint Committee on Health Problems in Education of the NEA and AMA, *Health Appraisal of School Children,* 4th ed., Washington, D.C., NEA and AMA, 1969.

2 *Ibid.*

3 *Ibid.*

4 *Vision Screening in Schools,* New York, N.Y., National Society for the Prevention of Blindness.

5 Joint Committee on Health Problems in Education of the NEA and AMA, *School Health Services,* 2nd ed., Washington, D.C., NEA and AMA, 1964, p. 82.

6 *Ibid.*

7 Orvis A. Harrelson *et al.,* "Comparison of Hearing Screening Methods," *Journal of School Health,* XXXIX, 3 (March 1969).

8 Norman C. Wetzel, "Physical Fitness in Terms of Physique, Development and Basal Metabolism," *Journal of the American Medical Association,* March 22, 1941, p. 1187.

9 ———, *Instruction Manual for Use of the Grid for Evaluating Physical Fitness,* Cleveland, NEA Service,

10 Joint Committee, *Health Appraisal of School Children, op. cit.*

11 Alfred Yankauer, Jr., *et al.,* "A Study of Case-Finding Methods in Elementary Schools," *American Journal of Public Health,* 52, 4. (April 1962), 656.

12 AMA, *Report of the Fourth National Conference on Physicians and Schools,* Chicago, AMA, 1953.

13 ———, *Report of the Fifth National Conference on Physicians and Schools,* Chicago, AMA, 1955.

CHAPTER 13
ADAPTATIONS

The success of a school health program can be judged on the basis of the effectiveness of its case finding, referral, and follow-up activities. However, an outstanding program is judged not only on the number of children whose health is improved through follow-up procedures, but also on the quality of information that returns to the school and the use to which the school district personnel put the data in providing appropriate educational environments for pupils.

Some health problems can be solved immediately, others over a period of time, and still others require long-term management when some residual deviation remains. Some situations are acute and short term, others are chronic and long term. No matter what the situation, a school health program strives to gain appropriate information concerning the child's health status and attempts to modify, in cooperation with school, parent, community, and child, the child's learning environment to his benefit. The success or failure of such a program depends almost entirely upon the quality of the information received from parent and community care sources.

Joy G. Cauffman has studied the factors relating to successful completion of school health referrals.[1] She has concluded that the most important factor in the success of a referral was the notification method used. "Parents who are notified about their child's defect by more than one contact technic (i.e. written notice, telephone call or home visit) are much more likely to secure attention for their children than are parents who are notified by only one contact technic."[2] It was also found that contact by more than one person led to success more often than when only one person was involved. Her findings indicate that the method of notification was eight times as powerful as the parents' rating of the urgency of the problem and three times as potent as social rank of the family in determining success of a referral. Presence of insurance, the ethnic or religious group, and the nature of the defect also play a role in determining the outcome of a referral, but these are minor in relation to the factors of notification, social rank, and the parents' perception of urgency.

Personal contact leads to referral success and also leads to the school receiving information as to the outcome of the treatment or examination. Parents who feel the school has a personal interest in their child are more apt to participate in helping plan needed school adaptations by providing adequate, accurate information.

It is often necessary to receive information from agencies and private practitioners. The first step in securing adequate cooperation from these out-of-school groups is to provide the care source with a release of confidential information signed by a parent. Information of any health, social, or medical nature is almost always confidential. An information release is necessary before a legal flow of information can be carried out between the school and community agency.

The quality of information received from community resources is most often determined by the nature and quality of the referral. A referral stating, "needs a complete physical exam" will most likely gain little specific information. A referral requesting an electroencephalogram and medicine for brain damage will most often reap antagonism and no information. A referral stating the nature of the problem that has brought about the referral, that asks specific questions, and that includes salient school-generated information such as classroom behavior, psychological evaluation, and achievement or aptitude scores will very likely generate a good response from the resource that cares for the child. If, in addition, time has been taken to involve the family in the planning process, good information is almost certain.

Adequate techniques of working with parents and community agencies reap information adequate for educational planning. Teachers, nurses, administrators, and special service personnel are all involved in the referral process and in the retrieval of information regarding referral success and recommendations as well. It is a prime function of the school health team (which, of course, includes the teacher) to gather health information and to distribute the data to appropriate school personnel so that educational adaptations can be planned and implemented. Such an information system must protect the privacy and sensitivity of the children involved. Adaptations in the school environment to meet the health needs of children must be based on good information shared by personnel at appropriate levels. Adaptations can then be made at the classroom and school district level to improve the educational opportunities of the pupils.

ADAPTATIONS IN THE CLASSROOM—ACTIVITY The most frequent adjustments made in the classroom by teachers trained in child growth and development, acting on the basis of their experience and with the guidance of information gleaned from referrals of pupils to outside care sources, are in the area of classroom activity and daily routine. The teacher knows there is an optimum activity load for each child that will help to promote optimum growth and development. She knows that this optimum varies widely even though most of the children in her classroom would be classified as normal or as mildly handicapped children. She explores all of the positive and negative aspects of the child's activities during his waking hours and attempts to develop a classroom routine for each child, a program of balanced activity that depends on the developmental level of the child, his sex, age, and whether or not he has a permanent or transitory physical condition. The teacher, in developing this balanced activity program for each child, does so from a knowledge of the factors in a child's activity load. This would include the time he spends in going to and from school and how he gets there; what kind of class and extraclass activities he participates in; and whether or not he is active at home with the family and in play activities. Does he have an outside job or work in which he participates? Does this child participate in community activities such as youth organizations and church groups? Not only will the teacher attempt to adjust the classroom activity on the basis of the knowledge gained and the knowledge she has of the factors in each child's activity load, but she will also attempt to work with the family to make sure that home and school activities are coordinated. Often this will mean an adjustment in the number of hours that a child sleeps or an improvement in the nutrition that he receives at home and at school. Sleep and nutrition factors can then be balanced with the classroom activity that takes place in the school.

Not only must the teacher attempt to provide a program of activity which is balanced with that of the home, she must also be able to adjust the school's schedule to meet the needs of the temporarily disabled child. Frequently children are disabled from having been ill or from having suffered a fracture, dislocation, or sprain. The teacher continues to be responsible for the optimum growth and development of this child even though he is temporarily disabled while attending school. Often times the temporarily disabled child forgets the limits that have been established for him during his period of disability. He may push himself in competition and may therefore experience avoidable hazards. It is the teacher's responsibility, and that of the whole school health team, to plan adequately for a proper activity prescription for the temporarily disabled child.[3]

In planning the school activity program the members of the school health team should have at their disposal all levels of activities ranging from rest to full activity. The health team should gain from the parent, and the provider of care to the temporarily disabled child, an activity prescription indicating the amount of energy the child should be able to spend and the kinds of activities in which he can participate without harm.

The best teachers arrange for adaptations on the basis of common sense and good teaching techniques. The child returning to school after absence with an illness is allowed to rest during recess or is given a task that is low in energy consumption to do for the teacher during the period when other children are actively exercising. The child with a cast or one limping from a sprain is given a special assignment so he will not feel left out of class activities. The shy pupil is placed in positions to be successful, whereas the brash, noisy pupil is given periods of exercise to relieve the pressure of his energy. Most of these activity adaptations are short term and are part of what the teacher does based on her knowledge of children and their health status. Nonetheless, this sort of classroom management is necessary for successful learning and for the good health of the children involved.[4]

Other adaptations in the activity of pupils are based on the age level and maturity of the children involved. Younger children have short attention spans and require alternation of quiet and active periods. As children grow older they require less exercise, but while in school they never give up the need for movement and energy release.

Districts that are aware of pupils' needs will carefully plan the daily routine. Where children ride busses to and from school, every effort will be made to keep portal to portal time at a minimum. When long bus rides are necessary, adjustments should be made in the activities at school to compensate for the energy spent in riding. The energy expenditure in daily routine is a very important part of school adaptation to meet the needs of children.

PHYSICAL EDUCATION Not only is it necessary for adaptations to be made in the daily routine of children who are temporarily disabled, but also it is important to develop adaptations for children by grouping for physical education. A physical education teacher is aware of the fact that not all children are fit for the normal, vigorous program but that all children should have some program constructed for them. Such differentiation requires assistance from physicians. Furthermore, the physical education program itself offers opportunity for health development and counseling and both should go forward in the light of the known condition of the student. Far less than half the schools in the nation are in a position to supply medical counsel for physical education or athletic purposes. There are not enough physicians employed or available to perform such services. Because of this, physical education teachers, including those who prepare competitive teams, have but two alternatives: to conduct their program in ignorance of the status of their charges or to do something themselves by way of screening. The latter seems altogether feasible. Excellent results can be obtained by physical education teachers who are qualified to interpret a carefully arranged health history and to make certain observations of high school or college students. Athletes may be screened and physical education students classified without the immediate services of a physician if those in charge will carefully study their task. This procedure, however, is not a substitute for adequate physician consultation when such is available.

Waiving a student's privilege of participation in physical education is a serious decision for a physician or physical educator, one that can profoundly influence the student's physical growth and emotional development. Unnecessary restriction can hamper personal development and interfere with group acceptance of a student.

There are four specific objectives of a classification of students for physical education:

1 To safeguard the health of participants
2 To group pupils for effective learning
3 To equalize competitive conditions
4 To facilitate progress and achievement[4]

The Committee on Exercise and Physical Fitness of the American Medical Association recommends four classifications:

1 Unrestricted activity to include full participation in athletics and physical education

2 Moderately restricted participation in prescribed physical education and athletics

3 Severe restriction and participation in a limited number of events at a low level of activity

4 Reconstruction or rehabilitative, that is participation in a program of corrective exercises and adaptive sports[5]

It is recognized that such recommendations need to be based on good communication among all interested parties and also require provision of all pertinent information, a strengthening of physical education programs, and an increased number of offerings from those that are now available. Although in most school districts at the present time the classification involves an unreachable goal in terms of the training of physical educators, the kinds of programs that are available, and the expertise of community resources, the classification should be used as a goal to reach in the constant quest to improve programs for the optimum growth and development of children.

ADAPTATION FOR THE GIFTED—COMPETITIVE ATHLETICS

In many communities a great deal of time and effort are being spent in organizing competitive sports for children thirteen years of age and younger. Whether or not this is a desirable practice depends entirely on the skill and sophistication of the program planners in adapting the sports and playing conditions to the growth and development of the level of the children involved. High quality athletic programs can be very beneficial to some children. However, the benefits of such programs do not occur without a high level of interest and knowledge on the part of the community people involved. Before a community considers the development of an athletic competition program there should be a physical education program available for all children and an adequate intramural program for children who are capable of participation in more skilled activities. Only after these two kinds of programs for all children are developed should a community begin to think of providing a narrow program for the child who is athletically gifted, well developed, or precocious.

Decisions about school or community competitive athletic programs should be made on the basis of guidelines established by a representative community group in which the teacher and the school health team should have a strong voice. Any decision about athletic programs for elementary school children should include consideration of eight points listed in a statement called, "Competitive Athletics for Children of Elementary School Age," prepared jointly by the American Academy of Pediatrics, the American Association for Health, Physical Education, and Recreation, the American Medical Association Committee on Medical Aspects of Sports, and the Society of State Directors of Health, Physical Education, and Recreation.

1 Proper physical conditioning
2 Conduct of the sport
   a Competent teaching and supervision with regard for the relative hazards of each particular sport
   b Modification of rules, game equipment, and facilities to suit the maturity level of the participants
   c Qualified officials

3 Careful grouping according to sex, weight, size, skill, and physical maturation when indicated

4 Good protective equipment, properly fitted

5 Well-maintained facilities suitable for the sport involved

6 Proper delineation of the spheres of authority and responsibility for school administration, family, sponsor, physician, coach, and athlete

7 Adequate medical care, including periodic health appraisal of children, a physician readily available during games and practices, established policies, procedures and responsibilities for first aid and referral of injured athletes, definitive treatment and follow-up, evaluation and certification for return following illness and injury, attention to matters of physical and emotional fatigue and stress, especially of a cumulative nature, and adequate reporting and analysis of injuries and illness

8 Salient educational and recreational considerations include programs for all children taking precedence over those having limited student clientele. No program should interfere with the regular school program either in hours or by the fatigue of children. There should be an avoidance of play-offs, bowl contests, all-star contests or other undesirable corollaries such as excessive publicity, pep squads, commercial promoting, victory celebrations, elaborate recognition ceremonies, paid admission, inappropriate spectator behavior, high pressure public contests, and exploitation of children in any form.[6,7]

The positive values of sports should be emphasized because of their important effects on stamina and physiologic functioning and because of their lifelong value as recreational activities. Children seek and can profit by competitive sports, but the benefits are not automatic.

COMMUNICATION

Although by far the greatest majority of adaptations made in the classroom have to do with the activity of the children, all members of the school health team have the responsibility for manipulation of the school and classroom environment for the promotion of communication. The teacher in particular has the opportunity to improve the child's education through promotion of conditions that improve vision and hearing in the classroom setting. This is important for all children but especially for those who have been found to have eye defects and on whom the teacher has information from the community care source.

– vision

Perhaps no function of human life has to make quite such a sharp adjustment to the unnaturalness of schooling as vision. The human eye is, fortunately, made of flexible and durable stuff. It seems able to weather surprisingly well the abuse it receives from inadequate school lighting systems and the demands of close work. Certainly there is no reason to believe the human eye, particularly the eye of a child, takes natively and easily to the environment and demands of a school.

Popular belief has it that one sees as much as one can see, but that may not be so. There is much reason to believe that through manipulation of the classroom environment vision can be improved.

In 1967 the program area committee on child health of the American Public Health Association and the National Society for the Prevention of Blindness described three rough classifications of children with vision handicaps:

1 *Sighted children with eye problems.* Have eye abnormalities or defects of vision which may be helped by medical treatment, may be corrected or compensated for by optical aids or may not be severe enough to be seriously handicapping. Most of the children in this group will need medical services and guidance at some period and perhaps minor or temporary adjustments in their educational program. For classification purposes these children have a visual acuity of more than 20/70 in the better eye after treatment and correction. A high percentage of individuals in this group have errors of refraction (myopia, hyperopia, astigmatism) or eye muscle imbalance (strabismus, heterophoria). Some have abnormalities such as inadequate color vision. Others have cataracts or ptosis or have some purely cosmetic defect of the eye. The occasional child who has lost one eye has not necessarily lost fifty percent of his sight if the other eye is normal, but more likely he has only from fifteen to twenty percent impairment in total visual acuity.

2 *Partially seeing children.* Have such marked visual difficulties that even after all medical and optical help has been provided, they require the aid of special educational services if they are to profit from many of the educational opportunities and experiences provided for children with normal vision. For classification purposes these children have a visual acuity of 20/70 or less in the better eye after the best correction possible, yet they have residual sight sufficient for use as one of their chief channels of learning. Also included in this group are children who, in the opinion of the eye physician or educator, can benefit from either temporary or long term use of special medical and educational services. They may have a progressive eye difficulty, or have had an accident or operation (removal of an eye, surgical correction of crossed eyes) which necessitates readaptation or re-education in the use of the eyes; or they may have an eye problem which has been intensified by some superimposed condition (accident, infection) or possibly there is an emotional difficulty associated with the eye problem that can be resolved with special help.

3 *Blind despite medical care and the best corrective measures.* Have such limited vision that they cannot use it as one of their channels of learning. Legal definition of blindness is a visual acuity of 20/100 or less in the better eye after correction or better than 20/100 with the visual field restricted to less than 20° in the widest

diameter. Many children classified as legally blind can read print. Some use large print, others use regular size print. These children should not be considered blind from the educational point of view. Some blind children can use their sight to a limited degree in getting about. Many have form, movement or light perception. A few must rely entirely on their other senses. They will all need special medical, educational, and social services. The differences between blind and partially seeing children are great. The educationally blind child depends largely upon the senses of touch and hearing for his education and for obtaining information about his physical and social environment. The partially seeing child should be educated chiefly through the sense of sight as are his normally seeing contemporaries with appropriate support from audio and other educational aids. He should be encouraged and helped to use the vision he has.[8]

Multiply-handicapped children with eye problems form a group particularly hard to define. The eye difficulty may represent an integral part of some serious general condition as in the postrubella syndrome or cerebral palsy; or the difficulty may be unrelated to the other handicapping conditions in etiology as an accidental eye injury in a child with rheumatic heart disease.

The nature and importance of the visual eye impairment will need to be evaluated for each child in relation to the overall problem and the child's other physical, emotional, social, and mental assets and liabilities. Treatment and correction for the eye condition must be carefully correlated with other phases of the rehabilitative program. For example, the blind child may exhibit a characteristic posture and gait that can be improved by orthopedic treatment and physical therapy.

The great majority of children with minor visual problems will have sufficient sight to enable them to follow a regular school curriculum with little need for additional help. They may benefit from optical aids, preferential seating in class, activities requiring a change of eye focus, and other simple modifications. A few will require more than slight adjustments in their educational program. Children classified as partially seeing should also use sight as a chief channel of learning. However, special materials, adjustments, and procedures will be needed to help each child use what vision he has to the best advantage.

– what the classroom teacher can do

There is much that the teacher can do to help maintain a classroom environment in which pupils can see with minimum effort and maximum comfort. Some teachers designate an illumination committee to check various aspects of the visual environment three or four times a day, rotating the duty each week. In regard to pupils the teacher can (1) permit pupils to arrange or change seats whenever this will promote better conditions for seeing; (2) arrange for pupils with eye difficulties to sit in places considered best from the standpoint of their specific defect; (3) arrange seats and desks so that no pupil will face the window or work in his own shadow; (4) try to alternate periods of close eye work with activities that are visually less demanding.[9]

In regard to materials and equipment the teacher can:

1 Insist that the minimum type size of textbooks be ten-point type. Young children should have books with larger type.

2 Make sure that all duplicated materials are of good quality.

3 Eliminate books, charts, and maps that have become so soiled that the contrast between print and paper is poor.

4 Use only matte-finished papers of high reflectance and a good degree of opacity for both work paper and printed material.

5 Encourage the use of nonglossy inks.

6 Write on chalk board in large, clear letters in the line of pupils' vision.

7 Keep chalk board clean; white chalk of good quality is preferable.

8 Stand or sit in positions that direct pupils' view away from windows.

9 Avoid hanging posters and charts between windows.

10 Make sure that electric lights are turned on whenever the illumination falls below standard in any part of the room. Some schools are equipped with photoelectric cells that do this automatically.

11 Report failed lamps and see that they are replaced immediately.

12 See that lighting equipment is cleaned periodically and thoroughly so that at least 70 foot candles illumination is maintained in all parts of the room.[10]

Through these procedures the classroom teacher helps to provide a healthful visual environment, one that increases the attractiveness of the classroom and enables pupils to see comfortably and clearly. Though the teacher has specific responsibility for carrying out these measures to improve the learning environment of the classroom, the whole school health team has the general responsibility for keeping the learning environment up to its visual optimum.

– hearing

Success in the classroom depends not only on the type of visual environment but also on the sonic environment and its effect on the learning process. A good deal of information has been accumulated on the engineering aspects of acoustics, including the manipulation of sound for desired effects. There is, on the other hand, a general lack of knowledge dealing with the relationship of the sound environment to the learning process. The deliberate use of sounds for communications is probably the most important single aspect of acoustics so far as learning is concerned. Recognition of this fact makes it imperative that the sonic portion of the total environment be optimized as far as is practical to facilitate the learning process.

Obviously humans can only function properly if the sound environment encompasses certain limits. Broadly speaking these limits can be expressed as "too much noise" or "too little noise" with noise being defined as unwanted sound.

There are many sources of noise in school—pupils and teachers, typewriters, motion picture projectors, mechanical ventilators, shop machines, activity in gymnasiums, activity in music rooms, and perhaps even dishwashing machines. Additional noises originate in the immediate vicinity of the school from automobiles and trucks on the road or planes roaring overhead. The problem of the school is to provide insulation against outside noises and to confine noises inside the building to particular areas.

Excessive exposure to noise may result in adverse physical and psychological manifestations. Hearing loss attributed to noise may occur in the uncontrolled industrial environment but is not likely within the school. Noise levels in schools, however, may very well produce detrimental psychologic effects and may also interfere with comprehension of the spoken word.[11]

In a school noise influences communication between pupils and teacher. Talking loudly in order to overcome the handicap of noise may produce tension and fatigue. It is acoustically advantageous that the speaker be located between the outside noise source and his listeners because, in that situation, the speakers will adjust the loudness of his voice to overcome interference and at the same time the listeners will be further away from the outside disturbance. For the same reasons a pupil with a hearing handicap should be so placed that, to the greatest degree possible, his better ear is on the side toward the source of speech he wants to hear.[12]

– classifications The Committee on Child Health of the American Public Health Association classifies impaired hearing in terms of everyday ability to hear speech as follows:

1 *Mild impairment* means difficulty in hearing speech under less than ideal acoustic conditions.

2 *Moderate impairment* means trouble hearing speech under most conditions.

3 *Severe impairment* means inability to hear speech unless amplified in some manner.

4 *Profound impairment* means inability to hear and appreciate speech by ear alone even with amplification of sound.

5 *Deafness* is a profound impairment in both ears which precludes any useful hearing.[13]

The committee further describes the two principal types of hearing impairments:

1 Conductive impairment is caused by obstruction of the passage of sound from the outer to the inner ear. It affects loudness of sounds, primarily. Many of the mild and moderate impairments are caused by conductive lesions. These lesions are often preventable and a considerable number respond well to medical treatment when discovered early.

2 Perceptive impairment is caused by degeneration, damage, or lack of development of the sensory cells of the internal ear, the acoustic branch of the eighth cranial nerve, or certain parts of the brain. It affects total clarity and sound discrimination (as well as loudness in certain cases). It is usually the perception of high tones which is most affected but when the loss is severe both high and low tones are involved and understanding as well as hearing is impaired. Medical treatment can, as yet, do little or nothing for perceptive impairment when it has become established. Prevention is therefore of prime importance.[14]

Physical facilities for the hard-of-hearing child in the regular classroom with normally hearing children may be the same as for any regular standard classroom. Great care should be taken to secure optimum illumination so the hard-of-hearing child can do speech reading readily. Flexible seating arrangements are desirable so the hard-of-hearing child can be seated advantageously. Typical qualities of such a room are sufficient space to allow for unhampered physical movement, adequate lighting, bulletin boards and chalk boards, and shades or other means for darkening the room for the use of visual aids.

Some children in regular classrooms will be children whose hearing handicap has been improved by a hearing aid to the point where they are able to participate in the regular classroom. The teacher has the responsibility for consulting with the person who prescribed the aid or with the school district audiologist in order to learn enough about the aid to help the child participate in regular classroom activities. The child may need encouragement to wear the aid regularly and to make sure the batteries are up to date and are providing adequate amplification.

It is estimated that there are some 14 million children in the United States who are handicapped or who deviate sufficiently in their makeup so as to present a special problem in their education. These include those with significantly impaired hearing or vision, the crippled children, and those with heart disease, epilepsy, or mental handicaps. This figure also includes the emotionally disturbed and those with other forms of nervous disease.

These unfortunate children, each forced to make adjustments to life in a seeing, hearing "normal" world, require the attention of school personnel in many ways. It is recognized at once that they must be provided for educationally. They are entitled to all that can be given them. They have the right under our conception of democracy in education to seek and gain from every part of the curriculum all that is available to them. To facilitate the process of educating the handicapped, schools are evolving a program with the following five features.

CASE FINDING A child is considered handicapped or exceptional or atypical if he cannot within limits play, learn, work, or do the things other children of his age can do—if he is hindered in achieving his full physical, mental, and social potentialities. The initial disability may be very mild and hardly noticeable, but potentially handicapping; or it may seriously involve several areas of function with the probability of lifelong impairment.

It is important that local school authorities develop a system of discovering handicapped children, because only after they are found can education extend its benefits to them. If the children remain unknown to school authorities, either they are left to grow up illiterate, ignorant, and unable to take their place in society or unintended hardship is placed upon them by asking them to adapt to a school program for which they are not fitted. Case-finding procedures have to be taken into the community and into the home, many times with the help of the local census office, to find the exceptional child. Other programs, developed within the school, rely upon various appraisal examinations to reveal those who seriously deviate from the normal. Of course, it is not ordinarily difficult to recognize the deaf child, the one seriously crippled, or the one with defective speech, but it is quite another matter to pick out the tuberculous, the heart deviate, or the epileptic. The screening programs in school have to be carefully effective; they have to utilize as much evidence as they can get by way of medical history and previous records from the family or agency physician. The school must share the evidence with the home and vice versa; thus cooperation can secure the best educational program possible. In instances of epilepsy, for example, unless the condition is recorded on the history, the school may know nothing of its existence and the child may be exposed not only to bodily harm in the event that a seizure occurs in the shop or in physical education, but also to great emotional distress if companions and teachers are not forewarned and ready to help and understand. A cumulative record from babyhood to date is an excellent means of transmitting such information to those who can use it to advantage. The school, therefore, should develop the best case-finding program possible.

MEDICAL TREATMENT Once the case-finding program gets under way, the extent of the problem in the community will become known. From this information, community and school officials can estimate the kind and extent of medical, social, and educational services needed, as well as determine the sort of vocational counseling that should be provided.

It is not, of course, the business of the school to provide medical treatment to handicapped children. It is important, however, that everything done in school be done in relation to any hopeful therapy that might alleviate the handicap. The school has several opportunities here. It can, in the first place, serve to bring children whose disabilities might be wholly or partially alleviated into contact with medical service, and it can help handicapped children learn to live as fully as possible with their problem—to compensate by developing talents and satisfactions within their means and abilities. Thousands of them, possibly millions, have never had the advantage of a medical examination, diagnosis, or care. It may have been that the child was always thought of as "weak," "spindly," "not bright," or was typed by some other homely characterization when actually there are underlying organic or psychological disturbances which need to be revealed. They might respond if appropriate therapy were provided. Through its screening and referral service the school should take great pains to see that whatever can be done medically is done.

School personnel also need to know of the medical problem involved in each case in order to recognize the limitations of the child as well as his possibilities. The personnel will not want to schedule the child for a school experience that will be harmful nor will they expect adherence to any standards when the current therapeutic treatment of the child is interfering. In short, the medical status of the child takes priority over his educational status. The school is in a position of wanting everything done that can be done medically before it imposes other requirements or opens other opportunities to the child.

THE SPECIAL EDUCATIONAL PROGRAM Modern education recognizes individual differences and tries to individualize educational programs as far as possible. The fact of individual differences is strikingly apparent with exceptional children. It becomes clear to all who deal with them that the more individual attention they receive, the greater educational progress they make. In planning to educate the partially sighted or the emotionally unstable, for example, the teacher, administrator, and nurse must understand as much as they can about each particular child and construct the educational program just as the therapeutic program would be prescribed—in relation to the need, capacities, and nature of that child.

That ideal is difficult to attain. The tendency is to group the children. Once they are grouped as "nutrition disabilities" or "heart cases," the temptation is to give them all the same program.

Around this question centers a major controversy in the education for the handicapped: Should the handicapped be educated in regular schools along with and in competition with normal children or should special schools be established for them? There are arguments for and successful demonstrations of both practices. Many specialists in the education of the deaf and blind believe strongly that the state should provide separate facilities where these people can be educated among their own kind and specialize in the development of those talents that are most likely to provide economic and social security for them. The many state schools for the blind and deaf are institutions devoted to this practice.

On the other hand, there are those who believe that because the blind must live in a seeing world and the palsied in a world of moving things they should learn as early as possible to adjust to others and meet them on their own ground. Their answer is to place the handicapped child in a regular school, give him the advantage of special techniques (speech-reading, Braille, hydrotherapy), and expect him to measure up as far as he can. The proponents of this plan not only claim a better adjustment on the part of the handicapped but cite the beneficial effect it has on the normal child in getting him accustomed to living with the less fortunate.

The fact is that education can go on successfully under either the mixed or the segregated plan. The determinant as to which place to send a handicapped child should be the child himself. Some children thrive in one situation but wilt in others. The educator and the physician must help the parent choose the environment and the program best suited to the individual.

But in either situation the educational program emphasizes the possibilities and not the limitations of the child. This is psychologically of the greatest importance. A cardiac case is helped to find what he can do and little emphasis is put upon what he cannot. The physical education teacher helps the blind to swim. He explores the possibility of bowling, fly-casting, or table tennis with the boy with the rheumatic heart. He assists the amputee to play golf, to fish, or to swim. The emphasis may be negative only in caution against injury; otherwise, it is positive—"This you can do." To help the blind to make progress academically; to aid the crippled, the tuberculous, the cardiac to learn; to experiment, to interpret, and to understand—these are opportunities that must be extended. The problem is not only a health one but a social one as well.

Educational programs for these children will develop only insofar as the community understands and is sympathetic to the problems. A fully developed program requires special facilities and services to provide for physical, speech, and occupational therapy, space in the school building, special teachers, special scheduling, and special services. All this requires not only capital outlay but added maintenance and salary provisions. The whole program becomes a cooperative venture between educational and medical personnel, with the medical phases being supervised by medical people and the educational phases being supervised by educators.

Not an inconsiderable feature of this educational program for the special child is the effort to inform the people of the community what the problem is and how it can be affected. School personnel working cooperatively with medical and social workers can, through various types of community groups, reveal the problem and make suggestions as to the program. Prevention should be emphasized and community groups should be made aware of programs that will aid in preventing or alleviating these handicaps.

FINDING COMPENSATIONS The handicapped frequently make extraordinary adjustments, physical and psychological, to their handicaps. Many of these adjustments revolve around the development of some compensation or compensatory device. The partially sighted wears heavy glasses and sees as well as the next child. The glasses compensate. The amputee masters the artificial limb and is proud when his gait approaches normal. The cardiac learns that he can play but one set of tennis and is content with being a spectator or official when that is done. The partially deaf wears a hearing aid, the stammerer finds satisfactions not in speech but in writing, the crippled child becomes more keenly aware of the world of nature. There are innumerable compensations that bring satisfactions in lieu of those which would come if the handicap did not exist. The teacher is in a strategic position to aid in the development of these satisfactions.

Next to the actual medical or psychological phases of the handicap, this development of appropriate compensations is perhaps the most important health problem for the handicapped. Children must be guided into them, helped to establish them, and rewarded for success in achieving them.

EMOTIONAL PROBLEMS Closely allied with the factor of compensation is the larger problem of total emotional and psychological adjustment to being different. Normal people who see, hear, speak, and move around probably cannot appreciate just what it means to be looked at, examined, pitied, given special attention, restricted, handicapped. Nevertheless, the educator must not only teach the skills of learning or earning a living; he must also exert every effort in helping the handicapped to become a "man among men"—a child accepted and not rejected—a person belonging to a group and not isolated from it. The elementary years are crucial in this regard. Let the palsied, the crippled, the cardiac be left out when sides are chosen, when the plan is outlined or the chorus formed, or when the physical education period comes, and the seeds of maladjustment are sown. The physical education teacher must be particularly alert. Throughout the school years from kindergarten through college the physical educator must make available to all, the handicapped as well as the normal, the opportunity to receive a physical education. None should be excluded. The program should be flexible enough to embrace all. The blind child and the crippled are both entitled to receive that contribution that an intelligent physical educator can make to their psychological adjustment to life.

Investigations of children with reading disabilities reveal that they are frequently isolated, lonely, and sometimes resentful. They hold themselves in low esteem and sometimes their group adjustment is virtually nonexistent. Although children with crippling conditions may be expected to have the same kinds of behavior and emotional patterns as their normal contemporaries, the burden of a handicap may add difficulties to the process of growing up. For some children the emotional and intellectual aspects of their special problem may be the most important. With each disabled child an attempt should be made to (1) understand how the awareness of his handicap affects his personality and behavior; (2) know the approximate level and quality of his mental capacity and liabilities, and the areas of strength and weakness in his personality; (3) estimate his ability to cooperate and profit from therapy and education; (4) learn the best ways of giving appropriate guidance to those who live, work, and play with him and who are responsible for his care and training; (5) determine whether or not brain damage is a factor underlying his behavior.

It must be realized that each child is different—different in personality, in ability, in aspiration. To aid each in identifying himself with the group, in compensating for the handicap that makes him different, in becoming poised and self-reliant—these are the aims of any educational program for the handicapped.

SPECIAL PROVISIONS The federal government and most states subsidize special education for the handicapped. Funds are usually administered through state departments of education and teachers should acquaint themselves with such resources as might be used locally to aid in the education of the handicapped. In every school there are pupils who deviate so far from what is called the "normal child" that they require special skills, services, and sometimes special placement in order to be educated and developed to the limit of their capabilities. The material that follows, taken from Special Education Program Planning Guidelines of the State of Washington, indicates the kinds of handicapping conditions for which special educational adaptations are made in many school districts of the United States.

> 1 Hard of hearing
>
> a Definition—Children who have impaired hearing severe enough to require special instructional methods, materials, supplies, and equipment.
>
> b Eligibility requirements—Children eligible to a program for the hard of hearing must be recommended by a qualified hearing specialist. The total evaluation should include examination by a physician who may prescribe medical treatment and with whom school personnel should cooperate closely.
>
> c Programming—Class load in a full day, hard of hearing special class would usually consist of six children but no more than eight at any one time. The class load in a regular classroom with normally hearing children would be reduced by about four fewer normally hearing children for each hard of hearing child in the class. Except in unusual circumstances not more than three hard of hearing children should be integrated into a single classroom with normally hearing children. Generally the specific techniques employed by teachers of the hard of hearing children include (1) speech training to improve articulation, (2) speech reading to develop improved ability at speech understanding (lip reading), (3) auditory training to enhance listening skills and to insure that the child makes maximum use of his residual hearing either with or without amplification, (4) special assistance in academic subjects, (5) appropriate counselling measures with the child, his parents, the regular classroom teacher and other persons who may be involved in the management of the child's problem.

A trial placement in a class for hard-of-hearing children would generally precede placement in a regular classroom with normally hearing children, but as the child's abilities permit, the major educational objective is integration with normal-hearing children in a regular classroom. However, it is expected that during his preschool, primary, and intermediate grades he will need special hearing training. Termination of the special program for the hard-of-hearing child should occur when evaluation indicates he is ready to continue his school program without special help or when he demonstrates that he has reached his maximum social, academic, and vocational potentials.

2 Deaf

a Definition—Children who have a hearing loss of 75 to 80 decibels (I.S.O. standards) or greater across the speech range in the better ear and who, even with amplification, are unable to develop adequate language and speech.

b Eligibility requirements—Children eligible for a school program for the deaf must be recommended by a qualified hearing specialist. The total evaluation should include examination by a physician who may prescribe medical treatment and with whom school personnel should cooperate closely.

c Programming—the class load in a regular classroom with normally hearing children would usually be reduced by four fewer normally hearing children for each deaf child in the class, depending on the competency of the child. Ordinarily, not more than three deaf children should be integrated into a single classroom of normally hearing children. The class load in a full day deaf special classroom would be made up of four children, but certainly no more than eight at any one time depending on the competencies of the children. The purpose of the special class for the deaf child is to teach him to communicate comfortably with his hearing peers. As soon as the child is able to communicate adequately he should be transferred into the regular school program with supportive training as needed to maintain him in this placement. Care should be taken, however, to be certain that the child is ready for such a transfer. Each deaf child in a regular class should be expected to achieve his level of academic work and should not be graded on social growth or on the basis of the degree of his handicap.

3 Partially seeing

a Definition—Children whose vision is limited to 20/70 or less in the better eye after correction. Included are children who have other medically certified conditions of the eye which require special instruction materials, equipment and services.

b Eligibility requirements—Children eligible for a school program for the partially seeing must be recommended by a licensed eye specialist.

c Programming—The class load of both the regular classroom and the special program for the partially seeing will depend on the grade and age level, the type and degree of visual disability. The following guidelines are recommended. In a regular classroom with normally seeing children the class load of the teacher would be reduced by one to three normally seeing children for each partially seeing child in the class. Not more than three partially seeing children should be integrated into a single classroom of normally seeing children. When the class consists all of partially seeing children the enrollment should range from six to twelve depending on the competencies of the children. Since the partially seeing child is usually able to participate in a regular classroom the following points are important: (1) The program for the partially seeing child is conducted on a cooperative plan with the special classroom teacher and the regular teacher sharing the responsibility. The standards of achievement for the partially seeing child are the same as for the regular classroom child. (2) All activities requiring close use of the eyes will require the utilization of special equipment and materials. The child should participate in the other usual activities of the classroom within the limits of his vision. (3) Special attention must be given to training the partially seeing child in correct habits of eye hygiene in order that he will understand his own eye difficulty in its relation to his successful school program.

4 Blind

a Definition—Children whose visual acuity is 20/100 or less in the better eye after correction. Included also are children who have been medically diagnosed with conditions of the eye that will certify them as legally blind.

b Eligibility requirements—Children eligible for school program for the blind must be recommended by a licensed eye specialist.

c Programming—Enrollment in special classes for the blind should not exceed six to ten children. The class load in the regular classroom for normally seeing children should be reduced by one to four fewer sighted children for each blind child in the class. As soon as it is feasible the blind child should be integrated into the regular classroom. The sequence of programming for the blind proceeds as follows: (1) Preschool readiness opportunities emphasizing development of aural and tactual skills. (2) Special classes for the blind preceeded by a trial period. (3) Special classes and special teachers available to the blind children who are being served in a combined program of placement in regular classes with seeing children and in special classes for the blind. (4) Integration into regular classes of seeing children with appropriate support from the special teacher of the blind children. (5) Reading service with the remainder of the day integrated into regular classes with seeing children.

Blind children in a regular classroom with normally seeing children should be encouraged by being provided with the following: (1) Physical education activities and free play with normally seeing children. (2) Opportunities to show sighted children how to assist them to take part in the regular school and classroom activities. (3) Adaptations in the classroom and on the playground to insure their safety. (4) Special and extra support for teachers in the regular classrooms who will be required to plan their programs. (5) Adequate assistance in the classroom so that the few special concessions that are needed can be given to the blind child.

5 Orthopedically handicapped

a Definition—Children who are handicapped through congenital or acquired motor defects or health problems requiring protective educational environment to a degree that they must have special services, materials, supplies, and equipment.

b Eligibility requirements—Children eligible for a school program for the orthopedically handicapped must have a recommendation by a physician. Some of the disabilities are: (1) Orthopedic, poliomyelitis, osteomyelitis, accident or other traumatic conditions, tuberculosis of the bones, cerebral palsy, congenital defects and anomalies. (2) Other health problems involving lowered vitality, restricted activity, or debilitation: heart disease, rheumatic fever, encephalitis, muscular dystrophy, cancer, birth injury, asthma, diabetes mellitus, allergy.

A child placed in a special classroom for orthopedically handicapped children will be terminated when any one of the following conditions has been met: is physically unable to continue in the program; is unable to return to the regular classroom with or without supportive services; graduates from high school; or the child can no longer profit from the services which the school is able to provide for the child's handicapped condition.

c Programming—(1) Integration of the orthopedically handicapped child is an essential part of a well-rounded program. The academic and therapy programs should be correlated to meet individual needs of the child. (2) Children enrolled in programs for orthopedically handicapped usually require additional services such as: (a) Physical therapy—The physical therapist must work with the classroom teacher as a member of the team. Physical therapy treatment is limited to that prescribed by a physician. The physical therapist should be registered with the American Physical Therapists Association and the state physical therapists association. (b) Occupational therapy—Occupational therapy is limited to that prescribed by the physician. The therapist should be registered in the American Occupational Therapists Association and the appropriate state association. (c) Speech therapy—The speech therapist is another member of the team which provides assistance to the orthopedically handicapped child. (d) Attendant—An attendant working under the direction of a certified staff member may be employed when the number of children requiring self-care assistance becomes too large for the teacher. Duties should include all of those self-care services required by children. Duties should not include full responsibility for the students.

6 Neurologically impaired

a Definition—Children who have central nervous system dysfunction so serious that they cannot adjust to a regular or other special education classroom without additional special services. These children demonstrate average or above average intelligence but exhibit impaired perceptual awareness and understanding of their learning environment.

b Eligibility—Children eligible in a school program for the neurologically impaired must have a medical and psychological evaluation.

c Programming—Class loads will vary in proportion to the severity of the problems within a particular class but the recommended size usually ranges from four to eight pupils. The needs of the neurologically impaired children can best be met in a carefully planned and arranged learning environment with limited visual and auditory distractions. These children often have such severe perceptual disabilities that teaching methods and materials must be specially adapted for them and their special problems. Much of the teaching will have to be on an individual basis. The program is aimed toward the adequate social adjustment of each child with the expectation that he will become a contributing member of his school group and work up to his capacity. For this reason, eventual integration, wherever possible, into a normal classroom is a major educational goal for these children. Some of these children may be on a program of prescribed medication related to their impairment. Special attention must be paid to the medical aspects of their handicaps. Frequent consultation with the school nurse and attending physician is necessary. Because gross communication disorders are frequently involved in neurological handicaps, speech, hearing consultation and therapy are necessary.

7 Trainable retarded.

a Definition—Children who because of retarded intellectual and social development are incapable of being educated in the programs for the educable mentally retarded. I.Q. criterion is not the primary consideration, however, the I.Q. will generally range below 51 on an individual test of intelligence as administered by a qualified psychologist.

b Eligibility—Children eligible for special classes for the trainable mentally retarded must be evaluated by a qualified psychologist.

c Programming—Class loads for the program for the trainable retarded generally will range from six to ten children in the class depending on the age and capabilities of the children. The program will be related to the degree of maturity of the children concerned. Emphasis will be in areas of intellectual, personal, social, communication, physical and occupational competencies.

8 Educable retarded

a Definition—Children who because of retarded intellectual and social development are incapable of being educated entirely through regular classroom instruction but who may profit from a special education setting designed to meet their needs. I.Q. criterion is not the primary consideration, however, the I.Q. will generally range between 51 and 75 on an individual test of intelligence administered by a qualified psychologist.

b Eligibility—Children eligible for special classes for the educable mentally retarded must be evaluated and recommended for such placement by a qualified psychologist.

c Programming—The class load will depend upon such factors as children's ages, degrees of intelligence, levels of educational achievement and difficulties of management, but in general will range from six to sixteen, depending on age. The program for the educable mentally retarded should concentrate on the social, intellectual, occupational, and physical development in terms of a child's age and ability. Association for part of the school day with peer groups in their regular school situation should be included where possible. The child properly selected for the program would not be expected to gain a normal grade placement expectation for age. If the child has been properly placed it will be anticipated that he will continue in the program throughout his school experience. Reconsideration of placement should be made periodically because of difficulties of accurate assessment.

9 Emotionally maladjusted

a Definition—Children whose emotional development results in incompatible learning behavior which cannot be adjusted or modified to regular classroom procedures without special services. This generally includes children who show the extremes of acting out or withdrawal behaviors included in the classification of personality disorders.

b Eligibility—Children eligible for this program must have had both a medical and a psychological evaluation.

c Programming—A school program for the emotionally maladjusted child recognizes the need for special organization of the school environment and requires adaptations of the regular school program for each child. This is necessary in order that positive personality and educational factors can be emphasized and stresses minimized. Although the class is generally therapeutic by nature, the school district must not assume primary responsibility for treatment or therapy. Since the degree of emotional maladjustment will vary widely among children, the school will need to develop an appropriate program for each child either by special class placement or by providing supportive services to the child and his regular class teacher. This often will take the form of support by a social worker trained in psychiatric group work and the clinical psychologist trained in learning theory.

10 Home and hospital instruction

a Definition—Children who because of medical restrictions (excluding normal pregnancies), must be confined at home or in hospitals for a minimal period of four weeks to warrant a continuing program of instruction. Must be medically certified.

b Eligibility—Children eligible for enrollment in a public school and unable to attend for four weeks or more because of a physical disability or illness may receive home or hospital instruction if they are so certified by a physician and approved by the school authorities. The parents must request these services in writing and agree to conditions of the service.

c Programming—The special home/hospital teacher will coordinate the lessons for the student with the teacher's regular classroom. Special arrangements must be made with an adult family member and the child to provide regular study periods and regular study space in the home or hospital situation, which are as free of distraction as possible.

11 The multiply-handicapped child

For the most part children are being placed under special instruction according to their major handicap. Concomitant handicaps are very often neglected, if not entirely overlooked in school, particularly if the teacher in charge is not well trained, if the plant is not well equipped, or if the school administration is not well oriented to the variety of disabilities and the need for specially designed programs. There is no area in special education that challenges the teacher to the degree that the field of the multiple handicapped does.

Actually, the number of children with multiple handicaps is very large if we consider the fact that they may be handicapped by two or more physical deviations. One may be marked, one may be minor, one or more may be allied to basic difficulties, and one or more may result from secondary deviations. Such handicaps may be permanent or temporary, incurable or curable. Multiple handicaps may stem from birth injuries, prenatal influences, accidents, infections, disabilities, maltreatment, maldiagnosis, heredity, or emotional factors.

Once again the type of educational environment provided to the child will be based on information regarding the child's capabilities and disabilities, but with accent on those things which he can do.[15]

THE ROLE OF THE SCHOOL HEALTH TEAM IN SPECIAL EDUCATION

The relationship among the members of the school health team and those who are organizing and implementing the program of special education for the exceptional child is extremely close. Most of the educational adaptations are based on information gathered by members of the school health team regarding the child's abilities and deviations. There is great need for complete evaluation of the child to be carried out by members of the school health team or on the basis of their referrals before a child is placed in special education. Follow-up and follow-through are also a necessary part of the school health team's work. Ordinarily they will function in several areas:

1 Early discovery of deformities in all children

2 Placing patients under immediate physical, surgical, and educational treatment

3 Engaging in a relentless and vigilant team approach involving the physician, teacher, psychologist, parent, nurse, social worker, and therapists

4 Following up at regular intervals with a testing and reevaluation program

5 Developing policies and procedures whereby a child can receive medication at school when it is so ordered by his physician

Special education and the school health team are closely related. Deep involvement in the special education process and the adaptations made in each child's learning environment are certainly a high priority in the functions of the school health team.

ARCHITECTURE AND THE HANDICAPPED

One out of ten persons has some disability that prevents him from using buildings and facilities designed only for the physically fit. Among this one-tenth of the population are over 2 million school children with various kinds of disabling handicaps. Many are forced to become backdoor citizens in order to use our schools. Often children cannot be placed in schools with their friends and neighbors because of handicaps that will not allow them to enter schools with architectural barriers. Parents also are kept from entering school buildings because of their disabilities. Some of these barriers are lack of proper parking facilities for the disabled, inaccessible entrances such as stairs, steep inclines, narrow doorways, hazardous doorways leading to dangerous areas with no sense of touch markings for the blind, restroom facilities not suitable for wheelchairs, and laboratories and classrooms that do not have spaces adaptable for those in wheelchairs or those who wear braces or crutches. Other barriers are too high telephones, drinking fountains, vending machines, light switches, and fire alarms.[17]

Members of the school health team have the opportunity to make the entire school district available to persons with handicapping conditions by working with architects and members of the school staff to add accessibility features in old buildings and to make sure new facilities are built to be available for all Americans. Such accessibility features include handrails, a ground level main entrance or ramp, steps that are rounded instead of squared at the edges, doors that open automatically, raised letters and numbers on doors and in elevators so that the blind can read them, danger signals equipped with light as well as sound so that the deaf will be warned, an open booth with a low-placed telephone, one or more side toilet stalls with grab rails, nonslip flooring, and elevators in any multiple storied buildings where the disabled can reach them easily from the main floor. The most authoritative guideline for architects and others planning school buildings is The United States of America Standards Institute, formerly called The American Standards Association, which has published "Specifications for Making Buildings and Facilities Accessible to and Usable by the Physically Handicapped." In almost every instance improved facilities for the handicapped help the able-bodied as well.

SUMMARY

The chapters of this book have described the process of school health services proceeding from the promotion of health to the knowledge of children's problems. The procedures of observation, screening, health appraisal, referral, and follow-up were described in order. This chapter on adaptations has stressed that while health care of the child is an important goal of school health education, the team members cannot allow their responsibilities to end there. They are charged with making sure that health information flows to the school and that appropriate adaptations are made in the child's learning environment at school. Most of the adjustments made on the basis of health information are made by the regular classroom teacher in regard to the activity programs and communication methods used. Frequently school districts have developed programs of special education for children who deviate from the "normal child" to the point where radically different educational environments and programs are necessary. The problem of architectural barriers to the disabled and handicapped was raised as another area where health information is valuable in planning the school environment. The close relationship between school health education, special education, and architectural planning for the exceptional child was stressed throughout.

NOTES AND REFERENCES

1 Joy G. Cauffman, Edward A. Warburton, and Carl S. Shultz, "Health Care of School Children: Effective Referral Patterns," *American Journal of Public Health,* 59, 1 (January 1969), 86.

2 Joy Cauffman, "Factors Affecting Outcome of School Health Referrals," *Journal of School Health,* XXXVIII, 6 (June 1968).

3 Tali Conine, and William T. Brennan, "Orthopedically Handicapped Children in Regular Classrooms," *Journal of School Health,* XXIX, 1 (January 1969).

4 Classification of Students for Physical Education," *Journal of Health, Physical Education and Recreation,* 38 (February 1967), 16 *passim.*

5 *Journal of the American Medical Association,* 199, 4 (January 1967).

6 "Competitive Athletics for Children of Elementary School Age," *Pediatrics,* 42 (October 1968).

7 "A Policy Statement on Competitive Athletics for Children of Elementary School Age," Washington, D.C., American Association for Health, Physical Education and Recreation, pamphlet copyright 1968.

8 American Public Health Association, "Services for Children with Eye Problems, A Guide for Public Health Personnel," New York, American Public Health Association, 1967.

9 AMA, *Healthful School Environment,* Washington, D.C. and Chicago, AMA, 1969

10 *Ibid.*

11 Peter Breysse, "Noise Investigation, Open Classroom Concept," Tacoma Public Schools, personal communication, April 30, 1970.

12 AMA, *op. cit.*

13 Committee on Child Health of the American Public Health Association, *Services for Children with Hearing Impairment,* New York, American Public Health Association, 1956.

14 Superintendent of Public Instruction, *Special Education Program Planning Guidelines,* Olympia, Wash. Superintendent of Public Instruction, 1969.

15 *Ibid.*

16 Leland M. Corliss, "Multiply Handicapped Children—Their Placement in the School Education Program," *Journal of School Health,* XXXVII, 3 (March 1967), 113.

17 "A Report of the National Commission on Architectural Barriers to Rehabilitation of the Handicapped—Design for All Americans," Washington, D.C., Rehabilitation Services Administration, Social and Rehabilitation Service Department of Health, Education and Welfare, Superintendent of Documents, Government Printing Office, 1967.

SELECTED READINGS

Cauffman, Jay G., Edward A. Warburton, and Carl S. Shultz, "Health Care of School Children: Effective Referral Patterns," *American Journal of Public Health,* 59:1, January 1969.

"Classification of Students for Physical Education," *Journal of Health, Physical Education and Recreation,* 38:16, February 1967; *Journal of the American Medical Association,* 199:4, Jan. 23, 1967.

"Desirable Athletic Competition for Children of Elementary School Age," American Association for Health, Physical Education and Recreation, National Education Association, Washington, D.C., 1968.

Healthful School Environment, Joint Committee on Health Problems in Education of the NEA and AMA, The Associations, Washington, D.C. and Chicago, 1969.

"Report of the National Commission on Architectural Barriers to Rehabilitation of the Handicapped—Design for all Americans," Rehabilitation Services Administration, Department of Health, Education, and Welfare, Washington, D.C. 1967.

"Services for Children with Eye Problems, A Guide for Public Health Personnel," American Public Health Association, New York, 1967.

"Services for Children with Hearing Impairment," American Public Health Association, New York, 1956.

CHAPTER 14 PROGRAMS FOR CONTROL OF PROBLEMS OF THE SCHOOL-AGE CHILD

The school health programs described so far are designed to provide optimum learning environments for individual students and to provide health services to children who have health problems. Case finding and referral activities and school adaptations to individual differences are examples of these.

School systems also develop health activities on the basis of a sense of responsibility for promoting the well-being of children and because of a desire to prevent health problems known to occur frequently and severely among school children. (See Chapter 10.) Programs of safety, communicable disease control, nutrition, and dental health are the most frequently found examples of school health plans to promote well-being and to prevent childhood problems.

THE SAFETY PROGRAM The accidental injury is a serious health problem. In 1968 there were 8,400 accidental deaths of school age children (ages 5 to 14). For the groups whose ages were 1 through 14 accidental death was the leading cause of mortality. Some of these deaths were due to failure on the part of school personnel to establish safety programs.

Not only are accidents the leading cause of death among children of school age but also they are one of the leading causes of disability among children. Only respiratory infections cause more disability in this age group. For every five school accidents two occur in unorganized activities, and three out of every five occur in organized activities. The classroom, the gymnasium, and the streets are the usual sites where accidents occur. The National Safety Council can inform any interested person on the frequency and location of school accidents.[1] The accident rate (number of accidents per one hundred thousand school days) is 10.6 for all grades compared to 5.0 for the nonschool jurisdictional accident.

Prevention of childhood accidents begins at home, of course, but an all school safety program is an essential element of school health education and will operate as follows:

1 An all school safety council, large or small depending on the size of the school, should include both teachers and students. Teachers of laboratory and shop classes, including physical education, should be represented as well as the nurse and physician if they are available. The principal should be a member ex officio. This safety council or committee would: (1) continuously analyze the cause and prevention of accidents in their own and other schools; (2) survey their own school for safety hazards; (3) recommend to the faculty and board of education ways to prevent the occurance of accidents; (4) provide teaching material in safety education for those giving health instruction anywhere in the school and assist in the continuous improvement of curriculum materials in safety; (5) arrange visual material for bulletin boards, plan assembly programs, and in every intelligent way promote safe living in the school environment; (6) formulate and supervise a program of safety for the school, including an emergency care program, fire drills, traffic supervision, and continuous inspection of building and grounds for danger spots and potential causes of accidents.

2 A thorough and modern program of traffic safety both within and outside the school is essential. Children must be brought to and from home safely, and local police authorities should be invited to assist in directing traffic, marking streets, installing traffic lights and signs, and discussing with children how to move in traffic. Traffic inside the school building must be regulated to assure the efficient flow of movement between classes. The school safety patrol can be organized to develop and maintain this traffic program.

3 The school bus program must leave nothing overlooked that contributes to safe practice. All state and local standards for school bus driving must be met completely and without exception. Drivers must be expert and without organic or psychological handicaps that would lower their efficiency as drivers and thus endanger the students. Buses must be equipped with safety exits, fire extinguishers, and first aid materials in sufficient quantity to care for a full load of children. No bus driver should ever allow more than the maximum number of passengers provided by law to board the bus. Warning lights, signals, and other paraphernalia

must be of the best according to local standards and checked regularly for efficient operation.

4 A program of laboratory, shop, and gymnasium safety must anticipate every contingency. Moving shop parts should be painted in danger colors. Gas jets should be of a different color than water outlets. Draft hoods for removing smoke and odors should be working whenever the laboratory is in use. Good housekeeping—everything in its place—should be the prevailing practice.

5 The entire staff should study and understand all local laws and ordinances pertaining to school safety and liability for accidents. This material might be provided by the safety committee. Prevention and liability are interesting topics for faculty meetings, and their discussion will go far in making a careless staff more alert to their responsibilities in the prevention of accidents.

6 Subcommittees on safety should be appointed from among the pupils in each room. These student committees should help to organize fire drills, be responsible for safe practice within the room, and provide discussion materials on safety for room use. The room committee can assume charge of room traffic and develop the safety program in shops, corridors, and physical education classes, both indoor and outdoor.

7 Programs for the regulation of vehicle travel and parking, school dances, night use of the building, smoking on the premises, handling of crowds at athletic contests and other gatherings should be worked out by the school safety council and their provisions made effective in the life of the school.

8 Courses for secondary students in driver training should be instituted wherever possible. Participation in driver education has been increasing steadily since 1960 according to figures supplied by the National Safety Council.[2] Figures for 1967–1968 indicate that 65 percent of eligible students participated in courses of high school driver's education whereas 81 percent of the eligible schools offered courses to the students. Such courses are a basic part of the school safety program and should be supported by school personnel.

EMERGENCY PROTECTION

The school has three responsibilities in regard to emergencies and accidents. One is to prevent accidents from happening in school; the second is to offer instruction in the curriculum regarding safety; and the third is to execute a program of action for emergencies that do happen at school. The latter is all too frequently neglected on the theory either that "accidents will not happen here" or that "when something does turn up it will be handled by common sense." Neither position is tenable. Accidents, fires, explosions, food poisoning, and emergencies of nearly every kind can and do happen at unexpected times and in unexpected places. And when they occur they are not always handled well because of the panic, excitement, forgetfulness, or lack of knowledge of one or more key persons. The unexpected must be prepared for. Every contingency must be met ahead of time.

There are many good and bad examples of meeting emergencies. In a medium-sized school known widely for its attention to the health of children, plans had been made for the unexpected. One day it occured. In an assembly children began to be nauseated. Within an hour over a hundred children were in various stages of collapse from food poisoning. At the first sign the school's emergency care program was in action and continued throughout the experience. Ambulances were called, physicians and nurses were summoned, parents were notified, family doctors were called, children were taken to a nearby hospital, and public health authorities were summoned. Later an investigation was held and corrections were made in the refrigeration of foods. Throughout the emergency all was done that could be done and without panic or noise. The teachers and principal knew what to do because they had planned for it. Eventualities had been anticipated and answers had been provided.

There are several steps to be taken toward the provision of complete plans for emergency care:

1 The faculty of the school must be made aware of the possibility of accident and emergency and must be responsive to the suggestion that they work out plans for any eventuality.

2 Every teacher in every room, shop, or gymnasium must think through what he would do in case of fire, explosion, or panic.

3 These plans must be correlated into a master plan, put in writing, and well studied and understood by all school personnel involved.

4 A roster of every pupil and staff person showing name, parents' names, address, home and business phones, name of family physician or physician of choice in case of emergency, hospital of choice, special directions for dealing with accidents, allergy sensitivities, and religion should be placed conveniently near a telephone in the main office. See the accompanying form. In case of accident the school, being morally responsible to give immediate care, would do so in accordance with practice agreed to and instructions received from parents.

5 First aid and emergency cabinets must be provided and placed at strategic spots around the school.[3,4] Their contents must be fresh, up to date, and in accordance with the best standards for first aid care. It is desirable for every teacher to be knowledgeable of first aid procedures. The physical education teacher, nurse, principal, and industrial arts and home economics teachers should be expert at first aid. School nurses make a great contribution to schools when they earn first aid instructor certificates and are then able to conduct classes for teachers within the school setting.

6 At the first indication of an emergency, code signals should be given throughout the school calling all first aiders, or calling all emergency drivers, or calling a general exodus from the building

SCHOOL ______________________ DATE ______________

NAME ______________________________________

In case of accident, sickness or death while at school the proper authorities are to notify the following:

Next of Kin (Relationship) ______________ Business Phone ________

Address ______________________ Home Phone ________

Other (Relationship - Friend) ______________ Business Phone ________

Address ____________ City ____________ Home Phone ________

Doctor ____________ Address ____________ Phone ________

Hospital Choice ______________________ Blood Type ________

Hospital Insurance: Blue Cross ______ Pierce County ______ Other ________

(*Optional*)
Religious Preference: Protestant ________ Catholic ________ Jewish ________

Minister ______________________ Phone ________

as in a fire drill. In one school Boy Scout and Camp Fire Girl first aid teams were called when needed; they were definitely needed one day when a flash storm knocked down high-tension wires and trapped several children.

7 Parents or guardians should be notified calmly and as early as possible, and every needed assistance should be given them in caring for their children.

8 The school medical adviser should prepare detailed instructions for the guidance of teachers and the school nurse with reference to the immediate treatment of such common school emergencies as abdominal pain, cuts, bruises, dog bites, suspected fractures, painful menstruation, and headache, as well as less frequent emergencies such as epileptic attacks or insulin shock. The school nurse is responsible for making sure that accident procedures and plans for immediate treatment of school emergencies are known and available to all school personnel.

9 Parents should be informed of every plan made by the school in anticipation of accidents and emergencies and be given the opportunity to state the kind of care they want their children to receive. They want to know that their child will be well cared for in case something unexpected happens. Informing parents of plans in advance gives them a chance to suggest modifications and obviates any criticism that might be leveled later if a parent did not approve the action taken.

10 The school should have stated plans for the handling of accidents occurring in athletic competition. These plans, in the form of either insurance or outright subsidy by the board of education in case of injury, should be well known to players and parents and should be given wide publicity in order to avoid misunderstanding after an accident. Insurance plans are receiving wide use, particularly in high school athletics, and experience with them so far has proved their value.

11 A report of each accident or other emergency situation should be kept on hand in the principal's office. This report should include names of persons concerned, time, location, nature of the accident, witnesses, and disposition of the case. Such records are frequently of great importance in later discussions of prevention or liability.

12 Plans for transporting children to home or hospital must be made. The school should provide for private cars, school buses, ambulances, or other means, with the method of calling drivers and means of paying for the trip all worked out in advance. Nothing should be left to after-the-accident argument. If insurance is carried on public conveyors, its coverage should be well known to all. If private cars are used at times of accidents, certain ones should be used and the insurance on them should be in force. It would be well to know what exits would be used in the event injured children had to be taken from the buildings to cars. Every conceivable detail should be thought out.

LIABILITY

In many communities it is common for parents or guardians of children injured in school to bring suit for damages against school personnel. In such instances it is alleged that the school personnel were responsible, perhaps through negligence, for the accidents. For protection against this practice as well as for the welfare of the children, school people should know as much as possible about the liability laws in their state.

There is a difference between responsibility and liability. Responsibility is a rather vague relationship established by school or community policy, but liability is described by law and can be established by the courts as they interpret the law. Teachers can be considered to be responsible for their pupils in the classrooms and on the playground, but whether they can be held liable for damages in case of an accident is quite another matter.

Liability can only be established if the teacher (or whoever is involved—bus driver, principal, or some other) can be proven negligent in the performance of duties ordinarily associated with the position or imprudent in the discharge of those responsibilities. The point is that negligence or imprudence has to be proven—usually in a court of law and to the satisfaction of a jury. If a teacher failed to warn pupils of dangers or to provide expected supervision, or if he knowingly conducted a class under unsafe conditions or committed any other imprudent act, then, in the event of accident, the offending teacher might be found liable and held for punitive damages.

Unfortunately there is some feeling among witnesses of accidents that to offer first aid treatment to the injured might make the Good Samaritan liable for suit if anything went wrong later that could be traced to the on-the-scene aid. So they refuse to help the injured person. Many states have enacted laws to protect the Good Samaritan, such as the one in the Ohio code (Sec. 2305.23, Revised Code, State of Ohio), which reads as follows:

> No person shall be liable in civil damages for administering emergency care or treatment at the scene of an emergency outside of a hospital, doctor's office, or other place having proper medical equipment, for acts performed at the scene of such emergency, unless such acts constitute willful or wanton misconduct.
>
> Nothing in this section applies to the administering of such care or treatment where the same is rendered for remuneration or with the expectation of remuneration.

Sometimes failure to provide first aid treatment or providing the wrong kind of first aid can be interpreted as negligence and grounds for the establishment of liability for damages. This is why all schools should have recognized first aiders (as certified by the American Red Cross) and a clear-cut first aid policy for everyone to read and understand. These policies should clearly state how far the school personnel can and will go in providing first aid; how and under what circumstances parents (or specified others) will be notified; how and under what circumstances children will be removed from school for treatment; and a statement concerning the financial arrangements involved.

INSURANCE

A complete safety program will offer to students, teachers, principals, and school secretaries accident insurance covering either the school-time hours or twenty-four hour activity. Many times these policies are administered by the Parent-Teacher Association or other parent organization with the endorsement and cooperation of the school board and school personnel. Such coverage usually includes accidental bodily injuries sustained by an insured person while: (1) traveling directly from home to school or from school to home each school day immediately prior to or following regular school hours or dismissal from an on-the-premises school activity that takes place immediately following regular school hours; (2) in or on buildings or other premises of the school at which enrolled or assigned during the time the student, while under direct supervision by members of the faculty, is attending a school sponsored and organized student activity; (3) the student is under direct supervision by members of the faculty participating in school sponsored and organized activities conducted off the school premises.

It is impossible to prevent all accidents from occurring at school; therefore it is wise to make insurance coverage available for a low fee to students and staff members who desire such coverage. Experience has shown that people who have insurance coverage are more likely to seek care for any disabilities which may be incurred in accidents.

A similar but different problem is insurance coverage for accidental injury incurred while participating in the school athletic program. In athletic activities students are at a greater risk of being injured than they are in the regular school situation. Coverage for injuries sustained in school athletics will be more expensive than regular accident insurance because of the increased risk. Many times insurance plans have been worked out by state high school activities associations or through medical society sponsored service programs or through group prepayment plans on competitive bid. It is impossible to develop standard insurance plans for all children in a state or in the United States so it is necessary for each community to work out its own arrangements to fit the local cost structure and supply of professional personnel. In any event, accident insurance is a desirable part of every school safety program, including not only regular activities but also all athletic endeavors.

THE DISEASE CONTROL PROGRAM

Schools and colleges are morally obligated to exert every effort to prevent the occurrence of disease among their students. School laws requiring attendance of children add to the obligation to have an adequate disease control program. Just as the school is required to have a fire control program to compensate in part for the unfavorable environment in which some children are forced to live during the day, it is also necessary to compensate for the increased exposure to disease.

The school environment is frequently conducive to the transmission of diseases of nearly all communicable kinds. A child may contract or develop a handicapping disease which, had he not been compelled to attend, he would not have contracted. Parents know this and expect the school to give children every protection against communicable disease. The school that operates under the authority of the compulsory attendance laws and does not accept the obligation to protect children against the disasters of, for example, poliomyelitis or tuberculosis is more than remiss; it is culpable.

What kinds of diseases afflict the school population? What exposures may a child meet? There are four principal kinds:

1 The respiratory group, including the familiar cold, mumps, measles, diptheria, tuberculosis, influenza, smallpox, chicken pox, and many others. Most of these, with the help of vaccines and drugs, are reasonably controllable, but some (mumps, chicken pox) still remain annoying.

2 Those entering through the skin or membranes, including impetigo, venereal diseases, pediculosis, ringworm, scabies, and others. Some are transmitted by microscopic organisms and others by insects.

3 The gastrointestinal diseases, including typhoid fever, food poisoning, and dysentery, acquired by ingesting contaminated food or water.

4 All others of less certain origin and presenting social problems, such as heart disease, rheumatic fever, muscular dystrophy, leukemia, and others.

One or more of these diseases is constantly present, sometimes in epidemic form, somewhere in the schools of the land. They are a cause of absence and sometimes of disability and death. Some merely cause inconvenience and retard learning. Because they are ever present, they require the establishment of policies and procedures to meet them.

– basic policies for control Although the control of communicable disease in the community is legally the responsibility of the board of health, there are several basic policies, concerning the control and prevention of disease, that should be familiar to everyone in education. These policies should serve as the basis for specific controls to be put into effect in every school. They should be understood and approved by boards of education and then made the subject for discussion at faculty meetings so that all personnel will be guided accordingly. All parents and children should be aware of the policies and understand that they are for the students' protection. These policies are as follows:

1 Principals and superintendents should have accurate and authoritative information concerning the legal status of vaccination and immunization in their state. State laws vary. Some require vaccination for smallpox as a condition for school entrance. Others do not. There are at least six variations of vaccination laws throughout the states, and administrators can go only so far as the state law permits. If a school desires to make satisfactory evidence of protection against smallpox, whooping cough, poliomyelitis, or any other disease for which effective vaccine is available, a condition of entrance, the right to do so must be established by law.

2 The practice of rewarding continuous attendance is not compatible with best protection against disease and should be discontinued. Infected pupils frequently may be sent to school for the sake of maintaining an attendance record and thus expose others to the disease. In localities where schools must rely on average daily attendance for financial support from the state a real problem is presented. Absences for any reason mean loss of revenues; attendance, however, may well mean more absences, and perhaps epidemics. A better solution to the problem of school support comes when reimbursement is based on average enrollment figures for a given period of time. In no instance should the school encourage the attendance of a sick child not only for his sake, but for the sake of others who may be exposed to a communicable disease.

3 No communicable disease program can be fully effective without the cooperation of parents. Schools should make every effort to acquaint parents with the disease problem and seek their active participation in the program to control disease.

4 Responsibility for the administration of exclusion and other control measures is vested by law in the board of health, but many procedures may need to be carried out by school authorities and personnel in cooperation with the board of health.

5 Home supervision of communicable diseases is necessarily carried out by the board of health. Therefore, school authorities must establish close cooperation with the health authorities in order to coordinate home and school procedures.

6 Whenever public schools administer their own communicable disease measures and private and parochial schools are served in similar capacity by the board of health, the program must be consistent and well coordinated to avoid community confusion, lack of cooperation, and resentments based upon real or fancied discriminations.

7 If the communicable disease program is administered by the board of health, it must be carefully coordinated with school schedules and operations of school plants, and there must be opportunities for classroom teachers to familiarize themselves with communicable disease control procedures and with their duties in relation thereto.

Plans for the administration of such policies vary. In some communities the board of health or health department assumes responsibility for all school health services, including, of course, the control of communicable diseases. In such instances the effective operation of the above policies is the obligation of the health department, which usually seeks and gets the active cooperation of the educational authorities.

In other instances the school authorities employ medical personnel who effectively operate disease control procedures in accordance with the regulations of the board of health; and in still a third pattern the matter of disease control becomes a joint responsibility.

– specific procedures in disease control

Eventually any good program of disease control must come down to dealing with specific children who have or have had a disease or who may be exposed to one. There are, of course, many things a school can do by way of maintaining standards of sanitation, ventilation and safety and these have been or will be mentioned in appropriate chapters. But to control the diseases as they occur or to prevent them requires a chain of procedures involving, in this order; immunization, case finding, isolation and exclusion, notification of parents and others, referrals to medical care, and readmission. Programs of immunization remain about the only concrete way to prevent specific diseases in specific people.

Immunization Program / The first step in any school effort to control communicable disease is to mobilize the forces within the community to prevent the occurrence of these diseases. This involves not only an educational program directed at children and parents to bring them into a receptive attitude towards such preventive measures, but also requires agreement upon and development of programs of action regarding the specific diseases. In view of the fact that science is constantly making progress in the control and prevention of these diseases, it behooves school authorities to avail themselves of the best current opinion and practice in their administration. Schools should consult local medical authorities about the utility, safety, and wisdom of every immunization procedure used.

Medical opinion of the day indicates that most of the immunizing that is to be done should be done before the child reaches school. If it is not done before entrance, then the school should maintain procedures that will accomplish immunization against these diseases in at least 80 percent of the school population. These procedures will include a history record for case-finding purposes and advice to all unimmunized children concerning the merits of protection. Parents should be urged to take their children to their own physician for immunization, and a record of such protection should be on file at the school. Many schools today are arranging for immunization at the school and as part of the school health education program. Children are being invited to avail themselves of this service at minimal cost (or free, in some instances). Before this is done, written requests from parents must be obtained, and the entire procedure must be placed in the hands of highly competent medical personnel.

However, some school systems do not sponsor the original or primary immunizations. They may administer booster shots, but they operate under the principle that the original immunizations should not wait until entrance to school. By declining to provide such service, the school encourages parents to use the services of private physicians or clinics.

When the immunization program in a school district is not regulated by the Board of Education of that district, but is required by state law, then, school authorities must know what the law is. Some states have compulsory programs with no exceptions. Some make allowances for those who conscientiously object to vaccination. Still others place the matter entirely in the hands of parents, to comply or not with the legislated recommendation.

Compulsory Immunization Law Requirements Before Entry to School

State	*Law*	*Year*	*Immunizations required*					
			Smallpox	*Measles*	*Polio-myelitis*	*Diphtheria*	*Pertussis*	*Tetanus*
Alabama[1]	No	–	–	–	–	–	–	–
Alaska[2]	No	–	–	–	–	–	–	–
Arizona	No	–	–	–	–	–	–	–
Arkansas	Yes	1967	No	Yes	Yes	Yes	Yes	Yes
California	Yes	1967	No	Yes	Yes	No	No	No
Colorado	No	–	–	–	–	–	–	–
Connecticut[3]	No	–	–	–	–	–	–	–
Delaware	No	–	–	–	–	–	–	–
District of Columbia	Yes	1906	Yes	No	No	No	No	No
Florida	No	–	–	–	–	–	–	–
Georgia	Yes	1968	Yes	Yes	Yes	Yes	Yes	Yes
Hawaii	Yes	1967	Yes	Yes	Yes	Yes	Yes	Yes
Idaho	No	–	–	–	–	–	–	–
Illinois	Yes	1968	Yes	Yes	Yes	Yes	Yes	Yes
Indiana[4]	No	–	–	–	–	–	–	–
Iowa	No	–	–	–	–	–	–	–
Kansas	Yes	1968	Yes	Yes	Yes	Yes	Yes	Yes
Kentucky	Yes	1967	Yes	Yes	Yes	Yes	Yes	Yes
Louisiana	Yes	1968	Yes	Yes	Yes	Yes	Yes	Yes
Maine	No	–	–	–		–	–	–
Maryland	Yes	1951	Yes	No	No	No	No	No
Massachusetts	Yes	1967	Yes	Yes	Yes	Yes	Yes	Yes
Michigan	Yes	1966	Yes	Yes	Yes	Yes	Yes	Yes
Minnesota	Yes	1967	No	Yes	No	No	No	No
Mississippi	Yes	1966	Yes	Yes	Yes	Yes	Yes	Yes
Missouri	Yes	1961	Yes	No	Yes	Yes	No	No
Montana	No	–	–	–	–	–	–	–
Nebraska[5]	No	–	–	–	–	–	–	–
Nevada	No	–	–	–	–	–	–	–
New Hampshire	Yes	1951	Yes	No	No	No	No	No
New Jersey	Yes	1967	Yes	Yes	Yes	Yes	No	No
New Mexico	Yes	1962	Yes	No	Yes	Yes	Yes	Yes
New York	Yes	1968	Yes	Yes	Yes	No	No	No
North Carolina	Yes	1957	Yes	No	Yes	Yes	Yes	Yes
North Dakota	No	–	–	–	–	–	–	–
Ohio	Yes	1959	Yes	No	Yes	Yes	Yes	Yes
Oklahoma	No	–	–	–	–	–	–	–
Oregon	No	–	–	–	–	–	–	–
Pennsylvania	Yes	1959	Yes	No	No	No	No	No
Rhode Island	Yes	1968	Yes	Yes	Yes	Yes	Yes	Yes

State	Law	Year	*Smallpox*	*Measles*	*Polio-myelitis*	*Diphtheria*	*Pertussis*	*Tetanus*
South Carolina	Yes	1952	Yes	No	No	No	No	No
South Dakota	No	–	–	–	–	–	–	–
Tennessee	Yes	1967	Yes	Yes	Yes	Yes	Yes	Yes
Texas[6]	No	–	–	–	–	–	–	–
Utah	No	–	–	–	–	–	–	–
Vermont	No	–	–	–	–	–	–	–
Virginia	Yes	1942	Yes	No	No	No	No	No
Washington	No	–	–	–	–	–	–	–
West Virginia	Yes	1967	Yes	Yes	Yes	Yes	Yes	Yes
Wisconsin	No	–	–	–	–	–	–	–
Wyoming	No	–	–	–	–	–	–	–

[1]*Montgomery County, Ala., requires diphtheria, tetanus, pertussis, smallpox, and poliomyelitis immunizations; not tested in court.*
[2]*Under special conditions, schoolchildren can be required to get immunizations.*
[3]*Compliance is a local option; majority of counties require compliance.* Source: *Public Health Reports,* 84:9, p. 789.
[4]*Kindergarten ordinance requires immunization in Marion County, Ind.*
[5]*School board resolutions require various immunization, but they are not considered binding.*
[6]*Local school boards may require immunizations.*

Source: *Public Health Reports,* 84, 9, September 1969.

The following provisions of the Ohio law are typical of a compulsory law that allows for certain exceptions:

> No pupil shall be admitted, at the time of his initial entry of each school year, to an elementary or high school, unless such pupil has presented written evidence, satisfactory to the person in charge of admission, that he has received, or is in the process of receiving immunization against poliomyelitis, smallpox, diphtheria, pertussis (whooping cough), and tetanus (lockjaw) by such means as may be approved by the Department of Health or unless such pupil has presented a written statement of his parent or guardian objecting to the immunization of such pupil against poliomyelitis, smallpox, diphtheria, pertussis and tetanus. The provisions of this section shall not limit or impair the right of a board of education to make and enforce rules or regulations to secure vaccination or immunization of the pupils under its jurisdiction.
>
> Boards of Health, legislative authorities of municipal corporations, and boards of township trustees on application of the Board of Education of the district or proper authority of any school affected by this section, at the public expense, without delay, shall provide the means of immunization against poliomyelitis, smallpox, diph-

theria, pertussis, and tetanus to such pupils as are not provided therewith by their parents or guardian.

The matter of exemptions is of some concern to educators because of the diversity in beliefs and practices in the population served by the school. There are three general types of exception allowed: those taken on religious grounds, those for personal reasons, and exceptions that are recommended for medical reasons. School administrators must know of any exemptions permitted by law and conduct the school program accordingly.

One of the strongest opportunities the school has to reinforce public policy is on the matter of immunization. Its program of health instruction should cover the complete story and facts about this phase of preventive medicine. School children become parents and as such will be responsible for their own children. Thus they should know fully the advantages and problems involved in the use of preventive vaccines. Rubeola is a case in point. It has taken the public far too long to make full use of the vaccines that are available.

Through the educational program parents can be informed of the desirability of keeping an accurate record of the vaccines received by their children and the dates received. Such records are of particular importance when children are moved from school to school and will save great inconvenience and unnecessary revaccination.

– medication at school In a very few cases of chronic disease such as epilepsy or hyperkinesis and in a smaller percent of acute illnesses, it is necessary for school health personnel, as substitute parents, to provide medication at school. Ordinarily it is possible to arrange for children to receive drugs at home, but on occasion it is necessary, particularly for young children, to receive medicine from an adult at school. When the giving of medication is necessary, it is mandatory that the parent request the school to carry out this service. In addition, a doctor's request should be received by the school which asks that the school give the medication at certain times. The form that the doctor fills out should describe the condition for which the child is receiving the medication and describe the effects to be expected from the drug. Also included should be directions as to the time of dosage and the length of time that the medication is to be used. School health personnel should screen thoroughly all requests and hold those accepted to an absolute minimum. Because school nurses are not in schools full time, the task of helping the child to remember to take the medication falls to a willing staff member. Ordinarily this is not held to be a part of the teaching task, but as a substitute parent the teacher often is willing to help the child with the control of his disease so that he can attend school with his peers.

An example of the medication policy in action is the case of a child who is severely allergic to bee stings. Should she be stung by a bee it is likely that she would have an acute allergic reaction with constriction of the respiratory passages and severe distress in breathing. In order for her to be able to attend school it is necessary that someone be available to inject medication immediately if she be stung. The parents' request and doctor's request to provide medication as needed should be received by the school and reviewed by the health services department. This unusual procedure must be approved and a willing staff member found. A school nurse may train the teacher to give the injection, the parents provide medication, and the child allowed to attend school.

– case finding The finding of a case of communicable disease begins at home with the parents. If parents would keep at home those children who show signs of fever, watery eyes, inflamed membranes, and indisposition, pending a diagnosis, there would be less communicable disease spread through the school. Children with signs of disease should be isolated from others immediately and either sent home or placed in a separate room to await medical diagnosis of their condition. School nurses, visiting teachers, and others should work with parents to give them an understanding of the value of this procedure. Pain, fever, cough, sore throat, rash, nausea, vomiting, lassitude, and pallor may be signs of illness. Teachers, nurses, parents, and administrators should all be on the lookout for them and, when they see them, know what to do to remove the child from association with others. This is case finding at the simplest level.

At the next level and conducted outside the school are the case-finding techniques used by a competent physician, perhaps a child specialist, as he reads and interprets the signs of growth and development during a physical examination. Here careful readings and diagnoses can be made, leading, in appropriate instances, to the prevention and control of communicable as well as other diseases. Occasionally, physicians serving in school health education programs recommend special case-finding procedures involving laboratory tests. These are unusual but necessary in some cases in order to facilitate growth or prevent illness. The school administration must be familiar with community facilities and other means for accomplishing these purposes.

Notification of parents and physicians if a child has been exposed to a contagious disease must be carried out on a selective basis. To notify parents of all children in a classroom whenever one of them has been diagnosed as having a contagious disease can cause considerable confusion by the frequency with which contagious diseases occur in the school classroom and also cause panic in the case of certain feared illnesses. School health personnel have the responsibility for notifying parents of those children who are at risk, for example, those with obvious disease or infirmity. Close observation of children who are in classrooms where children have been absent with communicable diseases and prompt notification of parents should symptoms occur is probably the best way to handle the case finding and notification procedure.

– isolation and exclusion The next step after case-finding is isolation and, if warranted, exclusion from school. In the procedures for teacher observation, it was suggested that each school should have an excluding authority (the nurse, the principal, or some other person of careful judgment) who can look at the children who have been sent from teachers and isolate them long enough for a judgment to be made. If it is deemed wise to exclude the child; then steps must be taken to see that he is safely delivered home. This procedure may break down if (1) no one is at home to receive the child, (2) parents do not want their children sent home, or (3) no transportation is available (sick children should not be sent home alone). Where those situations prevail the school should insist that parents designate other homes or places to receive their children. Transportation must be arranged by either the parent, the school, or some other means. The practice of sending children home because of illness should not be abandoned for want of means of getting them there.

School authorities, including all teachers, should be kept abreast of the latest and best practices among public health personnel in the control of the so-called children's diseases. Practices that were in the vogue twenty years ago no longer pertain today, and changes in the administration of disease control measures occur from time to time.

In any event, school policy and practice must be geared completely and cooperatively with those of the health department.

– notification Immediately after the decision to exclude is reached, machinery should be set in motion to notify several other people. First, of course, is the parent. The home should be called or in some other way it should be verified that the child will be received when he gets there. The first responsibility for receiving the child and caring for him lies with the parents. The parent should then be advised to call the family physician when there is one.

Second, the excluding authority should notify the teacher and the teachers of brothers and sisters of the child. These latter should be observed carefully for similar suspicious signs. Each additional exclusion should be reported to the school office.

Third, the local health authorities should be notified of any child excluded because of signs that may indicate a reportable disease.

All these routines must be in accordance with the regulations of local boards of health and thoroughly understood by all persons concerned.

– referrals What parents do with children suspected of having infectious diseases is largely a private matter. The school has accomplished its purpose when it has broken the contact between the child and other children in school. Many parents, however, have no physician and have never heard of the local health authorities. School personnel should be ready in any case to refer parents to physicians in their neighborhood or to the information bureau of the local medical society, to the local public health nursing office and the local health office, or to local social agencies or health agencies that can arrange for medical care in cases of indigence. These three referrals are important, and each school should be prepared to make them where necessary. Where school physicians or nurses are employed, they will be prepared to discuss the case with family physicians and local authorities.

– readmission Procedures for readmitting a child after illness must be worked out by the school authorities in conjunction with public health officials and in full accord with local and state public health law. Practices vary. In any event it is important to answer the following questions: (1) Is it safe for the child to return to school? and (2) Is it safe for other children to have the child back? The following procedures are recommended:

1 Pupils who have been isolated by the health department may be readmitted by certificate from the health department.

2 Pupils who have other diseases or who cannot obtain certificates from local health authorities because of distance, time, or some other factor may be readmitted by certificate or notice from their physician or from the physicians serving the schools.

3 Pupils may be readmitted by the principal on the basis of information received by a note from the parents.

These three provisions will not cover all cases. It is important that some competent authority have the readmitting responsibility. Children should not be permitted to resume their studies and their association with others merely on their own or their parents' wish.

– epidemic control Disease becomes epidemic when many more cases appear in a locality than would be considered normal or average for the month or season and pandemic when it crosses international or continental boundaries. There have been some notable pandemics in the world's history, and each nation or community can remember notable epidemics of poliomyelitis, diphtheria, measles, or any of a number of other diseases that are transmissible. Such epidemics are always periods of alarm and anxiety. People have been taught to fear disease. They fear its presence and they fear its consequences. To protect children in every way possible against epidemic diseases has become a part of our mores.

In times of epidemics the school finds itself in a strategic but somewhat confusing position. Unfortunately the public is slow to cast off some old ideas about the nature of epidemics. Many people persist in believing that all diseases are similar, that they are spread in the same manner, and that their causative organisms behave precisely alike. Furthermore, it remains in the minds of many that schools should forthwith be closed during epidemics to prevent the spread of the disease and that rooms and buildings and books should be fumigated afterward.

The more modern view (subject always to review and verification by the local health department) would include the following procedures:

1 Schools in communities where there are efficient public health facilities and personnel can generally remain open during epidemics but should strengthen their observational and exclusion practices to keep sick children out of school. Among large populations where school controls of disease are good, it is perhaps better that schools remain open.

2 When school controls are not adequate and it would be better for children to remain at home because they would be exposed to fewer contacts, then upon the advice of the health department the school might be closed.

3 If school and public health authorities close the schools during epidemics, they would insist that children be kept away from all public places and remain at home.

4 In view of the facts known about the transmissibility of disease, indicating that the vectors of the disease (microorganisms or other organisms) do not survive on dry, inanimate objects, the practice of fumigating books and classrooms has been discarded by most health authorities. If any such practices are followed, they should vary according to the resistance of the organisms rather than according to the severity of the disease in the individual attacked. The procedure of disinfecting or disposing of books at all is seriously questioned.

In recent years experimentation has been undertaken to determine whether room atmosphere can be purged of disease-producing organisms by the use of vapors or rays. Independent committees of the American Public Health Association and the National Research Council have reviewed the results of this work and concluded that the general use of ultraviolet irradiation or disinfectant vapors in schools, barracks, and industrial environments is not justified at the present time.

SPECIAL PROBLEMS

There are some particular and major problems of disease control that deserve special consideration.

– the common cold

Until scientists discover more about the etiology, means of transmission, and ways of prevention of the common cold, it will remain the most troublesome disease confronting the schools and by far the principal cause of absences. The cold is troublesome not only because of the discomfort and retardation caused by the disease itself, but because in its early stages it is barely distinguishable from the more serious infectious respiratory diseases. No school could send home every child presenting symptoms of the common cold, and yet if some control is not exercised, the so-called children's diseases run rampant through school systems. A consensus seems to show the following controls to be useful:

1 Parents should be encouraged to keep their children at home when the usual signs and symptoms of a cold are noticed.

2 They likewise should be advised to keep children with the beginning signs of a cold at home for the first two or three days as a precautionary measure not only against a worse cold but against any more serious disease.

3 Children with beginning and severe colds should be sent home from school with an escort.

4 It is not advisable to judge the communicability of a cold by the use of a clinical thermometer in the hands of a nonmedical person. Temperature above 98.6 may or may not be present in the early stages, and thus the nonmedical person cannot take an arbitrary standard of, say, 100 degrees as a point of exclusion.

– tuberculosis

The prevailing concept that tuberculosis in children is a disappearing disease is not, unfortunately, completely valid. Even with the sharp reduction in mortality rates, morbidity is still a serious problem. It is generally agreed that tuberculosis in children has not yet been mastered and that it remains a troublesome public health problem. In the United States alone, where tuberculosis is considered very rare in comparison with the incidence in the underdeveloped regions of the world, there are 800,000 contagious cases of tuberculosis.[5]

Many more persons are infected with the live organism than are diagnosed as having an active case of the disease. These persons remain threatened with the disease and thus need to be identified for their own protection and the protection of others. Location and identification of active cases and of the positive reactors (bacillus present) becomes the first step in a control program for schools. How much of this incidence is due to circumstances within the school is not accurately known, but assuredly some of it is. In the face of this, all schools can and should institute a full tuberculosis control program. No child should be permitted to contract tuberculosis because of the assumption of school authorities that tuberculosis is a problem for the home and for public health workers. Children and teachers bring tuberculosis to school with them; the school thus becomes a medium for its transmission to others. A control program is the only answer to date; the following are the essential steps in such a program:

1 Tuberculosis case-finding is the important primary step in school and college health programs. There are two principal ways of finding cases: by the tuberculin test or by X-ray screening. The choice between the two, for mass case-finding programs, is a matter for local medical authorities to decide. In low-prevalence populations tuberculin skin testing is likely to be the choice. If adequate safeguards are present, there is no present danger in using the X-ray (radiography) test. The amount of radiation to which the person is exposed under competent administration of the X-ray is negligible.

2 The decision whether to use the Tine test or the Mantoux intradermal test also belongs to the local medical authorities. The Mantoux intradermal test yields the most accurate reactor rate, whereas the Tine is less expensive and has better patient acceptance. Those who have a positive reaction to the Tine are rechecked with intermediate strength P.P.D. Although rates vary among local populations and among ages a reactor rate of 1 percent among children and 15 percent among adults would be expected at the present stage in the control of tuberculosis.

In any event, consensus seems to be that the test should be administered to all elementary school children at entrance and as often thereafter during their school years as the circumstances in their community warrant it. In high-prevalence areas tuberculin testing will be more frequent than in other areas. If a school employee in contact with children has active tuberculosis, tuberculin testing should become more frequent for a time. These are matters for medical decision and educational cooperation.

The tuberculin test tells who harbors the tubercle bacilli and, hence, who needs observation and treatment. It is highly useful in giving the lead to finding the active case of the disease.

3 All positive reactors should have an X-ray examination of the chest for further determination; if the disease, in either its primary or its reinfection form, is found, the child should be placed immediately under competent medical care.

4 The information on each child should be as complete and accurate as possible in regard to the tuberculosis history of close relatives.

5 Teachers in elementary schools should sharpen their continuous observations on the health of their pupils in order to be on the alert for any unusual behavior or complaint upon the part of students; when such deviations from the normal are observed, they should be promptly reported to parents and to school medical authorities.

6 Secondary school students (particularly upon reaching adolescence) should receive the same tests and observations. However, because of the higher rate of tuberculosis and the greater effectiveness of the X-ray in this age group, many schools are finding it profitable to dispense with tuberculin testing and go directly to the X-ray. Children who are known to be in contact with tuberculous persons should be examined frequently.

7 Every school employee should be required by the board of education to submit, before employment, evidence of freedom from tuberculosis and to submit the same evidence every two years thereafter. This required measure will stand up in the courts against those who view any such precautionary measures as an infringement of their personal rights. Courts have sustained boards of education who have required teachers and others to be X-rayed as a protection for children.

8 There should be a complete program of education that brings to the student population, to teachers, and to parents the full and accurate story of tuberculosis prevention, detection, and care. Only through education and scientific medical care can the disease be brought fully under control. People must know about the disease and act in accordance with what they know. Such a program must be geared completely with the efforts of local health authorities and must be aimed at ever more efficient case-finding programs.

9 The school program should be supplemented wherever possible by a complete community program of control aimed at a universal application of the chest X-ray to find every adult case and to remove him from public contact.

10 All personnel found to have tuberculosis should be removed from contact with others until, in the judgment of medical authorities, it is safe to allow them to return. The removal from duty of employees may work a hardship. In that event the board of education could well consider plans for extended sick leave with financial benefits to protect the employee against destitution.

In case anyone should become complacent about the transmissibility of tuberculosis or its presence in the population, the experience of one community will bring the facts sharply into focus. In this community a teacher was replaced at midyear by one of whom no demand was made for evidence of freedom from active tuberculosis. Actually the teacher had active tuberculosis, and it was not discovered until the tests of children in his room showed an abnormally high percentage of positive reactors. Of the 613 children tested, 66, or 10.8 percent, were positive reactors; of 19 adults tested, 6 were positive for a 32 percent reaction rate. In the tuberculous teacher's sixth grade, 100 percent were positive reactors, most of them with severe reactions. The school as a whole outside of this classroom then had 22 positive reactors out of 590 for a rate of 3.7 percent against the students in the teacher's room of 100 percent. Public health nurses visited the homes of every positive reactor child, explained the situation to the parent, and had all siblings checked either by tuberculin test or X-ray to see how far this epidemic had spread.

> *The score: July 20, 1962*
>
> 1 teacher with active primary TB
>
> 1 teacher hospitalized with active pulmonary TB
>
> 3 students hospitalized with active pulmonary TB
>
> 16 students diagnosed as having active, primary TB and placed under medication for at least one year
>
> 66 students to be checked every year the rest of their lives
>
> 6 adults to be checked every year for the rest of their lives[6]

It seems that parents have a right to be better assured that their children will not be infected because they attend school.

– skin diseases Schools are frequently, some constantly, beset with epidemics of skin diseases. Ringworm, impetigo, itch, and head lice or body lice are the most common communicable ones. Eczema, acne, and hives are common among the noncommunicable skin diseases. All of these require school controls, not because of their mortality but because their occurrence usually lead to absenteeism, embarrassment, social prejudice and ostracism, personal feelings of inadequacy, and in more than a few instances, secondary infections of a serious sort. Controls are suggested as follows:

1 There should be continuous observation of the skin of the hands, face, neck, and scalp of all pupils and, wherever possible, of the feet. This is as important in the secondary school as it is in the elementary school.

2 Children with communicable skin diseases should be excluded from all contact with other children; they should not use towels, shower rooms, swimming pools, mats, utensils, or books used by other children; they should be excluded from school completely unless they are dressed to prevent the spread of the disease.

3 Children excluded entirely should remain at home until they are medically approved to return.

4 Floors of gymnasiums, shower rooms, locker rooms, pool decks, training quarters, and all other floor areas likely to be moist and to come in contact with the skin should be cleaned and scrubbed thoroughly every day; they should also be aired or ventilated so as to be kept as dry as possible.

5 Whenever physical education, swimming, home economics, band, or other clothing is rented, it should be pasteurized (not

boiled) before being passed on to the next person. If gymnasium clothing (even socks and supporters) can be brought to the temperature of 180° F. three times in the washing, it will test out free of the communicable organisms of skin diseases.

6 All students should shower thoroughly before using pools and after physical education periods.

7 Students should be taught to dry off completely, hair and feet particularly, after using showers and pools.

8 Foot baths with disinfecting solutions are of less consequence in the control of ringworm of the feet than the controls just mentioned.

– venereal disease Figures or estimates on the amount of venereal disease among the school population are less reliable, perhaps, than for other diseases. (See Chapter 10.) Incidence of these diseases varies with the times; recent evidence indicates a dramatic increase in gonorrhea and syphilis among the school-age population. The venereal disease problem exists. It is pertinent to school health education. Its peculiar place in the public mind, related as it is to morals and taboos, seems to make venereal diseases a special problem. Actuallly, venereal diseases are clearly infectious and should be considered as such without fear, self-consciousness, or community opposition to the effort. Each of the principal venereal diseases is far too serious to keep adequate controls of these diseases off the agenda of a modern program of school health education. Such controls would include the following:

1 A full program of instruction about the venereal diseases should be given to produce an informed and enlightened school population. Information concerning the nature of venereal disease, means of communication, prevention, the problem of case finding, quackery, treatment, and relation to heredity and to congenital factors should be included.

2 A program of parental orientation with the problem of venereal disease is necessary. Not only should the school program be explained but also the information possessed by parents should be brought up to date.

3 A program of case finding, using the physical examination, personal counseling, blood serology tests, and any other techniques available, is essential. Although such programs of case finding are usually carried on by public health authorities, school programs can cooperate in the effort. Cases found in school should be reported to public health authorities.

4 If the school can obtain the cooperation of private physicians and of public health officials in reporting student cases to school authorities, the school not only can protect its other students by that knowledge, but also can assist the physicians in the educational program to which each case is usually submitted. In the instance of the venereal diseases, as in tuberculosis, a strong con-

trol program involving medicine, public health, and education offers an effective attack upon disease.

– epilepsy and seizures Information concerning epilepsy and seizures comes from many sources, principally the Epilepsy Foundation in Washington, D.C. Because of current public attitudes toward epilepsy, there are presumably a good number of childhood cases that are unknown to school authorities even though epilepsy is essentially a disease of childhood and youth. It is estimated that about 0.2 percent of school children have epilepsy, although teachers may not know of the individual cases in their classrooms. Parents are frequently reluctant to disclose the existence of the disease, or they may not actually know of it, or physicians knowing of the cases have not advised school authorities, so that frequently school personnel are not ready to aid the epileptic child at the time of a seizure.

A school program aimed at dealing with epileptic children in the best possible manner will contain the following features: (1) Teachers and other school officials will seek the best information available as to the nature, causes, type, prognosis, and recommended educational program for children so afflicted. (2) Information on cases will be sought from parents and physicians, so the school program can be adapted to the necessities involved, including the giving of medication in exceptional cases. (3) When cases are located, teachers will be on the alert for seizures taking place in school and will be able to do the appropriate thing. In view of the fact that the most severe convulsion or grand mal is different from petit mal—the simple and momentary black-out—and also from the psychomotor seizure, which is a brief period of automatic and sometimes unusual behavior, the following course of action is recommended: For petit mal and psychomotor attacks do nothing except explain the episode to other pupils. For a convulsion the following procedure is recommended:

1 Lay the pupil on his stomach with no pillow under his head and with the head turned to one side so that if there is vomiting, the vomit will not be drawn into the windpipe or lungs.

2 Loosen clothing about neck, wrists, and waist.

3 Do not try to restrain muscular contractions of the student. Try to prevent him from injuring himself.

4 Cover the pupil and keep him under constant observation.

5 Do not move him until he is quiet and relaxed.

6 Notify the parent and discuss the need for the pupil to be taken home or taken to the physician or to the hospital as soon as possible.[7]

The teacher should be calm and competent, even matter-of-fact, so that the other pupils are not unduly alarmed. She should give them an explanation of what occurred. For younger children it is usually sufficient to state simply that the attack is not serious and the child will be all right in a short while. Older children deserve a short explanation of the cause and treatment of seizures. The pupil is to be treated matter of factly. Ordinarily the fact of seizures will not alter the curriculum or activity of the child. Always subject to the advice of a physician, the child continues with the normal program, including physical education. Other pupils deserve the right to be informed of the nature of the seizures and to be encouraged to dispel any foolish and unscientific notions they may have about them. They should be encouraged to regard epileptic children with compassion, rather than fear or disdain, and to help them find a normal and compatible adjustment to school life. If the seizure is of the more serious type, resulting in extraordinary activity on the part of the child, distractibility and difficulty in perception, the teaching methods and materials may have to be altered to take into account these behavior and learning characteristics frequently displayed by children with brain injuries. Furthermore, the teacher will want to know what level of achievement to expect from these more seriously involved children.

– food-borne infections Although food handlers present no unique problems as contrasted to other employees, it is important that each person be certified as free from any communicable disease, notably tuberculosis, typhoid fever, and venereal disease.[8] Ordinarily city and state health departments have strict regulations concerning food handlers, but it is important that the school health education administration cooperate fully in the enforcement of these. The Joint Committee on Health Problems in Education has the following to say regarding food handlers:

> The nature of food-borne infection and poisoning requires daily attention to the health of workers. Workers should be trained to recognize danger signals in themselves and to take responsibility for protecting others. Some one person, however, should have authority within the school, or school system, to excuse from service any food handler who is a menace to the health of others. Provision should be made for substitute food service workers, and sick leave for the full-time food handler.
>
> Pre-employment and periodic medical examinations are desirable as preventive health measures for food handlers as for all school personnel. From the point of view of food handling, however, these measures are secondary in importance to daily supervision and in themselves may give a false sense of security.
>
> Clean personal habits are required for both hygienic and aesthetic reasons. Clean uniforms, hairnets, and trimmed nails are indicative of attention to careful grooming. Fingers should be kept from the hair, face and out of the mouth.[9]

Maintenance of healthful conditions requires close cooperation among health officers, school authorities, and school lunch personnel.

Ordinarily, the department of health establishes standards for food handling and sanitation. Periodic inspections should be made of facilities and procedures with written reports to the superintendent of schools or his delegate. Where possible it is desirable to have inspections made by sanitarians of the local health department.

– the child's return to school

Special problems may be presented by children and youth returning to school after prolonged or serious illness. These problems may be either psychological or physical or both. Teachers must remember that a disease or accident does not affect a child in fragments but involves the total being. The child may require specific rest periods, restriction of physical education activity, and in some cases special classes or special gear in regular classes. But it is equally important to guard against secondary handicaps. Morris Hamburg discusses this concern.

> Secondary handicaps which may emanate from a feeling of rejection can prove to be more harmful and crippling than the factor of the physical disability itself. Where teachers have an insight into such problems they can be of enormous help to both the child and his parents. To the child, she can extend a feeling of her acceptance of him on the same basis as other children. She can guide him toward self-understanding. She can work toward allaying any anxieties he may have developed, and can help him avoid developing compensatory characteristics that may create problems for himself and others.[10]

As early as possible it is desirable to reestablish a normal and acceptable relationship between the child who has been ill and his classmates.

NUTRITION

The school is interested in the nutritional status of its children because undernourished or malnourished children do not progress as well educationally as do children who are adequately nourished. Children suffering from protein calorie malnutrition show very low developmental scores. Where correctional diets are arranged for malnourished children, the disparity between their chronological ages and mental ages decreases. In severe cases, where there has been a damaging protein starvation, corrective measures will restore some balance, but there may remain a permanent handicap not only to physical growth but to mental capacity and personality development as well. Thought and action directed at the nutritional problem thus take the form of providing noon lunches, midmorning lunches, and deficiency meals for those undernourished and unable to secure adequate nourishment at home, and an instructional program in which the problems of nutrition are discussed. Attention is given to children whose nutritional status is subpar, and various educational and curriculum adjustments are made to cope with malnutrition.

– objectives of a nutrition program The school has a responsibility to accept in this area. It not only must discharge its traditional educational functions in regard to the problem, but because millions of children eat about one-fourth of their meals on school premises, the school must provide a good demonstration of food preparation and selection. The school is in a position to influence nutritional behavior even though it has stiff competition from commercial advertising, family customs, ignorance, and, perhaps above all, individual taste, which, when selection is limited, does not always lead a person to eat what is good for him.

The objectives of a school nutrition program are simple and clear. They are:

1 To inform the school population about the nutritional needs for best growth and development.

2 To provide an attractive and adequate variety of food in the school lunch program.

3 To seek correlation between home and school with reference to nutrition teaching and practice.

4 To solve individual problems of faulty practice, insufficiency, or malnutrition.

– the program of action To attain these objectives a program of action containing three principal features is instituted. These are a school lunch program that represents the best in nutritional practice, a program of instruction for all children in the best of nutritional information, and a program of appraisal and guidance for individual students in reference to their own nutritional status.

Malnutrition among school children in some communities is marked. Modern pediatricians and school physicians seek to identify it by determining the specific food deficiencies that produce it. Malnutrition produces fatigue, retards growth, development, and intellectual awareness, and lowers resistance to disease. It is a serious school problem in many localities and deserves the development of a program to combat it. Such a program would include these factors: Teachers should be prepared to note the signs of malnourishment or undernourishment as a part of the continuous observation of the health of their children. Teachers should be alert to paleness, irregularities in the steadily advancing weight curve, plateaus in weight, chronic fatigue, staring eyes and anxiety in the facial expression, decayed teeth, nervousness, restlessness, and inattention. When these observable signs present themselves, the teacher should report the situation to someone who can do something about it. The school nurse, the visiting teacher, a local social agency, or the local health department is in a position to visit the home to discover the causes of the malnutrition and to work out a program of restitution.

There are no tests of malnutrition yet developed that are diagnostically infallible. The age-height-weight averages are no longer considered useful. The diagnosis of malnutrition can best be arrived at only by a physician, preferably a pediatrician, who by examining for membrane color, skin texture, and signs at the corners of the mouth, as well as all the deviations noted above, can arrive at some conclusion.

Whatever the state of nutritional deficiency, something must be done about it. Obviously, we should begin by removing the cause. The possible causes of malnutrition among children are faulty diets, insufficient amounts of food at meals, no breakfasts, no lunches, too little of crucial foods such as milk and vegetables, too many sweets, too little sleep, overwork, fatigue, physical defects, and disease. The specific cause or causes must be found in each child. They will not be the same in every instance and thus the method of correction will vary. Much of the correction will depend upon a successful alteration of the home environment; meals, especially breakfasts, must be improved, the child must sleep better, and chronic infections must be removed. Because family rearrangements are frequently difficult to make, emphasis should be placed on the many things that can be done in the school program. Attention should be given to individual cases. Supplementary food midmorning, midday, and midafternoon can be supplied. Suggested menus may be supplied to the home. Placement in special classes may be necessary where feeding and rest schedules differ from those of other children. A constant check of nutritional status, noting improvement or retrogression, can be undertaken, and the medical services of the school may be used to examine and advise insofar as their limitations will permit.

THE LUNCH PROGRAM The school lunch program came into being as a result of forces that were partly humanitarian, partly economic, and partly political. Before the National School Lunch Act was signed by the President on June 4, 1946, it seemed implausible that the feeding of children in and by the schools would ever become a part of governmental activity, particularly at the federal level. To many this seemed the epitome of the welfare state.

However, communities had had experiences with feeding school children during the economic depression of 1929–1935, and the federal government, through its executive agencies such as the Children's Bureau, had given encouragement to the principle that where need existed official agencies should step in with aid. Surveys of the need were made. The nutritional state of school children was described in its true terms, and the public began to realize that there were literally millions of children who were badly nourished at home and that their growth, development, and educational progress were definitely being retarded. Should the school feed them? Should they be fed at school from funds provided elsewhere? Was this a private or a public matter? These were, and still are in some quarters, disturbing questions.

Coincident with the national awakening to the nutritional needs of children came the move to consolidate schools. One-room schoolhouses disappeared in some states at the rate of three or four hundred a year. New consolidated schools were built, children were brought to them by bus, and it was not feasible to have them return home for lunch. Because the children had to be fed at school, many rural and small city schools joined the metropolitan schools in establishing a school lunch service wherein meals were provided at cost.

At this time the nation was changing from a war economy to a peace economy, and it was not unusual to find surplus food supplies piling up, threatening a loss to the producers. What could be more reasonable than to have the government buy this food and redistribute it on a matching basis to communities? Economically this was a sound move, for it solved part of the farm problem, kept prices up, and helped to avert agricultural disaster. It thus became politically wise also, and neither political party could resist the double appeal—from the farmer and from needy school children.

So the lunch program became a part of our educational scene and has proved to be important nutritionally and significant educationally. Local authorities, directed by the Consumer and Marketing Services of the United States Department of Agriculture, are required to sponsor and be responsible for the program and to provide facilities, equipment, supervision, labor, and whatever additional funds are needed. Expenditures for such items may count toward the matching of federal funds. A reasonable value may be put on goods and services contributed to the program. A small amount may be charged for the lunches if the children are able to pay.

The school lunch should provide nutritive values as well as satisfaction and enjoyment to the student. The lunch should also help in the development of good eating habits. As an incentive for providing a wholesome lunch, the highest rate of reimbursement is given for the complete lunch. This is known as Type A and consists of the following foods:

1 One-half fluid pint of whole milk as a beverage

2 Two ounces of lean meat, poultry, fish, or cheese, or one egg, or one-half cup cooked dry beans or peas, or four tablespoons of peanut butter, or the equivalent combination of any of these

3 Three-fourths cup of two or more vegetables or fruits, or both

4 One or more portions of bread or muffins or other hot bread made of wholegrain cereal or enriched flour

5 Two teaspoons of butter or fortified margarine

If a school has limited lunchroom facilities, it may contract to serve a Type B lunch, which provides about two-thirds as much food as the Type A lunch. The Type B lunch should be supplemented by food brought from home. Schools that have no lunchroom facilities may wish to provide milk for the pupils. The Type C lunch consists of one-half pint of whole milk as a beverage.[11]

This program has made possible better lunches for children in nearly any school anywhere in the nation and supplements constructively the existing programs already established in thousands of schools.[12]

Since its inception, variations in the basic plan have appeared. Without lowering nutritional standards, some schools and some city systems have instituted breakfast plans. Others serve a la carte lunches; some do not serve a full lunch but supplement the home-packed lunch.

– special problems Much debate has centered around the serving of milk at both lunch hour and mid-sessions. Some schools have served skimmed milk because it is cheaper. The Joint Committee on Health Problems in Education has this to say on the matter:

> Whole milk is preferable to any other kind and may or may not be homogenized. Chocolate drink made from skim milk is less valuable from the nutritional viewpoint, because it has less butterfat and vitamin A than whole milk. It does, however, contain the same minerals, vitamin B, and protein, plus sugar and fat from the chocolate. The sweetness of chocolate milk or chocolate drink may lessen the appetite for other foods.[13]

Even more controversial is the matter of the sale of candy and soft drinks at school. Pressures of various kinds from commercial concerns, needy organizations, and students sometimes make it difficult to resist the installation of vending machines even though there is serious question as to the nutritional appropriateness of these foods.

Their deteriorating affect upon teeth is incontestable.[14]

To sell or not to sell sweets and soft drinks becomes a matter of school policy involving parents, board members, administration, faculty, and students. No edict or plan to prohibit the sale of these things will be particularly successful until the reasons for the prohibition are understood by all. If there is a disposition on the part of some to curb the sale, then the matter could well become a matter for study by the health council for recommendation to the school community. Such was the case in Minneapolis; the essential portions of the program adopted are as follows:

> 1 Nutritional education. That a sound program of health education be developed regarding the use of sweets and soft drinks. Our list of health goals includes understandings, attitudes, and skills directed toward this problem. These goals emphasize that excessive use of sweets, including candy, soft drinks, gum, and rich desserts, increases the amount of dental caries, and that excessive use of sweets prevents people from eating an adequate, nutritious diet. In our health education program, we try to develop on the part of students the desire to keep to a minimum the use of sweets in the diet, and try to develop skills in the selection of foods and drinks which serve nutritional needs.
>
> 2 Prohibitive measure. That the sale of soft drinks be eliminated during school hours.
>
> 3 School encouragement in the practice of nutritional health. That schools be encouraged to make every effort possible to substitute other beverages for soft drinks during afternoon and evening activities. This can be done by creating situations in which students see alternatives and make plans for their parties in terms of desirable health and social values.
>
> 4 Correct time for offering of sweets. That candy not be offered in competition with the noon meal in any school. The one exception applies only to senior high schools, where if candy is sold, it must be sold only through the lunchroom after the noon meal has been eaten.
>
> 5 Reduction of sweets in the diet. That candy sales, including candied apples, etc., mid-morning and mid-afternoon, be eliminated, as an excessive amount of candy interferes with appetites for the following meal and is injurious to teeth.[15]

– principles of operation Experience and research have shown the following to be good practices:

Balanced Meals / Every lunch served should be nutritionally balanced in accordance with the best in scientific menu planning. Millions of school children are inadequately or unwisely fed at home, and the school lunch has come to mean, in many places, the provision of at least one-half the caloric and vitamin need of these children. Making up for the deficiency in these home diets becomes as important a school enterprise as the establishment of special classes for children handicapped in other ways.

Minimum Standards Of Supply / In elementary schools serving one-half pint of whole pasteurized milk and a cracker is generally considered the minimum midmorning lunch. At noon one hot vegetable or meat dish is the minimum, but preferable is the full meal with choices of food as found in the larger school cafeterias.

Sanitation / The serving of food in school requires (but sometimes fails to get) perfection in food sanitation. Essentials include good refrigeration, nonporous and undamaged dishes, tables and counters without cracks and scrubbed clean after every using, and effective sterilization equipment for all eating utensils. Cooking and serving personnel must be free of communicable disease and must comply with the state and city sanitation codes for food handlers. State departments of health or of education frequently issue detailed standards for the sanitation of lunchrooms.

Personnel Sanitation / Hand-washing and toilet facilities should be liberally supplied and should be convenient for users of the lunchrooms. Children must be taught, even required, to use them before eating.

An Educational Opportunity / The school lunch can go far beyond the important function of feeding hungry children. It can influence the eating behavior of students and adults alike. If those in charge will devote thought and planning to the educational implications, courtesy, acceptable table manners, and polite living in the lunchroom will become an important part in the education of a citizen.

Increase in acceptance follows when school lunch menu planning is shared with pupils. One successful approach is through a school lunch committee of representatives from all grades, a teacher, and a school lunch worker. Through awareness of the attitudes and cultural patterns of their group and from what they are learning about foods and their contributions to health, the student representatives can plan a nutritious noon meal. Planning may begin with a pupil survey of the total food intake to learn how the school lunch can best contribute to a well-balanced diet. Classroom discussions and follow-up can be directed toward overcoming food dislikes. A census of discarded food may provide an additional basis for such discussions.[16]

Administration / Over three-fourths of the existing school lunch programs are controlled and run by the school administration. This is as it should be. In most places where the program has been tried, the use of catering concessions has been found to be an unsatisfactory arrangement.

In large schools it is necessary to employ specialized school lunch personnel. In small schools in which the employment of specialized professional personnel is not practicable, the responsibility should be shared by the various school departments. The home economics teacher or the teacher best suited to the job may be responsible for planning menus and possibly for general supervision of the program. Other school departments should make the kind of contribution they are qualified to make. For example, the commercial department may supervise the work at the cash register, keep the financial records, and make the deposits. The art department might contribute by helping to make the dining room attractive and by making necessary signs. Other staff members may eat with the children. In some schools upper grade or older pupils may take some special responsibilities. An active school lunch committee representing staff, parents, and students is an asset to any school lunch program.

The educational authorities should be responsible for the selection of the school lunch manager and other personnel. The school lunch manager is responsible for achieving a program that is an integral part of the school's curriculum and health services and that operates efficiently to provide an adequate and nutritious lunch under sanitary, attractive, and friendly conditions and at the lowest possible cost. The manager must also be able to train and supervise the other school lunch personnel that he has helped to select. With these responsibilities, the manager must have an understanding of nutrition, of food buying, and of food preparation. He should also have the ability to work with all other personnel in the school.

The size of the program determines the kind of school lunch manager to be employed. For a large school lunch program in a school system or in an individual school, the manager should have completed a four-year college curriculum with emphasis on food, health and nutrition, quantity food preparation, and school lunch management.

There are five principal sources of school lunch funds: (1) local tax funds, (2) state aid, (3) federal assistance through the Department of Agriculture, (4) receipts from sale of lunches, and (5) donations from local groups. In addition to these funds, substantial additional aid is provided through donations of agricultural commodities and other foods purchased by the Department of Agriculture in connection with the farm price support program. State aid earmarked for school lunches is provided in some states. Many school boards limit the contribution from school district general funds to provision of equipment and personnel, because the cost of food is generally paid from receipts from sales of lunches and funds from the federal government. Many school lunch programs are operated without federal assistance.

– the program of instruction in nutrition Matching the program of action just described to a program of instruction in the health classes, as well as in other curriculum areas where suitable, will materially strengthen the total program. Such instruction can be developed as part of the unit plan in direct health teaching or in correlation with such areas as home economics, science, or physical education. That there is need for such instruction is eloquently proved by observing the food buying and eating practices of many people. Dental decay, malnutrition, fatigue, and overweight are but a few of the maladies that can be attributed to inappropriate education in nutrition. The number of people who pursue dietary fads is alone sufficient to warrant some intelligent treatment of the subject in schools.

Hence a program of instruction that begins with the recognized problems of people and brings the evidence of science to bear upon those problems is a responsibility the school should not miss. Such a program would include appropriate experience at all levels with problems such as the balanced diet, the need for variety, selection of food, planning meals, food deficiencies, food and weight and disease, variations in national food habits, and food sanitation.

THE DENTAL PROGRAM Dental decay and loss of teeth are major health problems throughout every segment of the population. It is estimated that among the 600 million school children throughout the world 90 percent have one or more decayed teeth. In the United States many of the estimates report that over 90 percent of the population shows evidence of having dental disease. By the time children reach school age they average three or more primary teeth decayed, and many children show evidence of decay in the permanent teeth. By the time the child reaches the age of 16 he averages 7 teeth decayed, missing, or filled. According to the National Health Survey 28 percent of our nation's children from 5 to 14 years of age have never been to a dentist.[17] The majority of the rest of the population have had infrequent contact with the dentist, usually for emergency services only.

The severity of the problem is best illustrated by the following statement from J. W. Knutson.

> Tooth decay, or dental caries, may begin to attack the teeth of the child early in life, at the age of two or even younger. If neglected or untreated it may progress to pulp involvement, dental abscess, toothache, tooth loss, disfigurement, disturbed oral function, and to the need for progressively more complex and more expensive dental care services. Beginning at the age of six the permanent teeth are attacked at an average rate of approximately one tooth per person, per year, so that at age twenty the average person has fourteen decayed, missing, or filled permanent teeth. Attack on the supporting tissues of the teeth by periodontal diseases occurs later in life. Periodontal disease is not uncommon in children but is most prevalent and most destructive after the age of 30. It is

> estimated that 33 million people in the United States have periodontal disease.
>
> Between the ages of 10 to 60 years, loss of permanent teeth due to dental caries and later to periodontal disease proceeds at a rate of approximately two-fifths of a permanent tooth per person, per year. Fifty percent of our population past the age of 55 have lost all their natural teeth. A total of 23 million people are completely edentulous or without natural teeth—one in every eight persons. Roughly, half of our school children have evidence of malocclusion or a malrelationship of the teeth and of the jaws. Many of these are emotionally handicapped by disfiguring dento-facial deformities.[18]

These facts are an appalling commentary on our way of life. The situation deserves full attention in the program of health education. It should be well established, in every community, that adequate dental care should be available to all regardless of income or residence rather than providing limited services to large groups. Communities should support prevention and control of dental diseases through research activities. It should be realized that dental health is a responsibility of the individual, the family, and the community, in that order. A school, as a part of the community, is in a strategic position to organize within its scope a complete program of dental health education and to assume leadership in organizing resources for dental care for all children. As a part of its program a school should motivate children to go to their personal dentist or to a dental clinic of their choice.

– optimum services There are many variations possible in developing a school dental health program. Whatever plans are made, whatever local adaptations are necessary, all programs to include child dental health must, to be successful, meld three basic forms of activity—dental health education, prevention activity, and the treatment of dental disease. These three are inseparable. None can be undertaken successfully without decreasing the overall outcome. To quote Charles Hayden,

> Dental health education will lack a vital frame of reference unless children actually receive dental care and experience the benefits of personal preventive practices, for it is this kind of individual exposure which gives meaning to what is taught and supplies the motivation to further individual action. Dental treatment is also reduced in value unless the child assists in the maintenance of his own health through the knowledgeable practice of personal oral hygiene. Preventive procedures can be fully effective only if they, too, include good oral hygiene practices and regular dental care. Thus education, treatment and prevention are the three indispensable components in any concerted effort to overcome the dental problems of our children.[19]

– dental health instruction Efforts to help children learn ways of promoting their own dental health should follow the principals of health education found in the first chapters of this book. It is desirable to develop a sequential curriculum based on the conceptual abilities of the children involved. Not only should information concerning anatomy and physiology, nutrition, and dental hygiene be provided, but also children should have the opportunity to practice dental health at school.

Many school districts, in addition to a program of instruction in the traditional sense, have given children the opportunity to brush their teeth at school on arrival in the morning and again following the noon meal. Use of a fluoride-containing dentifrice or of a powder made by the children themselves as a part of the classroom activity adds further benefit to the program. Objections to the amount of time required for brushing at school have proven groundless. When brushing is done as a routine, the time required is minimal. What better way exists to establish the importance of tooth care than to allocate classroom time to do a good job of oral hygiene. What lesson could be more negative than to teach children that dental health is so unimportant that it deserves no time in the school schedule.

In those situations where running water is not available in the classroom or where the problems of logistics are prohibitive, good dental health education teaches children to cleanse their mouths after eating by swishing and swallowing—that is by using water or milk to rinse food debris from their teeth. Meals at school can be planned to include "nature's toothbrush," a piece of apple, celery, carrot, or other fibrous vegetable to help remove retained food debris.

A program of instruction relative to dental health in the prevention of dental problems is essential. Such a program should be designed to reach all children and their parents.

– further prevention measures In addition to toothbrushing at school two other procedures offer the opportunity for children to have personal dental experiences. These are annual dental examinations and direct fluoride applications.

Dental Examinations / Although some states require annual dental examinations and other school districts include thorough inspection as a part of the school dental health effort, there are some who question dental examinations at school. These people feel that examinations should be made in the offices of private dentists or public clinics rather than at school. They feel that all children should see a dentist because approximately 95 percent have dental disease and believe that the examiner should be able to go right from the inspection to therapeutic procedures. Some state, "Dental examinations are a waste of time and money unless treatment of problems found is carried out."

Those who promote dental exams at school feel that such activities support the teacher's dental education effort, bring children's dental health problems to the attention of school personnel, provide experiences with dentists in a familiar setting, thus allaying fears about dental treatment, and also provide data for the assessment of the overall school dental health problem.

On the other hand, examinations made in offices or clinics have the advantage of better equipment and parental presence, and more often lead to dental correction for the individual child.

Obviously, there are advantages to both procedures. School authorities should air the question with their own health education personnel, the local dental group, and parents of children before proceeding. The critical question seems to be how closely the examination effort is to be combined with other health education efforts.

Topical Fluoride / The value of periodic application of fluoride to the teeth is well substantiated. This procedure reduces tooth decay and may also serve as a positive educational experience for the child. Ordinarily fluoride is applied by school dental hygienists as a part of the dental health education program. On occasion topical fluoride is applied by using a therapeutic prophylaxis paste which cleans the child's teeth as well as supplying fluoride to the enamel. Inclusion of either of these processes in the school must be done on the basis of educational goals and priorities. However, either or both seem to fit into the treatment portion of the program rather than into educational activities.

In a few places a prophylaxis paste containing fluoride has been self-applied by children under professional direction in the school. This can be easily included as part of the regular classroom health education and when done twice a year offers benefit through reducing the number of new cavities that occur. A further desirable outcome is obtained when teachers and parents are invited to help with the "brush-in" because of the education they receive of the values of fluoride in dental health.

Fluoridation and Dietary Control / The dental health of children can also be improved through the provision of school menus that are low in the inclusion of fermentable carbohydrates and when harder, more detergent foods are incorporated as frequently as possible. As previously mentioned, the school should develop controls on vending machines at school so that the machines will be stocked with fruits and beverages that are low in carbohydrates. Though dietary control is not apt to produce a large decrease in the number of cavities in children, it certainly is consistent with the philosophy and implementation of a dental health education program.

The number of children who now are benefitting from the opportunity to drink fluoridated water from the local water supply is increasing year by year. Children who have this opportunity are fortunate, indeed. In localities that have not, for some reason, deemed it advisable to fluoridate their water supply it is incumbent on the school district to do all possible to make sure that children receive fluoride. Most often this will be in the form of topical fluoride through the treatment process or applied in the school as part of the educational process, but during the past few years an increasing number of school systems have found it possible to fluoridate the water supply of the school system. Though fluoridation of the school water supply will not have the same overall effect as fluoridating the water supply of the entire town or community, studies have indicated an overall cavity reduction of over 20 percent when fluoride is added to school water supplies in optimum amounts.[20]

Treatment / As with other school health services programs the dental health program is not complete until the school has made provision for dental care to children. Care is usually provided through private dental offices and local dental clinics. On some occasions care is provided through a school dental clinic sponsored either by the health department or by local federated financing. Whatever provision is to be made, the school should play a strong role in its development so that it meets the needs of the children in the school system. Where facilities do not exist in adequate amounts it is a further responsibility of the school system to bring this lack to the attention of the community and to aid in the development of adequate dental resources for children.

When it is agreed that all children should have the minimum complete dental service, thought must be given securing specific sources of funds. The extent to which the services are developed will depend upon the availability of public funds and on the local point of view about the extension of such services in the school. However, dental health is of utmost importance to children, and the school is in a key position to promote a dental program that combines the three elements of education, prevention, and treatment.

– principles of operation Any program such as the one in dental health needs to be conducted according to principle. Regardless of the extent to which dental services are rendered in schools, there are certain basic tenets of administration that, if followed, will make for more effective programs. These are:

1 The services of dentists and dental hygienists in school programs should be paid for. Free examinations or treatments at school or

charity work under school auspices should not be expected. "Payment to dentists participating in the examination or service phase of the program may be made on full time, part time, hourly or unit of service basis. Salaries for full time or part time dentists and fee schedules should be on a level consistent with provision of high grade dental service."[21] Nor should dentists or any dental supply offices be expected to supply materials for less than cost. The school dental program must be financially solvent for best results.

2 Local funds should be used in support of the program, but where they are not available, appeal can be made, usually through state departments of health (but sometimes through departments of education), for the use of state or federal subsidies. Many of the local voluntary agencies, such as local tuberculosis groups, frequently have funds available to augment tax funds for such health purposes.

3 In view of the fact that the years under 10 are the critical ones for dental health, school programs should be aimed to give as much service as possible in the primary years. Studies indicate that dental inspections at school which imperfectly locate carious teeth and which are followed by a casual notification of the findings to parents are a waste of money. Children seek and get adequate dental care only when the school examination is well and completely done (by dentists with mirrors and explorers) and accompanied by a complete program of dental treatment and dental education.

4 The teacher is an important figure in any program of dental health education. Beginning with case-finding, which is the least of the teacher's contributions because she is untrained to note caries or disease, and progressing through the various stages of educational work that can be done with pupils and parents, the teacher can stimulate dental care as perhaps no one else can. She can teach the value of good teeth in many different ways and once the need for dental care is established can work with the individual pupil and his parents until some action is obtained.

5 The public health or school nurse has important opportunities in a dental health program. They include serving as the go-between in the school-home follow-up relationship; coordinating the educational with the clinical services (so as to avoid inconsistencies and to secure better timing of educational materials); stimulating and helping teachers in the cultivation of their knowledge and interest in dental health problems; making home calls to encourage dental attention where needed; serving as a counselor to students, particularly older ones, about their dental problems; assisting the dentists on their school visitations; securing information about the personal and economic status of families so that dental care may be arranged with greater intelligence. In many of these functions a well prepared and well educated dental hygienist would be equally competent.

6 Agreement now exists among dental personnel to the effect that the administration of topical fluoride to the teeth of a child and the fluoridation of the water supply of a community will reduce the dental caries problem. There is no reason at present to believe that either usage will eliminate tooth decay entirely, but there is evidence to show that dental caries can be reduced materially in the population if the fluoride treatments are used. It becomes the clear responsibility of the school to inform children and parents of this and to urge the adoption of appropriate measures.

Investigations in recent years have established the desirability of adding fluorides to public water supplies where that material exists in the natural state in less than effective quantities. There is a large mass of evidence which demonstrates conclusively that there are approximately three times as many dental caries in children who use fluoride-free domestic water as there are in children who are born and reared in communities whose communal water contains 1 ppm or more of fluorine.[22]

> There is little, if any, dispute that children who drink water containing approximately one part per million of fluorine from birth until the age of eight or nine, while the teeth are being formed, will have fewer cavities than children drinking water containing no fluorine. The extent of the reduction of dental decay to be expected under such a program can only be approximated at this time, but estimates range from one-third to two-thirds reduction.[23]

Not only have these facts been established, but it is also agreed that the addition of fluoride compounds in the above-mentioned quantity presents no hazard to the public health. There is no evidence to support the antifluoridation view that the addition of fluorides will cause numerous diseases and ailments. Among the highly qualified and reputable professional organizations that have endorsed the fluoridation of public drinking water supplies are the American Medical Association, the National Research Council, the American Public Health Association, the American Dental Association, the Association of State and Territorial Health Officers, the United States Public Health Service, and the American School Health Association.

7 A program of instruction relative to dental problems is essential. Such a program should reach all children and their parents. There are two principal problems involved—the prevention of dental caries and the prevention of malocclusion of teeth.

SUMMARY

Accidents, communicable disease, nutrition, and dental cavities are major problems of childhood that affect all children at one time or another. Children are under the care and supervision of school districts for a good part of their lives. Schools, therefore, have the opportunity and the responsibility for developing programs of education and service to promote well-being and to control these problems. Such programs must be developed not only for the finding of treatment for these conditions when they arise, but also must include education for the promotion of health in these areas and in helping children learn responsibility for carrying out procedures of prevention designed to decrease the number of children suffering from these major conditions of childhood. In all of the discussion the close relationship between health education and health services, in fact their inseparability, has been stressed as has the concept that all members of the school staff are a part of the school health team with responsibilities for the health of children.

NOTES AND REFERENCES

1 National Safety Council, *National Safety Council Accident Facts,* Chicago, National Safety Council, 1969, pp. 89–93.

2 *Ibid.*

3 Joint Committee on Health Problems in Education, *Healthful School Environment,* Washington, D.C., NEA and AMA, 1969.

4 NEA, *School Health Services,* 2nd ed., Washington, D.C., NEA, 1964.

5 Thomas S. Bumbalo, "Tuberculosis in Children," *Journal of School Health,* XXXIII, 3 (March 1963), 111.

6 L. L. Taylor, "100% Is Not Always Good," *Journal of School Health,* XXXII, 10 (December 1962), 385.

7 Tacoma Public Schools, *Recommended Procedure for Sickness and Accidents Occurring at School,* Tacoma, Wash., Tacoma Public Schools, 1964.

8 National Safety Council, *op cit.*

9 Joint Committee on Health Problems in Education, *op. cit.*

10 Morris Hamburg, "The Educator's View of the Cardiac Child," *Journal of School Health,* XXVIII, 2 (February 1958), 46.

11 U. S. Dept. of Agriculture, Consumer and Marketing Service, *A Menu Planning Guide for Type A School Lunches,* bulletin PA no. 719, Washington, D.C., Government Printing Office, 1966.

12 Space does not permit description of scientifically planned school lunches. Interested readers should secure literature on the subject from the U.S. Department of Agriculture and from divisions of nutrition in local state health departments.

13 The Joint Committee on Health Problems in Education, *Healthful School Living,* Washington, D.C., NEA and AMA, 1957.

14 American Dental Association, "Dental Health Program for Children," *Journal of the American Dental Association,* 74 (February 1967), 330.

15 Minneapolis Public School, *Nutrition; The Sale of Candy and Soft Drinks in the School,* a school policy approved by the superintendent, August 1950.

16 The Joint Committee on Health Problems in Education of the NEA and the AMA *Health Aspects of the School Lunch Program,* 2nd ed., NEA and AMA, 1962, p. 12.

17 U. S. Public Health Service, Department of Health Education and Welfare, *Health Statistics from the U. S. National Health Survey: Dental Care Interval and Frequency of Visits, United States, July 1957 to June 1959,* Washington, D.C., Government Printing Office, 1960.

18 John W. Knutson, "The Gap Between Needs and Services," *Man in His Physical Environment,* Vol. 3, Philadelphia, International Conference on Health and Health Education, 1962, p. 299.

19 Charles H. Hayden, "Preventive Dental Procedures Adaptable to School Health Programs," *American Journal of Public Health,* 59, 3 (March 1969).

20 *Ibid.*

21 American Dental Association, *A Dental Health Program for Elementary and Secondary Schools,* Chicago, American Dental Association, 1947, p. 15.

22 "Fluorine and Dental Caries," *The Journal of the American Dental Association,* 74, 2 (January 1967).

SELECTED READINGS

Accident Facts, National Safety Council, Chicago, yearly.

"Dental Health Program for Children," *Journal of the American Dental Association,* 74:330, February 1967.

"Fluorine and Dental Caries," *The Journal of the American Dental Association,* 74:2, January 1967.

Healthful School Environment, The Joint Committee on Health Problems in Education of the NEA and AMA, The Associations, Washington, D.C. and Chicago, 1969.

Menu Planning Guide for Type A Lunches, U.S. Department of Agriculture, Consumer and Marketing Service, Bulletin P.A. #719, Washington, D.C.

School Health Services, Joint Committee on Health Problems in Education of the NEA and AMA, The Associations, Washington, D.C. and Chicago, 1964, 2nd. edition.

CHAPTER 15 ADMINISTRATIVE AND COMMUNITY RELATIONSHIPS

The development and execution of a program of school health education is not a one-man job. By its very nature it must be a shared responsibility requiring the cooperative effort and effective coordination of several professionally trained people willing to pool their knowledge and ability for a common beneficiary—the schoolchild.

A program of school health education can never develop in isolation from the community. The nature of the health problems of childhood, the traditional and accepted concept of family responsibility for the health of children, and the function of the physician and dentist in society make it altogether desirable that whatever efforts are expended by the school toward improving health be made in coordination with other community influences. The school, when it is best conceived, *is* a part of the community anyway. It cannot help but be concerned about and related to the factors in the community that bear upon the health of people. Only the outworn notion that the school is a classical, cloistered, and superior institution removed from the workaday problems of community life would justify a health program constructed without reference to persons and agencies outside the school who are concerned about child health.

The school health program deals realistically with improving the health of its constituents. It discovers the needs of childhood and institutes procedures within or outside the school that are necessary to meet those needs. In so doing, the school personnel rubs elbows with parents, private physicians and dentists, private and public health agencies, the worlds of legislation and politics, and with those who for various reasons oppose scientific health procedures. Such interrelationships can and sometimes do become confusing.

Once a school or school system decides that it must "do something" about the health of its children, it becomes committed to a planned development of interrelationship with persons and agencies from which there is no turning back. Generally speaking, it is in localities where this interrelationship has been explored and used to the fullest that the most intelligent and productive school health programs are found. The school that is concerned about its public relations and wants to gear its program as perfectly as possible into a position of leadership within the community will find such efforts rewarding in terms of better school programs. It is entirely possible to be responsive to local customs and local policies and yet lead the way to improved health conditions and health practices.

ORIGINS IN LAW

Authorization for any phase of school health education must be established in law. Public money may not be expended by local school systems without express enabling legislation.

In the main such laws pertaining to school health education emanate from state legislatures. Local municipal ordinances, school board regulations, standards and policies established by local boards and state departments of education, and occasionally federal legislation bear upon the development of school health education, and the administrator has to know them all.

– mandatory and permissive laws

Sometimes a state legislature will pass a law *requiring* vaccination for smallpox of all school children (Ohio and Kentucky, for example) or will *require* schools to offer health instruction. These are mandatory laws. Sometimes legislatures will enact legislation saying merely that schools may, if they wish, employ school physicians (for example, Ohio). This is called permissive or enabling legislation. Most of the time state laws take the form of legislation that allows state departments (or boards) of education or state boards of health to establish such programs, standards, or policies affecting the health of children as they deem wise. From this kind of legislation come most of the standards concerning time allotment for health education, teacher certification, frequency of medical examinations, and other similar matters.

– state laws and standards The state is the principal controlling agent in education in the United States. State legislatures are responsible for the passage of laws and appropriation of money in support of public education. The distributing agency that the state uses for this purpose is the state department of public instruction, or of education, as the case may be. In the operation of school health education that agency is supplemented in its work by the state department of health. The two work jointly in the development of school health education, frequently sharing personnel and extending joint services to communities in need of aid.

Such work as is done on the state level, emanating from state departments of health or education, in most of the states is directed by a supervisory staff in school health education and physical education. These supervisors and their assistants serve a variety of purposes, all aimed at the development of programs in health education and physical education. They establish minimum standards for program development, set standards for the training and certification of teachers and others who serve in school program, publish state courses of study for suggested use in communities, develop inservice improvement programs for personnel, give direct aid to communities in program development, and perform numberless other functions related to the promotion of the fields. The state laws require that such standards for program and personnel be established by state departments and be accepted by the schools of the state. Thus it may well be said that the quality and quantity of local programs will depend upon the leadership exerted at the state level.

There are contrasting ways in which the framework within which this leadership can work is set. Some states (Pennsylvania, Florida, Illinois) have extended laws specifying in great detail the character of the program that is expected. These laws indicate how many minutes a week must be devoted to health instruction, the frequency with which examinations are to be held, which types of immunization are mandatory and which optional, and in many other ways describe an optimal program in law. Other states (Wisconsin, Ohio) rely more upon state standards. The law will briefly declare that there must or may be programs of health education and physical education in the schools of the state and vest the authority for developing the details in the state department of education. This department then develops a program of standards that is accepted by local schools wishing to become accredited. Such a plan allows for greater flexibility in the improvement of the minimum level of programs in that standards may be altered by the official state agency without raising the complicated problem of legislative action. Furthermore, the acceptance of standard is, to many school systems, a more palatable process than adherence to law. Whether the state operates principally by law or by standards, the personnel of a local system will want to know the full detail of what is expected of them and what the mandated and permitted features are in school health education in their state. There being no standard school law used in all states, a study must be made locally to determine the scope of the law or standards.

The trend, in recent years, is toward centralizing the responsibility for many related areas in one state bureau, division, or department, whatever local term is used. Thus physical education, health education, driver education, safety education, school recreation, lunch programs, and sometimes special education and civil defense education have all been brought together under one head. Whether, in such a large organization, effective consultation and development can be given to school health education depends of course upon the quantity and quality of personnel in the department.

For many years the federal government has subsidized health education in state departments of health, usually through the work in maternity and child health.

This program has served well the effort in school health education by supplying supplementary counseling personnel who have given important aid to schools in many of the states where such programs exist. To combine the efforts of people from education and from public health is an interesting exercise in cooperation and understanding.

Whatever the state statute, standard, or policy may be, the local administrator *and teacher* should know what it is. Possibly the law exempts certain students from compulsory health instruction (religious objectors). The teacher must know of this and be prepared to receive and dispose of such cases. Perhaps the law gives boards of education the right to employ physicians whose judgment must be taken as final in all matters of health eligibility for athletics. Exercise of this provision will solve occasional troublesome disputes. State laws frequently require boards to require evidence of freedom from tuberculosis and venereal disease before employment, or laws may set other health standards regarding emotional health or physical examinations. Local authorities must know of these laws and enforce them.

Laws regarding handicapped (or exceptional) children, aid to partially sighted or hearing children, vaccination requirements, exclusion and readmission in connection with disease, and care of emergency illness or injury are frequently passed by legislatures, and they must be enforced locally by boards of education or boards of health. Local personnel in health education would be well advised to be thoroughly familiar with such state laws and standards as may affect their work.

FEDERAL PARTICIPATION

Increasingly the federal influence is being felt in education. Principally this influence has been expressed through Congressional subsidies of work for the handicapped, for the federal school lunch program, for supervisory and consultative service through state boards, through the President's Council on Physical Fitness, through legislation in the areas of mental health, loans to students, building construction, and notably through the support of the Office of Child Development, the Office of Nutrition and Health Service in the United States Office of Education, and the Public Health Service. Federal assistance is consultative and, in addition, through subsidization may aid programs at state and local levels. Local authorities should keep informed of opportunities from these sources. Two pieces of legislation have had a major effect on school health education for the last five years. These are the Elementary and Secondary Education Act of 1965 and the Economic Opportunity Act of 1964.

The Elementary and Secondary Education Act[1] was designed to strengthen and improve the educational quality and educational opportunity in the nation's elementary and secondary schools. This act was originally divided into five Titles, and in 1967 a sixth Title was added.

Of the Titles, I, III, and VI have made the most effect on school health education. Title I recognized the close relationship between poverty and lack of educational development and poor academic performance. Money was appropriated through this section of the act to provide for improvement of elementary schools located in poverty areas. There was financial support for a great number of services to be located in the schools. Notable among these was support for guidance, supplementary health and food services, school health, and psychological and psychiatric services. On the basis of this emphasis many schools have been able to mount health service programs and school health education programs which previously had not been able to do so. Many schools have brought nurses into the school system to provide health services at the local school level. In some instances it has been possible to spend Title I funds for direct case services.

In the Tacoma, Washington schools it was possible to develop a health education resource teacher position and three teachers were hired. The duties of these teachers included going from school to school in the poverty areas of the town and working with teachers to promote the health education of the children in the area. These teachers were able to tailor lesson plans to the particular needs of disadvantaged children and help them to develop skills that would help them to be more healthy in spite of their disadvantaged environment.

Title III of the Elementary and Secondary Education Act was designed to support supplementary educational centers and services of a model or exemplary nature. It was through the support of this Title that many schools were able to develop innovative and exemplary school health programs to demonstrate the values of good school health education to those who still doubt the effectiveness of such programs.

Title VI, the most recent addition to the act, supports programs for handicapped children. The support is for special education classes and for all manner of supportive services. In some instances the money has gone for case-finding procedures. Included among these have been screening programs for children who are visually or hearing handicapped.

The other Titles included Title II, which was designed to support school library resources, Title IV, which supported a cooperative research project in which national and regional educational research facilities have been developed, and Title V, which has allowed for the strengthening of state departments of education. In a few instances Title V money has been spent to hire health education supervisors in state departments of education.

Although mistakes have been made and on occasion enthusiasm overrode common sense, the overall effect of the Elementary and Secondary Education Act on School Health Education has been stimulating and beneficial. School districts that have not deemed it wise to use Elementary and Secondary Education Act funds for school health education would be advised to look into the possibilities. Many school districts have found great benefits from the use of the monies in health services and health education.

The Economic Opportunity Act of 1964 had the effect of plunging school health programs into the field of early childhood education and particularly preschool health services and health education. Many school districts became delegate agencies for the operation of Project Headstart programs. The health goals of Project Headstart are as follows:

I To improve a child's present function by:

A Finding all existing health defects through:

1 Accumulating records of past health and immunization status

2 Considering the observations of classroom teachers and other staff

3 Performing screening tests, including tuberculin, hematocrit or hemoglobin, urinalysis, vision testing, hearing testing

4 Interviewing the child and his parents about his current and past health and function

5 Performing a physical examination as part of a complete health evaluation

B Remedying any existing defects through:

1 Applying whatever medical or dental treatments are necessary

2 Arranging for rehabilitative services, special education, and other forms of continuing care

II To ensure a child's future health by:

A Providing preventive services including:

1 Immunization against infectious diseases

2 Fluoride treatment to prevent dental decay

3 Health education for children and parents

4 Introduction of the child to a physician and dentist that will be responsible for his continuing health care

B Improving the health of all members of the child's family through:

1 Calling attention to family health needs

2 Introducing the family to health care services and to sources of funds for these services

C Improving the health of the community in which the child lives through:

1 Increasing the awareness and concern of professionals, and the general population with the health problems of poor children

2 Stimulating and providing new resources for health care

3 Making existing health resources more responsive to the special needs of the poor

4 Demonstrating new skills, techniques, and patterns of care to health professionals

5 Acquiring new knowledge through research[2]

These goals essentially are the goals of school health programs and so were easy to incorporate into the school health field. Subsequently, as federal funds have come along for the support of Parent-Child Centers and for Follow Through, the goals of Project Headstart have been incorporated in the newer programs. Many long time health personnel have found a great feeling of success through Headstart and Follow Through because of the emphasis on health education and on health services. It has been particularly helpful to have case-service money available through Headstart to pay for care for disadvantaged children who previously had found it difficult to receive service. As a result of the federal programs for the disadvantaged child, particularly the preschooler, many children will be entering school with fewer health handicaps than ever before.

Although Parent-Child Centers, Headstart, and Follow Through programs and the Titles of the Elementary and Secondary Education Act have been administered separately, there is at the writing of this book a considerable effort to bring about coordination among the programs listed above. The emphasis at the federal level will be developing programs of continuous comprehensive health care for children with the school and with the federally funded programs serving as the entry point into the health-care system. Such coordination is deemed desirable starting from the Parent-Child Centers and going through Headstart, Follow Through, and Title I supported classes.

If recent experience is any indicator, there will continue to be administrative changes and changes in the titles of the offices administering federal programs in school health and school health education. Whatever the changes in the names and the acts supporting school health, it is predicted that the federal commitment for health care to children is increasing and will continue to increase in the near future. Hopefully, it will be possible to maintain a balance between federally written guidelines and complete local autonomy. All must work for increasing mutual confidence and flexibility so that the unique needs of children in each community can be better met.

LOCAL POLICY

The system we have in American education gives virtual autonomy to the community in determining the kind and quality of educational program it shall have. State departments of education lead, encourage, illuminate, and enforce minimum standards. Departments of health can enforce state laws representing minimum standards of performance in sanitation, safety or disease control. As we have seen, there is, so far, some small relationship between the federal government and the community. But by and large the program in health education and physical education is a local matter and dependent almost wholly upon the willingness and ability of local administrators and teachers. To offer health instruction well, poorly, or not at all is in most states a local matter. To employ a physician, or to organize special education for the handicapped, to install adequate lighting and sanitary facilities—these are local problems mainly. *School health education and physical education are well or poorly given according to the extent to which local school, health, and municipal authorities exercise their prerogatives under the law.* The responsibility falls most heavily upon the local superintendent of schools. The quality of the health program in the school reflects his professional attitude toward and skill in developing adequate programs for the health of the children of his community. Others share with him, but leadership should come from the chief administrator as he works within the framework of the laws and standards that his state and board have established.

Once state legislatures or state departments of education or health have laid down the basic principles upon which such programs shall operate or have established the permissive or enabling legistlation, then the details of operation are usually left up to the local board of education or board of health. And their jurisdiction is final. If, for example, state law gives local boards the right to require a physical examination of employed personnel, then the local group may specify whatever health standards it wishes. Even further, if public funds may be expended for such a program (a right usually reserved for legislatures to decide), then local boards may or may not establish that examination requirement as they see fit. Local boards may have autonomy in the curriculum so long as they meet state standards; thus they might, if they saw fit, prohibit the teaching of sex education, or require a six-week unit of work on alcoholism and tobacco. Their word is usually definitive and final.

This is why local policy and regulations in health education are so important. Who pays what amounts for injuries incurred in high school athletics? How much sick leave may teachers have? What prerogatives belong to the family physician? What health excuses from physical education are admissible? Is health instruction to be carried on in segregated or mixed classes? Are parental permissions required for participation in athletics? How much freedom does the health teacher have in dealing with controversial matters?

All these are matters of policy. They require some predetermined judgment. Once the policy is established and given full notice throughout the community, such problems as may be covered by the policy are usually handled without difficulty.

From where does such policy emanate? How is it developed? Sometimes policy comes from the top down. The board of education formulates the policy without consultation or hearing. Sometimes the board will ask a committee of interested personnel to study the matter and make a recommendation to it. Sometimes a committee of teachers or the school principal will work out a policy and submit it to the board for ratification.

Perhaps the best way to have policy evolve is to have it come upon recommendation of the school-community health council. This sort of organization has proven its usefulness in hundreds of communities in the country and is described more fully later in this chapter. Through its subcommittees or individual members, councils discover problems, discuss solutions, and formulate policies. These policies are then recommended to the board of education or the board of health, as the case may be, for adoption.

There should be a policy for everything. Who shall render first aid? Who shall teach? Shall parents be notified in case of injury? How? By whom? There are hundreds of such questions involved in a program of school health education, the answers to which ought not to be left to spur-of-the-moment decision.

ADMINISTRATIVE ORGANIZATION

In view of the multitude of laws and standards which regulate the school health education program, it is apparent that administrative organization can become somewhat complex. And yet, as state and local programs have developed, certain agreements on points of view have been reached, and, although there is little standard practice in local organization, some similarities in the placement of responsibility are beginning to appear.

– at the local level

By virtue of school law the superintendent of the school district and the principal of the school (or executive head, or whatever term is used to designate the administrative officer) is responsible for all the health activity, of whatever nature, that goes on in that school or jurisdiction. The only exceptions to this must be and are specified by laws that give health officers the right to affect school procedure in the control of epidemics or other dangers to school personnel, fire marshals the right to condemn or order changes in school construction, and building or sanitary inspectors the right to judge parts or all of the school plant unfit for use.

But aside from these, the school administrator bears the responsibility for the organization and conduct of the school health education program, for its personnel, its supervision, its operation, and its outcomes. There should be no misapprehension about this. Any curriculum development, any testing or screening program, any examinations, any health policies are subject to the administration of the school administrator and the board of education legally established to conduct the program of education. Neither the board of health nor any other official or nonofficial community agency has the legal responsibility for developing any phase of school health education. When noneducation personnel bring their talent to bear upon the school health program, it is by invitation of the educational authorities.

Depending upon the size of the program—and the school district—the school administrator employs health education personnel in the persons of teachers, supervisors (consultants), dentists, physicians, nurses, dental hygienists, and others to work within the program. In larger districts (Minneapolis, Los Angeles, Denver, New York, for example) there usually is a central office staff of educators, physicians, nurses, and specialists of one kind or another working together to evolve policy, advise on curriculum, supervise personnel practice, deal with budget and finance, and in every way enhance the program.

Teachers in the schools benefit from such central office activity and would do well to use the services and assistance provided.

In an excellent brochure entitled *Teamwork in School Health* the American Association for Health, Physical Education and Recreation and the National Health Council have cited several patterns for coordinated local administration of the school health program, among them being:

Informal procedure—the utilization of day-to-day contacts for solution of problems and administrative decisions.
Ad hoc problem-solving—the solution of problems as they arise by ad hoc special purpose committees.
The continuing committee or council—a permanent organization whose business it is to discuss and solve school health problems.
Special advisory committees—useful on many technical matters, similar to the ad hoc committees.
Combinations of the above.[3]

In some communities there persists the problem of locating the final authority for the administration of school health services (for example, screening, health examinations, immunization programs). Shall the administrative control of these be vested in the board of education or the board of health? To many people the answer is clearly the school health council as described below. But some public health workers believe that with the development of a modern program of health education, including both health instruction and health service phases, this framework of administration has to be reexamined to see if the job of health education can get done within it. As soon as schools began to employ physicians and nurses, as soon as physical examinations, immunization programs, and screening and referral systems were established, the question arose as to whether all that sort of activity did not belong under the administrative jurisdiction of boards of health rather than boards of education. Should physicians and nurses be employed as school personnel and work in schools and communities without any official relationship to the official health agency, or should the local health authority supervise and conduct all of the activities going on within the school?

The problem has never been completely solved in all states. Three patterns of administration have emerged: one in which the schools operate their own health program, that is, under the administrative jurisdiction of the board of education; another in which the board of health has administrative responsibility; and a third in which there is a joint administration.

A 1965 study of such arrangements showed that 64 percent of the health services in cities were under the board of education, 30 percent under boards of health, and 6 percent under joint administration.[4]

Characteristically, the health services producing the fullest services are found in the large cities and under the jurisdiction of the boards of education.

In this connection it is always helpful for school personnel to remember that the scope of activity for local health authorities is usually prescribed by law and thus their duties impinge upon the school population. Children are children first and schoolchildren second. Health authorities see children as part of the public for whose health they are responsible, and thus it is entirely essential that school and health personnel cooperate so as to get *both* jobs done. School people should realize that health officers are charged by law to:

1 Enforce all state health laws and regulations.

2 Prepare and enforce regulations for the control of communicable disease.

3 Record incidence and instances of communicable disease.

4 Investigate all instances of disease carriers and contacts.

5 Under some conditions, supply and administer vaccines and serums.

Those and many other legal and traditional functions of boards of health bring them in close contact with school problems.

At all events, regardless of where the final budgetary and administrative jurisdiction lies, the following features of a smooth-running and adequate school program should be preserved and maintained:

1 Joint planning for school and community programs between boards of education and health should be a constant feature of any system.

2 School personnel should welcome the advice and consultation of health or medical personnel at each stage of program development.

3 Medical personnel should learn to work with school people, to understand their problems, and cooperate within rather than dominate the program.

4 Health departments should be constantly ready to improve the inservice preparation of teachers.

5 School and community health councils should invariably carry adequate representation from both health and education administrative offices.

6 In any given school building the administrative authority of the principal over all activities, including health service, must remain.

7 Medical, nursing, and dental personnel who have some preparation in the field of professional education have an advantage in working in an educational setting.

8 Boards of education, charged as they are with the responsibility for the education of the children of the community and recognizing the basic *educational* character of school health education,

can be encouraged to work cooperatively with boards of health on mutual problems without relinquishing administrative jurisdiction over any part of the educational program.

– qualifications of the administrator

Some localities and some states are perplexed over the problem of qualifications of the administrative personnel for the program. Should a physician or an educator be chosen to administer, supervise, "head up" the program?

There is no standard practice. Good work is being done under both. Whether a physician should head the school health program or whether an educator should be its principal officer depends almost wholly upon the administrative skill and personal qualifications of the persons in question. In cities or counties large enough to have a staff of supervisors or consultants at work in this field, the medical or educational background of the person is of less importance than his conception of the program and his organizing ability. In smaller school systems where there may be one supervisor of health education in a county or a small city or village, the possibilities are that the position will be held by a specialist in health education or in health and physical education. Physicians are rare in these positions not because they are disqualified on professional grounds but merely because there are not enough of them available to serve communities in that way.

These central office supervisors or consultants, working directly under the superintendent, are helpful in assisting elementary teachers with instructional plans and materials, providing teaching aids and demonstrations, aiding in the appraisal programs, supplying new materials for teaching, coordinating school and community effort, and facilitating in every way the development of school health education in the communities and in the individual schools. In many rural areas the consultant becomes a traveling teacher and may be on the staff of six or seven schools, teaching in each one and conducting health service activities in them all.

THE SCHOOL HEALTH COUNCIL

The formation of a school and community health council (or committee), with a council chairman chosen from available trained personnel, seems to be an excellent device for developing a school health program in a single school or group of schools. Experience is proving the soundness of such a plan. The council gives various interests a chance to participate in the formation and conduct of the program. It assures many an opportunity to be heard. Under an able school principal many fine school health programs have come into being as a result of this cooperative effort.

In some places the council does not include representatives of community interests but confines its membership to school personnel and its activities to school matters. It serves in this way as a school committee on the health program. Current thought, however, favors a broadening of scope to include community interests and thus gives tangible recognition to the fact that the health of the schoolchild is the concern of many and not only of school personnel.

The health council or committee plan is adaptive to any school, large or small, rural or urban. The work of each is planned in relation to local needs. A survey may be made, needs established, and committees invited to undertake the work. The list of activities to be undertaken will depend largely upon the imagination, insight, and conscience of the members of the council.

For effective action, the organization of such a body either wholly within the school or joining forces with the community should remain as simple as possible. The officers could well be only a chairman, a secretary, and perhaps an editor for whatever publications the council chooses to issue. Subcommittees can be appointed for continuous function and reporting to the council on emergencies and accidents, the school environment, disease control, appraisals and screening, school-home relationships, athletics and physical education, research, or any other large area of health interest. The membership on committees and officers of the council may be rotated every two or three years for variety and to sustain community interest.

The membership of the council should include persons interested in child health and willing to work cooperatively for its betterment. The list of potential members of such a council usually includes:

From the School	*From the Community*
The principal	Physicians
Physical education teachers	Dentists
The nurse	Ministers
The physician and dentist	A PTA representative
The psychologist	Representatives from service clubs
Teachers	The public health officer and nurse
The custodian	Any appropriate civic leaders
Students	The mayor or a councilman
The dental hygienist	Specialists in contributing fields
The guidance counselor	

Such a school and community health council could be small or very large. If the latter, it should have a strong program committee to guide the work, a competent chairman, and a well-conceived plan of action. Individual schools within the community where such large councils exist would want individual school committees chosen from school personnel only.

Business that comes before such councils is described by the National Conference as:

1 Delineation of the various aspects of the school health program.
2 Interpretation of these functions to member agencies and the public.
3 Definition of the health responsibilities of the school and other community agencies.
4 Determination of local school health strengths and needs.
5 Identification of resources to meet recognized needs.
6 Recommendations of related policies and programs.
7 Evaluation of progress made and detection of unmet needs.
8 Initiation of follow-up projects and programs.[5]

There are hundreds of effective school and community health councils in action throughout the nation. We quote the principles which guide one of the better ones, that of the Grand Rapids-Kent County Health Departments:

– principles

The following principles are basic to the effectiveness of a school health council:

1 It should bring together the efforts, the thinking, the resources and the interest of all organizations and individuals working in the cause of good health for the schoolchild.
2 It should encompass the whole range of health needs of the school child and should utilize all available resources—governmental and voluntary, local, state and national—for serving these needs, including a close and effective relationship with other community councils or welfare planning bodies.
3 It should focus on the needs of schoolchildren rather than on the operation of individual agency programs and should undertake to coordinate efforts to meet those needs as effectively as possible.
4 It should have a democratic base with responsibility resting in a delegate body designated by autonomous groups, plus members at large chosen to provide broad representation of all community interests.
The delegate body should consist of official delegates from health, education, and related agencies, and institutions; professional health organizations; civic groups with demonstrated interest in health; and members-at-large who are broadly representative of the community.
5 It should have no administrative authority over participating agencies or organizations but should strive to achieve its purpose through group discussion and education.
6 Its members should share responsibility and credit for planning and should also share for accomplishment, without domination by any groups, whether constituent organization, fund-raising groups or national agencies.

7 Its decisions and action should be based upon facts obtained through objective, accurate, and comprehensive research into the nature of needs of people and the most effective means of serving them.

8 Its program should be primarily one of coordinating and planning rather than the direct operation of services for people. Certain common services for agencies and the community may be operated, however, when its member agencies agree that these services can be best done by united effort rather than by individual agency efforts. Certain short-time demonstration projects may also be carried on by agreement of member agencies.

9 It should emphasize long-range programs with specified short-term goals, which can be carried to successful conclusion.

10 It should develop effective channels of communication and opportunities for producing interaction with statewide and nationwide planning groups.

11 It should concern itself with adequate financing of health and social welfare services for the school age child, whether from governmental or voluntary sources.

12 It should have a staff qualified to execute the work program adopted by its members and a budget adequate for that purpose.[6]

There is no suggestion, however, that these councils, whether for one building or one school only, or for schools and community, are in positions of administrative authority or responsibility. They are advisory only; exploratory, research, promotional, and fund-raising activities may come within their scope, but they do not usurp administrative responsibility legally invested in the board of education.

ROLE OF THE STATE GOVERNMENT

Most states have active programs in school health education operating out of state departments of public instruction or state departments of health, or both. These departments are the instruments used by the state legislatures for the execution of whatever legislation is passed benefiting the health of the schoolchild. It becomes exceedingly important to all local personnel in school health education and physical education to know the limitations and possibilities of program development as established by state law.

State supervisory programs not only interpret existing statutes for the benefit of communities but extend a great deal of consultative service as well. These programs are ordinarily located in departments of public instruction and are thus under the administrative direction of the state superintendent. In some states, however, the office is located in the department of health and in others the two share the work. The most fortunate states are those that not only have such programs established but have the two principal departments—health and education—working in complete harmony and in enthusiastic support of each other in school health education.

The Council of Chief State School Officers suggests the following as the principal responsibilities for state departments of education in the development of school health programs:

1 Orienting new school health personnel to their responsibilities through publications, consultations, and group and area conferences.

2 Orienting schools employing health services for the first time to the best practices in administering and providing for health services.

3 Assisting teacher-training institutions in the development of curriculums which define the total health responsibilities of teachers, administrators, and specialists.

4 Recommending minimum standards of competence for school health personnel, for the maintenance of healthful school environments, and for school health practices.

5 Orienting boards of education, through appropriate channels, to the desirability of providing appropriate health services for children.[7]

ROLE OF FEDERAL GOVERNMENT

The federal government has little or no administrative control over local school procedures and programs. Except in those instances when federal money is appropriated (for example, for school lunches or for vocational agriculture), the government exercises merely an advisory and research function in relation to education in general and to school health education in particular. Where federal money is appropriated for the support of educational enterprises, Congress has usually established minimum standards for local acceptance and left the enforcement of those standards to an appropriate executive branch. Otherwise, the tradition of local autonomy in education persists, and states are reluctant to give up their rights in determining the kind of education their people should have. As time goes on, however, and the movement for equalizing educational opportunity over the nation gains more popularity, it is entirely possible that the federal government will have increasing control over the administration of local programs because of the use of federal funds in their support.

Furthermore, Congress may someday become interested in legislation specifically directed at school and college health and physical education and may be willing to subsidize much of the school health education program as it is now known. Bills drawn up for that purpose will probably call for the acknowledgment of basic minimum standards in program and personnel. Depending entirely upon the state and local administration thereof, such bills may have a salutary effect upon the extension of the benefits of school health education to more and more children.

The chief executive agencies in the government having influence in school health education are the Department of Health, Education and Welfare (in which will be found the Office of Education, the Public Health Service, and the Office of Child Development) and the Department of Agriculture. There are many others. At one time it was determined that over seventy bureaus or agencies within the government had something to do with the health or recreation of the people! But the above-named offices are the principal ones. The Office of Education provides assistance in the form of information, field consultation service, research data, and information on trends that is of use to local and state groups. The other three agencies are likewise of great assistance to local groups in providing information. They operate together in giving suggestions on policy and standards that guide school systems over the nation in the development of health education. Teachers and administrators will find all these agencies available for consultation through field representatives or by correspondence.

COMMUNITY INVOLVEMENT

School health programs develop with greater facility when various agencies and people in the community become involved than if their development was attempted in isolation. There are many persons who either personally or professionally or both have an interest and equity in the health of children. It is quite reasonable, therefore, that a school health program should relate to their interests and capitalize, if possible, upon their talent and wisdom.

– boards of health and public clinics

A school health education program comes into its greatest fulfillment only when completely cooperative and constructive relationships have been established with local boards of health and other medical, dental, and public health facilities. The use of personnel, funds, and public clinics for indigent school children in need of dental or medical care is a case in point. Health officers do, of course, have their legal responsibility for certain aspects of health care, and schools will want to cooperate fully in the exercise of those functions.

State laws will indicate whether the local or state health officer may close the schools in case of epidemics, whether he may require vaccination of all those attending school, and whether he has the power to "abate any nuisance" or remove any hazard to the public health.

These are powers usually vested in boards of health, and boards of education should cooperate fully in their execution.

On the other hand, local health officers, when serving the school, should approach their tasks not as medical but as educational ones. They should make every effort to conform to the school schedule and the school's purpose and resist any effort to dictate curriculum content or method in health instruction. Their services are best used in a cooperative relationship, functioning in school health education in the way any other physician might function.

– relation to parents The home-school relationship should be the closest of all. Through every known device the parents should be encouraged to accept their crucial part in improving the health status and the health practices of their children.

> Parents should be acquainted with the health needs of their children as revealed in school health records in order to seek needed medical care, plan diet changes, make alterations in daily routine, and take any other necessary steps for improving the child's health. To this end the school should regularly report to parents their observations about the child's health status and make immediate notification of serious deviations. In many schools parents are invited to come to the school at an appointed time to discuss their child's health needs with the teacher, school physician, nurse, or other qualified health service personnel. Conferences of this type should be considered part of the normal working load of the school staff, and time for such conferences should be budgeted. If the parents do not come to the school, the school nurse or a teacher should visit them to interpret the child's urgent health needs.[8]

Parents should be given a chance to express themselves concerning any phase of the school health program. Parent study groups on problems of child health can be organized. The parent-teacher group can devote time to studying improvements in school health education. The program can become the subject of public forum and debate. For without parental action or hampered by parental apathy or distrust, the health program cannot help the individual students in need of assistance. It must be clear to parents that the interest of the school in the health of children is a valid one, for educational as well as developmental and protective purposes, and that the school is prepared to go far in serving its objectives in health education.

Many parents, for reasons of indigence, neglect, or ignorance, are unable or unwilling to play their part in the plans outlined to improve their children's health. In such instances the school is justified in going to considerable lengths to mobilize community resources in aid to the indigent and in acting through the courts when child health is being willfully neglected or jeopardized. Mindful of its limitations, the school itself cannot supply or perform medical aid; it cannot, in many states, enforce vaccination. It can, however, play its part in making medical aid available; it can help parents choose physicians and dentists; and it can establish vaccination and other protective measures as conditions of entrance in order to protect the school population.

Basic to any intelligent relationships with parents is the need for keeping them informed of school policies and action. Parents cannot be expected to react with very much interest or to be very helpful if they do not know what the program of the school is or the principles upon which it is based. Parents are naturally concerned about the welfare of their own children, and when the schools deal in any way with the health of these children, the parents want to know all about it.

For those reasons the schools should develop a plan for getting information to parents. Occasional announcements in parent groups are not enough. Bulletins should be issued periodically, policies should be stated in writing, and each household should have a copy. Full notice should be given of every move in the health education program. The parents should have full access to information about such things as athletic insurance, policies for dealing with injuries incurred under school auspices, emergency and accident care, immunization requirements and programs, the purpose and nature of the physical examination programs, vision and hearing testing, policies regarding exclusion, absences, and readmission on account of illness, and the functions of all personnel in school relating to the health of children.

– the school as a community center

Perhaps future years will see even more fruitful relationships between schools and parents than are now practical in many places. The school is increasingly becoming a great community center where families gather for social purposes and at the same time participate in those activities that make for healthful living. Precedent for this is set in many current institutions like YMCAs, YWCAs, and Turnvereins. This tendency finds complete expression in an English effort that, although not centering in a school, nevertheless indicates how a well-planned school could be used for healthful family living:

> The new center, built to service 2,000 families, was opened in 1935. It offered consultative services as before, but in addition it provided the facilities for the exercise of the physical, mental, and social capacities so necessary for health. It was a physical structure of steel and concrete, but more important it was a social structure based upon a new unit. . . .
>
> The plan of action was patterned after a family club, with periodic health overhauls for all members and with the various auxiliary services for infants, children, and parents. . . . The Peckham

> community had been selected because it was an average community, and yet 90 percent of the individuals (3,911 had been examined) were not healthy. . . . In the center of the building was a 35-by-75 foot swimming pool, visible from each floor through a continuous band of glass. On the ground floor were the nursery, gymnasium, playground, theater, storerooms, and service rooms. The second floor housed the main recreation and dance floor, the cafeteria, and several small activity rooms. On the third floor were the laboratories and consultation rooms, a recreation room, work room, band room, and committee room. The building was properly insulated and soundproofed. Most of the facilities were designed for self-service.
>
> At different times of the day one may see children in the nursery, waders in the pool, toddlers on the swings and slides, and any one or several of the following activities in progress: sewing, handicraft, games, bicycling, keep-fit classes, swimming, billiards, dancing, band, drama, chess, public speaking, tap dancing, boxing, tumbling, roller skating, parties, hiking, luncheon in the cafeteria and study groups. More recently the center has acquired a farm and camp which provide many week-end activities in the open. The center often accommodates 1,200 persons on Saturday nights. It is open from 2 to 10 p.m. daily except Sunday. . . .
>
> All the activity within the center is voluntary and spontaneous. There is no center hostess, no one to make introductions, very little programming, no herding, coaxing, or guiding to action. Earlier attempts at promotion have been abandoned. . . . This is the reason for membership on the family basis, the unit of living. In the presence of a vertical age grouping, where youth is surrounded by every stage of maturity and every degree of skill, there are present and natural incentives to development. The children are growing up in families which are expanding their physical, social, and intellectual contacts because of the activities of the center. As the parents penetrate the active society which surrounds them and the child shares their experiences, his confidence expands and he reaches for new forms of activity. This can only come about where the young are in contact with a society which includes people of varying degrees of maturity, possessing varying degrees of accomplishment.[9]

An experiment like this would not be out of the question for American communities. There are many present school buildings which could be immediately used for such purposes. The buildings of the future should surely be planned with such things in mind. If schools are interested in people's health, school personnel should fully correlate their efforts with those of interested citizens to bring opportunities for living healthfully closer to home.

– medical and dental societies

There is a reciprocal relationship possible between the school health program and private physicians, dentists, and medical and dental societies. Fully developed, such a relationship would enhance the position and programs of all concerned. It has taken many years to bring about a mutual understanding between the educator and the physician and dentist. The following suggestions are made with the idea of deepening that understanding in communities:

1 Schools should invite local physicians and dentists to serve on school health committees and on health councils in city systems. They should share in the planning and problem-solving which occupies the time of such councils. Invitations for such service should be extended through the local medical and dental societies. If a particular physician or dentist is wanted for a specific purpose, he may be invited directly, but generally it is best to allow the local professional groups to pick their own representatives.

2 In recent years, particularly as a result of the encouragement given local medical societies by the parent organization, the American Medical Association, and with the assistance also of the American Dental Association, the state and local medical and dental societies have been appointing school health committees. These become usually very effective liaison groups with school programs. They serve as intermediaries and can very effectively make the task of cooperation between medical and educational groups easier.

The function of such school health committees in medical and dental societies has been described as (1) to stimulate cooperation by individual physicians in the school health program, (2) to keep the profession informed on school health problems, (3) to encourage sanction by the medical profession of a sound school health program, and (4) to report to the profession on progress. The medical society committee can perform these functions most effectively, within the framework of the community, by developing reciprocal relations with the dental society, school system, health department, parent groups, and other appropriate organizations. Specifically such a committee of the medical society could:

a Aid in the establishment of health appraisal standards, including standards for physical examinations, observation, and screening.

b Assist in the development of adequate cumulative health records and facilitation of the proper interchange of appropriate data among schools, family medical advisor, and parents.

c Help formulate policies for handling of confidential medical information relating to the health problems of pupils and school personnel.

d Assist in the development of follow-up procedures including effective methods of referring children needing attention to the family physician and dentist or other community resources and evaluation of the effectiveness of such follow-up.

e Advise on the health and medical aspects of school administration, such as health counseling done by nonmedical personnel and the formulation of a plan for the prompt handling of school medical emergencies.

f Provide counsel on communicable disease control, including immunization procedures, exclusion and readmission policies, quarantine regulations, and specific disease detection.

g Help in the establishment of health and safety measures to protect participants in physical education and athletics.

h Aid in the development of standards for safety and sanitation in the general school environment, including procedures for inspection and methods of improving dietary standards in the school lunchroom and other food services.

i Advise and counsel on the emotional factors in the school environment and their implications for pupils and school personnel.

j Provide advice concerning the health problems of the handicapped child, especially in regard to adjustment to irremediable handicaps and interpretation of the emotional implications of the school environment for such children.

k Aid in the evaluation and selection of health education materials with particular reference to their scientific accuracy.

l Encourage utilization of the private physician as a resource person in the health instruction program.

m Assist in intelligent understanding and utilization of the health resources of the community.

n Help formulate standards for the qualification of various personnel involved in health education and health services in the schools.

o Assist in establishing sound policies and procedures to guide the health and medical supervision of school personnel.

p Advise the medical society on legislative and financial needs of the school health program.[10]

In addition, the medical or dental committees can supply students with materials and opportunities with which to study current problems of medical and dental care of the public. Considerable misunderstanding exists in the minds of the general public about dentistry and medicine because the groups representing those sciences have rarely supplied the school health education programs with appropriate educational materials. Furthermore, in view of the fact that these professional societies and their national organizations are significant in the national scene, their policies and activities should be known to schools. A study of the American Dental Association, the American Medical Association, the American Public Health Association, and all other professional agencies or associations dealing with the health of people could well become not only a study for health council personnel, but a unit of work in the health instruction of high school and college students.

3 Schools and medical societies should cooperate in supplying to indigent people, or to those who have never selected a family physician, a panel of names from which to pick when the need arises.

4 Where no physician serves the school and thus no adequate program of classification or appraisal of pupils is established, schools should confer with local physicians to determine whether they would examine their own pupil-patients as well as others for a fee, and make such reports to school personnel as will be useful in guiding the educational program of the child. Such procedures have been successful and neighborhood physicians are usually pleased to meet new patients and to cooperate with school personnel.

PRIVATE HEALTH AGENCIES

The private health agencies and other civic or social groups having an interest in health are generally anxious to foster the development of school health education any way they can. Organizations such as the American Heart Association, the National Tuberculosis Association, the American Cancer Society, and others in the health agency field, as well as the parent-teacher associations, American Legion, labor organizations, and others with child health committees, are available for assistance in many ways if the proper representations are made. On local, state, and national levels those organizations are ready to assist in school health education because they recognize in the school one of the most effective media for attaining their own educational objectives. Conversely schools are in a position to help the private agencies.

Such reciprocal relationships are mutually profitable. Whether from private or official agencies, the students can profit educationally and healthfully from such community contacts. The possibilities are many and varied. Here follow some citations of actual projects developed in schools:

1 Held a conference on cancer education sponsored jointly by school and local chapter of American Cancer Society

2 Stimulated the establishment of a cancer clinic by local health authorities

3 Organized and provided the site for a baby clinic for low-income families in the community

4 Cooperated fully in the preschool round-up of the Parent-Teacher Association

5 Acquainted students by field trips and discussion with the operation of all civic functions relating to health

6 Made possible the use of the X-ray machine donated to the county health department by the Tuberculosis Association in surveying all young people in the district

7 Helped in the selection of worthy cases for a charitable summer camp

8 Received from the Junior Chamber of Commerce the benefits of a dental health program and from the American Legion an athletic program during summer months

9 Received from a local service club funds for aiding the treatment of crippled children and from another service club money for shoes for indigent children

10 Used the local theater and projection equipment for the showing of health motion pictures

These are but ten of hundreds of projects that strengthen the programs of both the community organizations and the school. They can be easily thought of and planned by an imaginative and energetic health council.

There are, of course, principles that underlie such school-agency cooperative relationships. A Committee of the Health Education Division of the American Association for Health, Physical Education and Recreation working in cooperation with representatives from the private agencies evolved these:

Guiding Principles

1 Recognition of common goals is essential.

2 Mutual understanding of purposes and procedures is necessary.

3 Mutual projects are best when planned and undertaken jointly.

4 New health activities should be an integral part of the school health education program.

5 Fund-raising activities may have value for education.

Recommended Agency Activities

1 Make available to the school personnel the latest health information.

2 Provide teaching aids.

3 Help in the preparation of resource units.

4 Help with special short-term projects.

5 Help with in-service education of teachers.

6 Participate in the recruitment and pre-service education of school health personnel.

7 Provide the means for demonstrations and studies.

8 Enrich the curriculum.

9 Interpret the school health program and unmet needs to the community.

10 Help in interpretation to parents.[11]

PROFESSIONAL ASSOCIATIONS

There are a great many professional organizations on the national and International level (see the Selected Readings Section of Chapter 8) that have some bearing upon local programs and that may influence policy formation and occasionally distribute funds. Some of the more prominent and influential of these are:

The American Medical Association
The American Public Health Association
The American School Health Association
The American College Health Association
The American Association for Health, Physical Education and Recreation
The Society of Public Health Educators
The American Nurses Association
The National League for Nursing

At the international level the following organizations are influential:

The Health Division of the United Nations Educational, Scientific and Cultural Organization
The World Health Organization
The International Union for Health Education

These agencies function in school health education in a variety of ways. Some have funds for local use and others do not. Some of them will supply teaching materials or other data of local interest, and school health personnel should be familiar with the available resources of these organizations.

COMMERCIAL ORGANIZATIONS

There is a wealth of health education material now offered by business enterprises for use in school health education. Some life insurance companies publish teaching aids, teachers' bulletins, actuarial data, and research studies that are of great value. Food manufacturers issue attractive materials on diet and nutrition. Soap companies and pharmaceutical corporations make available posters and brochures on cleanliness and disease prevention. Advertising agencies and publishers frequently call the attention of schools to usable materials on nearly every subject pertaining to health programs. Much of this material is good. Some of it is unscientific. Some of it is frankly biased advertising and as such is unsuitable for use in public institutions. Teachers and administrators should (1) preview all material from commercial organizations to determine whether it contains offensive advertising, (2) have the scientific accuracy of the material established by medical or other scientific personnel on the school health council, (3) conform to whatever state laws or local policies have been established regarding the use of such material, (4) determine if it is educationally sound.

OPPOSITION GROUPS

In probably every community there are small groups, or individuals, who do not believe in the merit or propriety of a school health program. They oppose the health care or instruction of children in school on personal, religious, or other grounds and insist on their right to be heard and to have their wishes respected. Many state laws recognize the existence of such opposition by providing that no child shall be examined, for example, whose parents object thereto. Other states make the teaching in controversial areas like sex and reproduction, animal experimentation, or evolution illegal. Locally, such groups may protest certain phases of a complete program and stir up enough public opposition to destroy that segment of it.

In all such instances the school, perhaps through its health council, and with the official sanction of the board of education, should have a carefully thought-out policy that will make its position clear to the public. The board must recognize its obligation to protect its pupils and staff from communicable disease. It must recognize the existence of the health needs of the community and of the nation. At the same time, it will observe the rights of parents and children to their own religious beliefs as long as the exercise of them does not jeopardize the public welfare.

In health teaching there are always controversial areas. Not all material in these areas is suitable for classroom use. Whatever *is* used should be accurate and inoffensively presented, and it would be well for the teacher to keep accurate notes himself on what he has taught in the event of protest about it later. It is common experience among teachers that a frank and public declaration of intent, with an opportunity given to explore the pros and cons in advance of the actual teaching, will bring about a better understanding of the problem and, perhaps, avoid any public protest. In other instances teachers will find it desirable to visit doubting or protesting citizens to explain to them the necessity for the program and to give them the details of its operation. Frequently, this is greatly appreciated and alleviates any apprehension upon the part of the prospective opponent.

PERSONNEL INTERRELATIONSHIPS

It is axiomatic that the success of any enterprise as complex as a program of school health education depends upon the qualifications of the personnel involved and the way in which they work together. Friction, animosity, professional jealousy or incompetence, provincialism, or ignorance can retard the development of any program to the ultimate disservice of the children or youth involved. School health education is actually a fascinating and massive experiment in group cooperation. Each person within the program relies to some extent upon someone else or upon many others, and unless all are well prepared for their tasks and fulfill their responsibilities effectively the total program falls short of its goals.

THE HEALTH OF EMPLOYED PERSONNEL Of basic significance to any health education program is the health of the teacher.[12] It is obvious that the teacher affects the pupil or student in many ways—by personal example, as a purveyor of knowledge, but also as a potential carrier of disease. For this reason, and because the teacher is in a profession which is not without its own hazards, the health of the teacher is of fundamental concern. It is not possible to discuss here in detail the provisions that should be made for teachers, but the following are the principal elements of health activitiy that have a bearing upon the life of a teacher:

1 The teacher should be given every protection possible from communicable disease by being provided with recent immunization against poliomyelitis, mumps, smallpox, diphtheria, and any other disease against which science has a reasonably effective protection.

2 The teacher should be required to present satisfactory evidence of freedom from tuberculosis as a condition for annual employment.

3 Teachers who develop physical or mental incapacity should receive sympathetic treatment from boards of education in terms of continuance of salary, pensions, insurance, or other benefits, and ought not to be removed from employment until the handicap is proven irreversible and harmful to the children in the classroom.

4 "Good administration attempts to guard school personnel from pressures. Administrators have obligations to see that pressures both internal and external are not so great as to affect the health and proper functioning of the teacher."[13]

5 The following provisions by school administration would also be of significance:

A healthful and attractive physical environment
The absence of excessive mental-emotional pressures
Rational teaching load and extended day assignments
Reasonable tenure and security
A healthful school-community social climate
Adequate sick leave provisions
Sabbatical and retirement provisions
Appropriate insurance programs
Pupil-teacher-parent-administrator interaction
Community recognition and respect[14]

6 Responsibility for maintaining good health is, of course, the teacher's own. Adjusting to the problems of the classroom, to interrelationships with colleagues and parents, to recalcitrant children, and to the tedium of school routines, requires conscious effort and self-control.

Maladjustment can easily develop among teachers who refuse to take or cannot take responsibility for their own actions.

7 The serious problem of sick leave for teachers confronts most boards of education. It is basic to the morale of the teaching staff. What is an adequate arrangement for teachers who are ill during the school year? Can a system be devised that will neither penalize teachers nor be abused by them? It would be wise for teachers to remain away from school when they have respiratory diseases or are otherwise seriously incapacitated. And yet if such absences are costly to them in income, many teachers will prefer to inflict themselves upon the children. If sick leave is financially attractive, some malingerers will stay away longer than is their due. The American Association of School Administrators has this to say about the problem:

– sick leave Although it is humanitarian to provide sick leave for school employees, the primary justification for a liberal sick-leave policy is the protection and benefits that accrue to pupils. Without sick-leave provisions, classroom teachers and other employees who cannot afford to lose even one day's salary may remain in school in direct contact with pupils when they are suffering from illness. A teacher who is ill cannot do a good job of teaching, and if the illness is contagious it is a direct hazard to the health of pupils.

State laws creating minimum sick-leave plans are becoming more and more numerous. Half the states now provide a minimum number of days of sick leave with pay. Many local school boards provide sick leave even though they are not required to do so and many grant additional leave beyond the state's minimum requirement. In numerous school systems, however, sick-leave provisions still are totally lacking or are far from adequate.

Where sick leave is authorized by state law or local regulations, the time allowed may vary from five to twenty days. Accumulated sick leave may vary from twenty to ninety days or more and school boards sometimes allow more than the stipulated number of accumulated sick-leave days to teachers who have rendered long and faithful service. Although a few employees probably take advantage of sick-leave provisions, the great majority do not avail themselves of the provisions as frequently as would be justified for both their own benefit and that of the pupils.

Medical examinations before school employees return to work after being ill are a safeguard to both pupils and teachers. Compensation for periods of absence frequently depends upon presentation of a certificate issued by a physician—a practice that appears to be justifiable.[15]

DISTRIBUTION OF COSTS

The development of school health education is not, at the moment, a costly enterprise compared with the cost of public health endeavors in the United States today.[16] It is estimated that the latter figure is $6.32 per person per year, whereas the average cost of school health education per pupils per year is roughly $2.70 (the cost for elementary health education is always larger than the program in the secondary school). These figures are based on data from 40 states, using the average daily attendance base rather than enrollment.

From where does this support come? For the most part it comes from the normal school budget as prepared by the local board of education. There are, however, other sources from which all or part of the needed money may come. Not every dollar spent by schools has been raised by the local school tax. Some money has come from state and federal taxes and from more than one agency and bureau within the state and federal government. Some may have been provided by a nonofficial agency and given to the schools for some specific purpose. The following sources are apparent today:

1 Congress has from time to time been asked to appropriate federal money for school health purposes. The School Lunch Law is a case in point: in a matching plan states and communities are allowed to share the support of a lunch program for children whose need can be demonstrated. Other proposals have requested federal subsidy for local physical examinations and immunization programs, although they have not yet become law. As many as twenty bills related in some way to school health are presented to Congress each session, and although few of them are passed, the trend seems to be toward federal subsidies for services or supervision.

2 Every state has some law pertaining to school health. Many states are rather fully provided with the legislation needed to operate a school health program in the community. Education equalization laws frequently provide money for employing health personnel, and other laws permit the community to spend its income on such programs and personnel as it deems wise. Some states have enacted legislation to provide money directly to communities for school health purposes.

3 In certain states funds may be transferred outright from boards of health to boards of education for the support of specified health activities. Or, more commonly, such activities may be financed by the board of health. This situation requires a high degree of cooperation for efficient administration when public health money is spent in the school. The quality of service should be no less than if it were contracted for from private physicians. School authorities should not expect good service if they ask the local health officer to visit the

school, perform fifty examinations an hour, immunize all the first-grade children who need immunization, and attend to any other necessities of the moment. Such services by colleagues in public welfare should be rendered well or not at all, and the school should exercise its right to refuse anything less than the best. The health officer should refuse to perform the perfunctory job sometimes asked of him.

4 In the last analysis, most school health funds must originate in or be disbursed by local boards of education. The budgeting for disease control programs, special classes for the partially sighted, testing programs, in fact anything having to do with school health education, must be done locally. Physicians and nurses must be paid for their work and will be listed as salaried employees of the board. Every element of a school health program must be approved and paid for ultimately by the board of education. That is why school administrators must know a great deal about health education in order to supply the board with appropriate recommendations.

5 A practice has been established in recent years by voluntary health agencies and foundations of granting funds or providing services to schools. Books have been bought, salaries paid, indigents cared for, audiometers purchased, nursing and medical salaries paid, courses of study underwritten, and scholarships provided by these organizations as they seek to improve the health of people through the medium of the school. Much of the pioneer work, the frontier development in school health education, has been made possible by grants given directly to local or state boards of education from these private agencies. School health educators should be familiar with such potential resources in their own communities.

COSTS IN SALARIES For health personnel other than teachers, standard salary scales have not generally been in vogue in school health education. School nurses, dental hygienists, and some others in larger centers may have been employed on the teachers' salary schedule, but generally speaking the salary for nonteaching personnel becomes a matter of local negotiation. The amount paid depends on the current supply and demand for such services. Nurses and physicians are best paid by annual contract in terms of a fair appraisal of the value of their time in relation to the services offered. As more and more nurses are hired by boards of education, and as they become qualified for school nursing by obtaining both nursing and education training as well as experience, the trend should be toward hiring nurses on the same salary conditions as teachers.

How many specialists should be employed? The answer to this question is problematical, but it has a great bearing upon the total cost of a health program. Certainly 1 nurse to every 1500 elementary pupils, a standard sometimes given, is too high a ratio; 1 to every 1000 or less would be better. However, planning for the numbers of personnel to be hired cannot be based on a static, nationally prescribed ratio. Program planners in school health education must know the nature of the population to be served, the kinds of health problems that are present, the amount of health education to be carried out, and the aims of the school district and/or health department involved. Only on the basis of stated goals and health goals in relation to a given population is it possible to predict the number of nurses and other personnel necessary to carry on the activities that will lead to the attainment of the goals. The number of psychologists, dental hygienists, nutritionists or full-or part-time dentists and physicians is determined by the scope and quality of work expected of them. Costs for services can be figured only in terms of the prevailing salaries or income.

NOTES AND REFERENCES

1 U.S., Congress, House, Report No. 143, *Elementary and Secondary Education Act of 1965,* 89th Cong., 1st sess., H. Rept. 143.

2 Office of Economic Opportunity, *Project Headstart, Health Services, A Guide for Project Directors and Health Personnel,* Washington, D.C., Government Printing Office, 1967.

3 American Association for Health, Physical Education and Recreation, *Teamwork in School Health,* A Report of the National Conference on Coordination of the School Health Program, Washington, D.C., American Association for Health, Physical Education and Recreation, 1962.

4 James M. Wolf and Howard C. Pritham, "Administrative Patterns of School Health Services," *Journal of the American Medical Association,* 193, (July 1965).

5 American Association for Health, Physical Education and Recreation, *op. cit.*

6 Reproduced with permission of W. B. Prothro, M.D., Public Health Director, and adapted from the Conference for Health Council Work, May 1965, Grand Rapids, Mich.

7 Council of Chief State School Officers, "Coordination of Pupil Personnel Services—School Health Services," Pupil Personnel Services, 1960, p. 14.

8 National Committee on School Health Policies of the National Conference for Cooperation in School Health, *Suggested School Health Policies,* 3rd ed., Health Education Council, 1956, pp. 19–20.

9 Innes Pearse and Lucy Crocker, *The Peckham Experiment,* New Haven, Conn., Yale University Press, 1945. Reviewed by D. M. Hall in *Research Quarterly* (October 1947), p. 232.

10 Fred V. Hein and Donald A. Dukelow (eds.), *Physicians and Schools,* Report of the Fourth National Conference on Physicians and Schools, Chicago, AMA, 1953, pp. 56–57.

11 "How Schools and Voluntary Agencies Can Work Together To Improve School Health Programs," *Journal of Health, Physical Education and Recreation* (October 1955), pp. 35, 36. See also American School Health Association, *A Directory of National Organizations Concerned With School Health,* Kent, Ohio, American School Health Association, 1970.

12 See the excellent yearbook of the American Association for Health, Physical Education and Recreation, *Fit To Teach,* Washington, D.C., NEA, 1957.

13 W. W. Bauer (ed.), *Physicians and Schools,* Report of the Sixth National Conference on Physicians and Schools, Chicago, AMA, 1957.

14 *Ibid.*

15 American Association of School Administrators, *Health in Schools,* rev. ed., Washington, D.C., American Association of School Administrators, 1951, p. 61.

16 For an illuminating article on comparative costs, the reader is referred to an article by Dr. Elena M. Sliepcevich entitled "Should Public Health Be Interested in School Health?" in *Journal of School Health,* XXXIII, 4 (April 1963), 145.

SELECTED READINGS

Directory of National Organizations with Interest in School Health, U.S. Public Health Service, June 1968.

Health is a Community Affair, National Commission on Community Health Services, Harvard University Press, Cambridge, Mass., 1966.

Knutson, Audie L., *The Individual, Society, and Health Behavior,* Russell Sage Foundation, New York, 1965.

Mayshark, Cyrus, and Donald Shaw, *Administration of School Health Programs,* Mosby, St. Louis, 1967.

Project Headstart Health Services, A Guide for Project Directors and Health Personnel, U.S. Office of Economic Opportunity, Washington, D.C., 1967.

Teamwork in School Health, Report of the National Conference on Coordination of the School Health Program, American Association for Health, Physical Education and Recreation, Washington, D.C., 1962.

CHAPTER 16
EVALUATION

Evaluating school health services and activities is similar to appraising health instruction. (See Chapter 6).

The chapters of Part Two, Foundations of Administration and Organization, have been written from a planning point of view. The child and his needs in health and illness were described as the basis for planning. Subsequently there were chapters containing descriptions of the personnel, activities, and programs designed to improve the health of the child at school. And, finally, the administrative and community relationships necessary to support the school health program were detailed.

Evaluation is viewed as part of the planning-implementing-evaluating cycle. Evaluation is a special kind of information processing by which judgments are made about past activities in order to determine future action. It is the mirror image of planning in that it involves looking back upon action and making a judgment about it in order to provide the necessary information for planning.[1]

Vernon E. Weckworth states that evaluation by definition is value laden, requiring selection of certain attributes, qualities, or conditions, measurement of these qualities; and comparison of results with the underlying value system.[2] More simply put, evaluation attempts to describe something and to indicate its perceived merits and shortcomings.[3] In other words, how good is the program that has been implemented? How effective was it in accomplishing the objectives for which it was designed? Do the procedures produce satisfactory results in terms of improving the health of children? Is what is done up to date? Should anything new be tried?

Likewise, the health educator wants to know whether the patrons of the school understand what is being done and whether they believe it to be worthwhile. Are the purposes of the school health program clear? Do they make sense? Do people generally understand what the total school health education program contains?

WHO EVALUATES?

Everyone associated with a program makes at least an informal evaluation. Depending on the knowledge of the evaluator, the criteria he selects as signs of success, and the data he uses to measure the criteria, the outcomes will differ. There is, then, no one correct evaluation of any program. However, it is critical that the value of a program be decided upon the basis of the objectives chosen by the operatives of the program. The outcomes that the administrators and implementors have chosen are the basis for determining whether or not they have been successful.

Most often evaluations are done by the personnel operating an activity—in this case, school personnel. On other occasions a panel of experts may be called in. Occasionally evaluation is used as a learning opportunity involving district staff, outside experts, and community representatives. All work together in the development of instruments, the selection of priorities, measurement of selected criteria, and determination of recommendations for the future. Evaluation should be a cooperative enterprise, including at least all who are directly affected.

APPROACHES TO EVALUATION

There are at least three approaches to the evaluation of school health: structure, process, and outcomes.

1 The evaluation of *structure* requires assessment of the organization and resources used in school health education. This approach is concerned with facilities, manpower, equipment, and financing. Usually instruments are used that specify certain requirements and are similar to those used by certifying or accrediting agencies. This approach presumes that when certain conditions are met, good school health programs will follow. This may often be a false presumption.

2 Auditing of *process* is not satisfied with presumption. In this approach procedures are subjected to professional judgment as to their adequacy and competence.

3 Evaluation by *outcomes* consists of assessment of end results. This approach answers the question What good are we doing? in terms of the well being of the client or the solution of a problem.[4]

A well rounded program evaluation more often than not will include some aspects of each of these approaches to the extent that it is possible to observe and measure under the limitations inherent in the school setting. The present state of the art of evaluation technology also presents limits.

For example, those planning a school health program generally feel poor vision to be a problem of school age children and institute a screening program. Often, as described previously, the Snellen procedure is used. Evaluation of the structure of such a program would assess the number of persons doing screening, their training, the physical facilities available, the type of equipment used, the frequency of screening and the procedure to be used. These data might be compared with standards recommended by the National Society for the Prevention of Blindness. Determination of the value of the program would be based on the interpretation of differences between data and standards.

The evaluation of process most often would consist of peer review and observation of procedures used in screening to determine whether the elements of good practice were present and to what degree. Did the screener follow procedure? Was the orientation of pupils adequate? When screening monocular vision, was one eye truly covered? Was the screener able to adjust her techniques to individual children? Does she screen more children than she can actually follow through to care? The answers to these or similar questions provide the basis for judgment of the screening process.

Those to whom outcomes are most important would list the objectives of a vision testing program and collect data to measure the degree of accomplishment of each. For example the outcomes of vision screening might be listed as follows: (1) to get preliminary but accurate screening of all children every other year, (2) to screen out all children with 20/40 vision or worse, (3) to arrange teacher-nurse-parent conferences where necessary to assure recommended corrective or compensatory action, (4) to secure correction in every needed case, (5) to adjust room environment for benefit of vision, (6) to provide needed special sight saving training. The key question is: How near does the vision program come to attaining these six objectives?

Thorough evaluation of vision screening in schools will assess elements of structure, process, and outcomes.

WHEN TO EVALUATE The current climate is very favorable toward evaluation. More and more funding agencies by law and by regulation are requiring program proposals to include assessment plans in the original write-up. Favorable evaluation gives great personal satisfaction. It gives one confidence that previous program decisions were wise. In addition evaluation provides those supporting or financing programs confidence in giving and continuing such support. And, of course, evaluative information guides the action of the administrator and the practitioner in improving their operation.

Evaluation, however, is costly and time consuming and can steal resources from the activities leading to the desired outcomes. It is a mixed blessing and should not be accepted as desirable without adequate consideration. There are times when one should not evaluate. Mary Arnold lists four:

> 1 When the cost of rigorous evaluation is higher than the cost of the program.
> This requires assessment of the cost of evaluation and the cost of not evaluating. In an individual school or district the costs of a complete evaluation would be quite high. However, if this were done for one school or district the results might be extremely valuable to the total program and be considered worth the cost.
>
> 2 When the current program is the only strategy available and there is some evidence the program is having some effect.
> This is a tricky situation in that it should not be used merely as a rationalization for not evaluating. One should look for alternative approaches to the current program before concluding dire consequences should the present method be dropped.
>
> 3 When the program is desired by the community regardless of effectiveness.
> Current smoking and health or alcohol education programs might not stand up to evaluation of efficiency and effectiveness. Public demands make it unlikely they would be discontinued no matter what the evaluation.
>
> 4 When change of activity would be too disruptive to other programs.
> Evaluation might lead to a recommendation for reallocation of program personnel. If such a change would lead to sanctions or a strike, the costs of change would likely outweigh the benefits.[5]

At the present time, too few school health programs are adequately evaluated. If an error is to be made, it should be made on the side of evaluating. School health has much to offer and must be able to document this fact.

THE ESTABLISHMENT OF PRINCIPLES

To evaluate all aspects of a school health program requires tests, surveys, checks, follow-ups, retests, and other measuring devices. To date the available technology does not provide means to accomplish an evaluation complete in every respect. New techniques are continuously being developed through research and experience.

When the decision is made to evaluate, those charged with the responsibility must first seek to establish principles. The following have proved worthwhile:

1 Evaluation should be continuous and concurrent with program activities.

2 It should embrace all the important functions of the school health program including instruction, services, and activities.

3 It should be concerned with outcomes, process, and structure.

4 Evaluation should be cooperative. All who are effected by the evaluation should participate. This includes administrators, teachers, pupils, parents, physicians, nurses, hygienists, nutritionists, and community representatives.

5 Evaluation should be focused upon the important values that underlie the health program of the school. Those values are best expressed in terms of program objectives and goals stated during the program planning period.

6 A long-range evaluation program should be planned so that no one year would involve a complete study of every aspect of school health education.

7 Data gathering and record keeping should be performed to aid in the evaluation of the functions of school health education and not as ends in themselves.

With the establishment of principles the program evaluation may proceed to the selection of techniques and processes. Evaluation, whenever possible, should be based on objectives, principles, and procedures established during program planning. As a matter of practicality it must be remembered that many programs do not now include evaluation, and it is necessary to break into the cycle of planning and implementing to include evaluating. This will require after-the-fact evaluation.

THE SELECTION OF EVALUATION TECHNIQUES

Evaluation techniques are selected in relation to the program element to be appraised. The procedures used successfully to find answers for a vision program would not be applicable, perhaps, in evaluating the school lunch. The evaluators will choose from statistical analyses, surveys, testimony of participants or observers, rating scales, or other devices and will attempt to be sure that the measurements attained reflect proper scientific evaluation procedures.

There are many criteria for evaluation of program success besides the relatively simple one of how much effort was expended. For example, an educational or health program may be judged on the basis of at least five criteria:

1 Appropriateness—this is related to value, the good-bad continuum. Is the program desirable or undesirable? If desirable what is its priority ranking in relation to other programs? Is it as desirable for the future as it has been in the past?

2 Effectiveness—is this program attaining the goals established? Are the desired outcomes occurring?

3 Adequacy—to what extent are the outcomes affecting the total problem which it has been designed to prevent or eliminate.

4 Efficiency—is the cost in resources in relation to effectiveness reasonable? Are there less expensive ways to accomplish the same result?

5 Side effects—are there program effects good or bad which are different from the intended or projected ones? A program requiring physical examination of athletes might get the exams done but could have the side effect of reducing the number of boys participating if a financial hardship were caused or there was a lack of physicians available.[6]

All of these approaches are valid and the techniques and instruments of evaluation must be selected to reflect the major approach or approaches used.

An example of one evaluating process in chart form for a school health program is shown on page 422. Note that the objectives, the hoped for changes and outcomes, and the appraisal techniques all point toward interpretation and replanning, which are the major reasons for evaluation.

Often those charged with assessment may create and develop a process that could specifically pinpoint strengths and weaknesses of a program. This is a common evaluation tool, and, when accompanied by an estimate of the degree or quality of the practice or provision being evaluated plus an opportunity to make notations of the changes needed and recommended steps to be taken, can be extremely valuable. An example of a list of general criteria expressed in terms of desirable practices and used to evaluate health services in an elementary school follows. Omitted here are the specific points listed under each general statement.

A A health service guide is provided by the school district or by the office of the county superintendent of schools.

B A health service committee, preferably a subcommittee of the health council or committee, has advisory responsibility for health services.

C Health services are provided in accordance with the provisions of the guide, provided, however, that the advice of the health services committee is an important consideration in decisions regarding adaptations that are required to meet special needs of individuals and of the total school population.

D The school health services are of sufficient scope to provide school personnel the information and assistance needed to determine status of, protect, and promote the health of pupils.

E School health personnel encourage and guide teacher observation of pupils' health characteristics and accept referrals of pupils whose characteristics are unlike those of the well child.

F School personnel inform and advise parents regarding medical examinations their children should have and assist in making provision for the medical examinations as necessary.

G School personnel inform parents of the importance of eye examinations for children prior to school entrance, maintain a vision screening program, and inform and advise parents regarding eye conditions of their children that require the attention of a specialist.

H School health personnel provide for all pupils to have hearing tests at regular intervals, individual tests for pupils discovered with hearing difficulties; inform and advise parents regarding their children's need for examinations by ear specialists; and recommend classroom adjustments for children with hearing difficulties.

I Health services provide for parents to be informed regarding their children's need for regular dental examinations beginning prior to the children's entrance to school, and for parents of children who have defective dental conditions to be informed regarding the undesirable effects of the conditions and advised regarding essential treatment.

J Pupil's growth characteristics are observed to determine deviations in growth patterns that merit special attention.

K Follow-up procedures are taken as necessary—begin when pupils with health difficulties are identified and conclude when the health difficulties have been corrected or their effects minimized.

L Health counseling and guidance is provided.

M Provisions are made for supplying teachers with health information concerning handicapped pupils and for recommending cases for whom home teaching may be necessary.

N The health service program includes provisions for the prevention and control of communicable diseases.

O The health service program provides emergency service for injury and sudden illness and for disasters.[7]

REPORT OF EVALUATION

No evaluation process is complete until a report is written and disseminated to appropriate people. Those receiving the report should include, but not be limited to, those who participated in the evaluation and those expected to implement the recommendations and future program activities. The party responsible for allocation of resources to the program must be included. In addition, efforts must be made to explain the report and to receive feedback from the consumers and/or clients of the program.

The report should include the following:

1 A clear description of the program or program element that was appraised including a description of the context in which it was carried on.

2 A description of how evaluation was made, including revelation of the techniques and instruments used.

3 The detailed findings, with the original data available on request.

4 A statement of general conclusions from the evaluation. This will include strengths as well as weaknesses and the inferred "causes" of each.

5 A series of specific recommendations (and suggested alternatives) for improvement of the program, arranged from the simple to the complex and from those now possible to those possible only in the future.

EVALUATION AND THE FUTURE

We are living in a time of rapidly expanding capability to perform meaningful evaluation. Decision-making theory and policy-making science are becoming available to the local practitioner. The techniques of comprehensive planning, systems analysis, operations research, P.E.R.T. (Program Evaluation Review Technique) and P.P.B.S. (Program Planning Budgeting System) are diffusing rapidly through our society. Within the next decade this intellectual technology will be available to all.

Growing in parallel fashion to the development of this technology and its diffusion is the political demand on the part of the public for accountability. The voters want to know if their money is being wisely spent. They demand effectiveness and efficiency as well and are asking for proof of each.

Programs of health education that have not been formally evaluated or that have been evaluated by statistical compilation of inputs, that is, dollars spent, training programs, qualifications of personnel, children screened, and nurse/pupil ratios, will have to become more sophisticated. The key to the assessment of school health programs will be the identification of the impact of the services and instruction on the health of the children served, the costs, and comparison of actual impacts with those desired by professionals *and consumers,* who establish the goals.

Where money is being spent, where time is being consumed, and where the health of children is at stake, program activities must be proved useful, and they must be plainly related to a clearly stated

Appraisal of School Health Program Activities

School Health Program, School X	*Changes in Whom or What*	*Kind of Changes Sought*	*Means of Appraisal*	*Interpretation of Findings*	*Replanning*
Established policies School health council	Administrators Teachers Parents Program activities	Understanding of program Participation in program activities	Check lists Participation records	Analysis of strengths and weaknesses	Improved program activities Mutual understanding—cooperation
Objectives: School health services Teacher observation Medical exam Health guidance Communicable disease control	Doctors Nurses Teachers Health coordinator Students Procedures	Discovering student needs School health services made educational	A check list of school health services	Analysis of strengths and weaknesses	Health needs through improved appraisals and follow-up
Objectives: Healthful school living School site and plant Lighting, heating, and ventilation School food services Mental-emotional tone	Teachers Students Facilities	Safe, sanitary school environment; improved faculty-student relationships, faculty-custodial relationships	State Department of Education check list for healthful and safe school environment	Analysis of strengths and weaknesses	More healthful environment Use of environmental factors in health training
Objectives: Health instruction Content areas Teaching methods Scientific materials	Administrators Teachers Students Parents	Student behavioral changes Knowledge Attitudes Practices Teacher understanding	Tests Inventories Observations Examination records	Analysis of strengths and weaknesses	Functional planned health instruction
Objectives: Community resources Utilization of community resources Joint program planning School contribution to community program	Administrators Teachers Students Community leaders Citizens	Understanding the educational point of view Mutual understanding	Community health evaluation forms	Analysis of strengths and weaknesses	Better school-community cooperation

Source: Los Angeles City Schools, Division of Educational Services, *Evaluation of the Health Program in Los Angeles City Schools, 1954–1961*, school publication no. 673, Los Angeles, Los Angeles City Schools, 1962, p. 18.

aim. Planning, evaluation and accountability are the waves of the future.

NOTES AND REFERENCES

1 Mary Arnold, "Evaluation, a Feedback Model," in Henrik L. Blum, *Health Planning 1969,* San Francisco, American Public Health Association, 1969.

2 Vernon E. Weckworth, "An Evaluation: A Tool or a Tyranny—II," Systems Development Project, Comment Series, Minneapolis, University of Minnesota, n.d.

3 Robert E. Stake, and Terry Denny, "Needed Concepts and Techniques for Utilizing More Fully the Potential of Evaluation," *The Sixty-eighth Yearbook of the National Society for the Study of Education, Part II,* Chicago, University of Chicago Press, 1969.

4 Avedis Donabedian, "Some Issues in Evaluating the Quality of Nursing Care," *American Journal of Public Health,* 59, 10 (October 1969), 1833.

5 Arnold, *op. cit.*

6 O. Lynn Deniston, and I. M. Rosenstock, "Evaluating Health Programs," *Public Health Reports,* 85, 9 (September 1970), 835.

7 *Criteria for Evaluating the Elementary School Health Program,* Sacramento, California State Department of Education, 1962, pp. 8–14.

SELECTED READINGS

Blum, Henrik, L., *Health Planning 1969,* American Public Health Association Western Regional Office, San Francisco, 1969.

Churchman, C. West, *The Systems Approach,* Delacorte Press, New York, 1968.

Health Program Implementation Through PERT, American Public Health Association Western Regional Office, October 1966.

Novick, David, *Program Budgeting,* Harvard University Press, Cambridge, Mass., 1965.

"Planning—Programming—Budgeting System: A Symposium," *Public Administration Review,* 26:4, December 1966.

Sixty-Eighth Yearbook of the National Society for the Study of Education, Part II, The University of Chicago Press, Chicago, 1969.

Weckworth, Vernon, *Systems Development Project,* Comment Series, University of Minnesota, Minneapolis (n.d.).

INDEXES

INDEX OF NAMES

INDEX OF SUBJECTS

72 73 74 7 6 5 4 3 2 1